Physiology of the Fetal and Neonatal Lung

Proceedings of the International Symposium
on Physiology and Pathophysiology of the Fetal
and Neonatal Lung,
held in Brussels, June 6–8, 1985

Edited by

Dr D. V. Walters and **Prof. L. B. Strang,**
Department of Paediatrics,
University College Hospital Medical School,
The Rayne Institute, London

and

Prof. F. Geubelle
Clinique des Maladies de l'Enfance,
Université de Liege,
Belgium

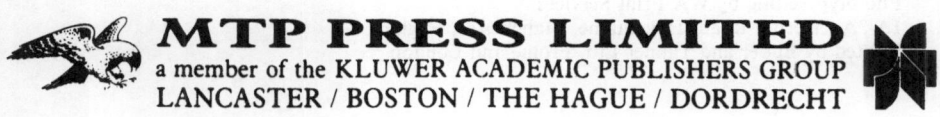

MTP PRESS LIMITED
a member of the KLUWER ACADEMIC PUBLISHERS GROUP
LANCASTER / BOSTON / THE HAGUE / DORDRECHT

Published in the UK and Europe by
MTP Press Limited
Falcon House
Lancaster, England

British Library Cataloguing in Publication Data

International Symposium on Physiology and
  Pathophysiology of the Fetal and Neonatal Lung.
  (1985 : Brussels)
  Physiology of the fetal and neonatal lung: proceedings of
  the International Symposium on Physiology and
  Pathology of the Fetal and Neonatal Lung, held in
  Brussels, June 6–8, 1985.
  1. Infants (Newborn)—Physiology   2. Respiratory
  organs
  I. Title   II. Walter, D. V.   III. Strang, L. B.
  IV. Geubelle, F.
  612^{1}.2   RG620

ISBN-13: 978-94-010-8344-7   e-ISBN-13: 978-94-009-4155-7
DOI: 10.1007/978-94-009-4155-7

A division of Kluwer Academic Publishers
101 Philip Drive
Norwell, MA 02061, USA

Library of Congress Cataloging in Publication Data

International Symposium on Physiology and Pathophysiology of the Fetal and Neonatal Lung (1985 : Brussels,
  Belgium) Physiology of the fetal and neonatal lung.

  Includes bibliographies and index.
  1. Lungs—Congresses.   2. Fetus—Physiology—
Congresses.   3. Infants (Newborn)—Physiology—
Congresses.   I. Walters, D. V. (Dafydd Vaughan)
II. Strang, L. B.   III. Geubelle, F.   IV. Title.
[DNLM: 1. Lung—physiology—congresses.   2. Peri-
natology—congresses. WF 600 I6115 1985]
RG620.I58 1985   612^{1}.640124   86-21505
ISBN-13: 978-94-010-8344-7

Phototypesetting by WA Print Services
1A-3A Tiverton Road, Davyhulme, Manchester, England
Printed by Butler and Tanner Ltd, Frome and London

Contents

CONTENTS

Physiology of the Fetal and Neonatal Lung

CONTENTS

List of Contributors

J. J. BATENBURG
Department of Veterinary
  Biochemistry
State University of Utrecht
PO Box 80177
3508 TD Utrecht
The Netherlands

R. C. BOUCHER
Department of Medicine
School of Medicine
University of North Carolina
Chapel Hill
NC 27514
USA

C. A. R. BOYD
Department of Human Anatomy
University of Oxford
South Parks Road
Oxford OX1 3QX
UK

A. C. BRYAN
Department of Respiratory
  Physiology
Hospital for Sick Children
555 University Avenue
Toronto, M5G 1XB
Ontario
Canada

R. BURKHARDT
Medizinische Poliklinik
Klinikum der Phillips-Universität
Balderingerstrasse
3550 Marburg
West Germany

P. H. BURRI
Section of Developmental Biology
Institute of Anatomy
University of Berne
Buehlstrasse 26
CH 3012 Berne
Switzerland

J. CLEAVE
Department of Mathematics
University of Bristol
Senate House
Tyndall Ave
Bristol BS8 1TH

J. A. CLEMENTS
Cardiovascular Research Institute
University of California
  San Francisco
Moffitt 1327
San Francisco, CA 94143
USA

C. U. COTTON
Department of Physiology and
Biophysics
Medical Branch
University of Texas
Galveston, TX 77550
USA

H. De CROO
Professor and Chairman
The Princess Marie-Christine Foundation
for Paediatric Research

E. A. EGAN
Department of Pediatrics and
  Physiology
University at Buffalo SUNY
New York
USA

G. ENHORNING
Department of Gynecology and
  Obstetrics
Children's Hospital of Buffalo
219 Bryant Street
Buffalo, New York 14222
USA

P. J. FLEMING
Department of Child Health
University of Bristol
Bristol Maternity Hospital
Southwell Street
Bristol BS2 8EG
England

J. FLOROS
Department of Pediatrics
Harvard Medical School
75 Francis Street
Boston, MA 02115
USA

J. T. GATZY
Department of Pharmacology
School of Medicine
University of North Carolina
Chapel Hill, NC 27514
USA

Cl. GAULTIER
Laboratory of Physiology
Hopital Antoine Béclère
92141 Clamart
France

F. GEUBELLE
Clinique de Pédiatrie
Hôpital de Bavière
Université de Liège
66 blvd de la Constitution
B-4020 Liège
Belgium

L. M. G. VAN GOLDE
Department of Veterinary
  Biochemistry
State University of Utrecht
PO Box 80177
3508 TD Utrecht
The Netherlands

C. W. GOWEN
Department of Pediatrics
School of Medicine
East Carolina University
Pitt County Hospital
Greenville, NC 27834
USA

M. HALLMAN
Department of Pediatrics
Children's Hospital, University of
  Helsinki
Stenbäckinkatu 11
00290 Helsinki
Finland

M. R. KNOWLES
Department of Medicine
School of Medicine
University of North Carolina
Chapel Hill
NC 27514
USA

M. S. KWONG
Children's Hospital of Buffalo
219 Bryant Street
Buffalo
New York 14222
USA

D. LAGNEAUX
Physiologie Humaine, Normale et
  Pathologique
Institut Léon Fredericq
Université de Liège
17, Place Delcour
B-4020 Liège
Belgium

M. LEVINE
Department of Physiology
University of Bristol
Bristol Maternity Hospital
Southwell Street
Bristol BS2 8EG
England

A. M. LONG
Department of Child Health
University of Bristol
Bristol Maternity Hospital
Southwell Street
Bristol BS2 8EG

L. MARIN
Unite INSERM U29
Hopital Port Royal
123 Boulevard de Port Royal
75674 Paris Cedex 14
France

C. MORLEY
University of Cambridge
Department of Paediatrics
Addenbrookes Hospital
Cambridge CB2 2QQ
UK

J. P. MORTOLA
Department of Physiology
McGill University
3655 Drummond Street
Montreal, Quebec
H3G 1Y6
Canada

H. NEUHOF
Medizinische Klinik
Klinikstrasse 36
D-63 Giessen
West Germany

R. H. NOTTER
Division of Neonatology
Strong Memorial Hospital
601 Elmwood Avenue
Rochester, New York 14642
USA

M. POST
Research Institute
The Hospital for Sick Children
555 University Ave
Toronto, Ontario
Canada M5G 1X8

C. A. RAMSDEN
Department of Paediatrics
Clinical Sciences
University College London
5 University Street
London WC1E 6JJ

B. ROBERTSON
Departments of Pediatrics and
  Pediatric Pathology
St Göran's Children's Hospital
S-112 81 Stockholm
Sweden

W. SEEGER
Medizinsche Klinik
Klinikstrasse 36
D-63 Giessen
West Germany

B. T. SMITH
Department of Neonatology
The Hospital for Sick Children
555 University Ave
Toronto, Ontario
Canada M5G 1X8

G. STÖHR
Medizinische Klinik
Klinikstrasse 36
D-63 Giessen
West Germany

L. B. STRANG
Department of Paediatrics
University College London
5 University Street
London WC1E 6JJ
UK

A. C. J. DE VRIES
Department of Veterinary
Biochemistry
State University of Utrecht
PO Box 80177
3508 TD Utrecht
The Netherlands

D. V. WALTERS
Department of Paediatrics
Clinical Sciences
University College London
5 University Street
London WC1E 6JJ

M. R. WARD
Department of Physiology
University of Dundee
Dundee DD1 4HN
Scotland

J. S. WIGGLESWORTH
Department of Paediatrics &
  Neonatal Medicine
Royal Postgraduate Medical
  School
Hammersmith Hospital
Du Cane Road
London W12 0HS
UK

The Princess Marie-Christine Foundation

Fondation de Recherche Pediatrique Princess Marie-Christine
Sicutuig Voor Pediatrisch Onderzoek Princess-Marie-Christine

The Princess Marie-Christine Foundation was founded in 1975 by the enlightened and generous initiative of H..M.. King Leopold and H.R.H. Princess Lilian of Belgium with the purpose of creating a scientific basis for the University Hospital for Children in Brussels. Part of its activity is to organize international symposia on subjects of importance to the prevention and treatment of childhood disease.

It was in this context that in June, 1985, the Foundation organized a symposium on the physiology and pathophysiology of the fetal and neonatal lung. It was attended by leading scientists from several European countries, Canada and the USA. The symposium was chaired throughout by Professor Leonard Strang to whom I would like to express grateful thanks on behalf of the Board of Trustees of the Princess Marie-Christine Foundation. Professor F. Geubelle and Dr D. V. Walters in collaboration with Professor Strang undertook the task of editing the papers and discussions which are presented here. To them and to all our distinguished guests I wish to express, likewise, our heartfelt thanks.

H. de Croo

Introduction

L. B. STRANG

The past 25 years have seen a remarkable growth in our knowledge of lung development in its structural, physiological and biochemical dimensions. Much of the impetus for research leading to new knowledge has derived from the perception that many respiratory disorders in the newborn infant are due to defective development or maladaption of some component or components of the respiratory system. Thus, to cite one example, surfactant deficiency is clearly seen to be the cause of atelectasis in hyaline membrane disease; and to cite another, it is widely accepted that the mechanisms controlling patency of the ductus arteriosus and pulmonary vascular resistance also determine the right-to-left or left-to-right shunting frequently observed in the course of neonatal respiratory disorders. There are, however, areas of physiological knowledge – such as those relating to respiratory control and to liquid formation and absorption – which are clearly of great relevance to lung adaptation at birth but where it has not yet proved possible to link a specific clinical state to the malfunction of a particular mechanism.

In planning this symposium an attempt was made to organize the material in an orderly manner, starting with the embryonic and fetal stages of growth and development, continuing with respiratory control and the role of surfactant in lung aeration at birth, and ending with the treatment of neonatal respiratory disorders. Within this framework, special attention was given to matters of current interest without attempting any kind of balanced representation of the whole subject. A bias towards matters of current interest is most evident in the last section in which three of the four papers deal with surfactant replacement and the fourth with high frequency ventilation.

On behalf of the International Scientific Council of the Foundation Princess Marie-Christine, I would like to express my thanks to the many colleagues and friends who contributed to this symposium and made of it such a happy occasion. All the contributors owe a debt of gratitude to Prof. F. Geubelle and Prof. G. Lyon who played an all-important role in initiating and organizing this symposium. I would also like to thank Prof. Herman de Croo and the Board of the Foundation for their comprehensive support; and most particularly, HRH Princess Lilian for the great interest she showed in our work and for the generosity, warmth and simplicity with which she received us.

1
Lung Embryogenesis and Differentiation

L. MARIN

INTRODUCTION

The subject of this chapter, 'Lung embryogenesis and differentiation', represents an immense field which covers the whole history of lung development, starting from early fetal stages and continuing after birth. This can be recounted in a number of ways. One of these would be to describe the appearance and evolution of the various features – anatomical, histological, biochemical, etc. – specific for functional lung. Another one would be to try to understand these events and to consider the mechanisms underlying lung development, i.e. the mechanisms leading from a small group of uniformly undifferentiated prelung cells to the highly heterogeneous functional lung tissue.

In fact, efforts to analyse experimentally lung development, especially its early stages, were made years ago, even though normal development was not yet fully described. These efforts met a renewed and sustained interest when respiratory problems of prematurely born babies were first correlated with the immaturity of the surfactant system[1,2]. This explains, at least partly, why experimental data gained so far are still restricted mostly to two domains: at one end, the mechanisms involved in the control of the branching mechanisms of the epithelial network, which characterize the first stages of lung development; at the other end of fetal lung history, the factors controlling the differentiation of the respiratory epithelium, and, more specifically, the differentiation of type II cells.

In this chapter, early lung morphogenesis will be briefly surveyed first. Then some results gained from our own work concerning the factors involved in the control of type II cell differentiation will be discussed.

EARLY LUNG DEVELOPMENT, BRANCHING PROCESSES, EPITHELIOMESENCHYMAL INTERACTIONS

Like many other organs, lung tissue originates from two distinct cell layers: the endoderm and the mesoderm. Prelung endodermal and mesodermal

1

cells have been traced in the chicken embryo by means of thymidine labelling and subsequent transplantation[3]. At the earliest stage investigated, the medium-streak stage, the endodermal and mesodermal prelung cells are not yet in contact: the first are located medially, in the anterior third of the primitive streak, while the second lie laterally, at a more caudal level. As the embryo develops, endodermal and mesodermal prelung cells migrate from their original location and finally reach the ventrolateral walls of the newly appearing primitive gut. Once they have reached this region, lung primordia proper first appear as endodermal outgrowths which extend in the surrounding mesoderm. This is the first morphologically recognizable stage in lung morphogenesis. From then on the endodermal component starts to grow and, by branching repeatedly, develops into the epithelial network characteristic of functional lung. This aspect of lung morphogenesis was actively investigated about 20 years ago in a number of species. It was then clearly demonstrated that the endodermal budding activity depends on the presence of homologous mesenchyme[4-7].

The inductive effect of lung mesenchyme has been reanalysed more recently. It was thus shown that mesodermal cells act by enhancing endodermal cell multiplication at precise sites[8,9], by acting upon the organization of intracellular microfilaments[9] and by modifying spatial distribution of basement membrane components[10,11]. As in other tissues of dual origin, the differentiation of the various cell types of the epithelial network depends also on the associated mesoderm[7].

The inductive influence is organ-specific, but not species-specific[6]. For instance, as seen from Fig. 1.1a, normal type II cells can differentiate from fetal rat epithelial cells which have been associated with chicken lung mesenchyme. Reciprocally (Fig. 1.1b), chicken lung epithelium associated with rat lung mesenchyme also gives rise to type II cells.

As will be seen in Chapter 2, interactions between cells of endodermal and mesodermal origin remain essential factors throughout lung development[12,13]. Although new cell types gradually differentiate, their spatial relationships change[14], and systemic factors eventually take part in the control of lung maturation.

ROLE OF THE FETAL 'MILIEU INTÉRIEUR' IN THE CONTROL OF LUNG DEVELOPMENT

It is now widely accepted that fetal hormones, especially corticosteroids, play a major role in the control of lung maturation[15,16]. Indeed, the regulatory function of hormones has been largely proved in the period after distal epithelial cells have started to differentiate into type II pneumonocytes. But the role of the hormones as factors initiating differentiation still remains controversial[17,18]. We investigated this problem using two culture methods:

1. an in vivo culture system, the intraembryonic graft method;
2. a classical in vitro technique.

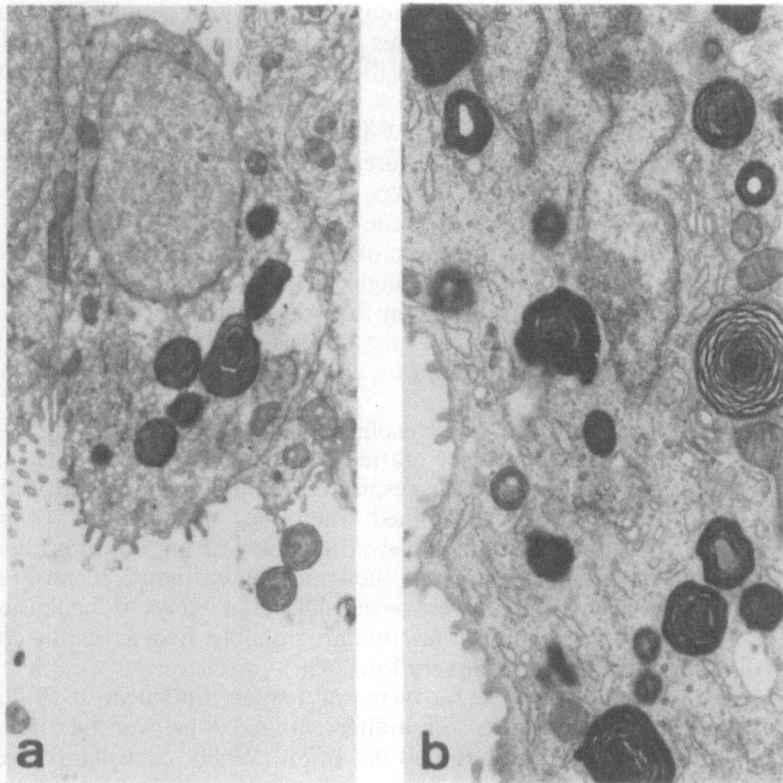

Figure 1.1 (a) Rat lung epithelium originating from a 13-day-old fetus, associated with lung mesenchyme originating from a 4.5-day-old chick embryo, and grafted for 13 days. Type II cells have differentiated ($\times$ 5625); (b) Chick lung epithelium, originating from a 4.5-day-old embryo, associated with rat lung mesenchyme, and grafted for 13 days, differentiated into type II cells ($\times$ 10500)

INTRAEMBRYONIC GRAFTING

The intraembryonic graft method offers a number of advantages: the transplanted fetal tissues start development in a living environment; the relationships between the various cell types are maintained, and the grafted tissues are rapidly colonized by the recipient's circulation. Therefore all systemic factors provided by the host reach the differentiating cells through a normal pathway, i.e. via the blood stream.

In a first series of experiments, lungs were dissected from 13-day-old rat fetuses, a short time after lung bud appearance. Each lung was inserted into the flank of a 3.5-day-old chick embryo, at a stage when the vascular network is already well developed and when possible circulating hormones are still at a very low level[20-24]. The eggs containing the graft-bearing embryos were further incubated for 7 or 13 days. The embryos were then sacrificed, the grafts recovered and processed for electron microscopy.

The lungs that had been grafted for 7 days had theoretically reached a stage equivalent to 20 days of gestation, and therefore should have contained differentiated type II cells. In fact, as shown in Fig. 1.2a, the epithelium was loaded with glycogen, as in the course of normal development, but no type II cell had differentiated.

When lungs had been grafted for 13 days they were examined at a time when type II cells were actively differentiating in the epithelium of the host's lung. As seen from Fig. 2.2b, type II cells, containing normal lamellar bodies, had also differentiated in the grafted rat lungs.

So, when grafted rat lung primordia originated from 13-day-old fetuses, they were able to differentiate, although slower than normally. In addition, type II cells seemed to appear in the grafted tissue when these cells were appearing in the lungs of the host. It was therefore concluded that systemic factors – possibly hormones – are necessary for type II cell differentiation to be initiated.

In another set of graftings we transplanted lung tissue originating from older rat fetuses. Lung tissue to be grafted was dissected from 16-, 17- and 18-day-old fetuses. In all these the respiratory epithelium was still undifferentiated. The grafts were examined when they had reached a stage equivalent to 19, 20 and 21 days of gestation; the grafting duration therefore depended on the initial stage of the transplanted tissue. It never exceeded 5 days, so that the hosts were never older than 8 days of incubation, and the level of circulating hormones that are possibly involved in the control of lung maturation was still very low[20-24].

When the grafted lungs were recovered at a stage equivalent to 19 days of gestation the epithelium was still undifferentiated, whatever the original stage of the grafted tissue (Fig. 1.3a, b, c). When transplants were recovered at a stage equivalent to 20 days of gestation, if grafts originated from 16-day-old fetuses, the epithelium was still tall, but sometimes small lamellar bodies were observed. In the transplants which originated from 17- and 18-day-old fetuses, differentiated type II cells were more numerous and contained more lamellar bodies. Finally, when transplants were recovered at a stage equivalent to 21 days of gestation, in those which originated from 16-day-old fetuses, type II cells were more easily found (Fig. 1.4a). This was also true when transplants originated from 17- and 18-day-old rat fetuses (Fig. 1.4b, c). In addition, free lamellar bodies were observed in the lumina.

These results show that when lung tissue originated from fetuses which were at 16 days of gestation, or more, although differentiation was delayed as compared to normal development, type II cells did appear in conditions in which hormones are practically absent. Therefore, as already suggested by others[17,18], hormonal factors might not be involved in the initiation of type II cell differentiation.

IN VITRO CULTURE

In order to further investigate this problem, we started to study lung epithelial differentiation *in vitro*. In the preliminary experiments which

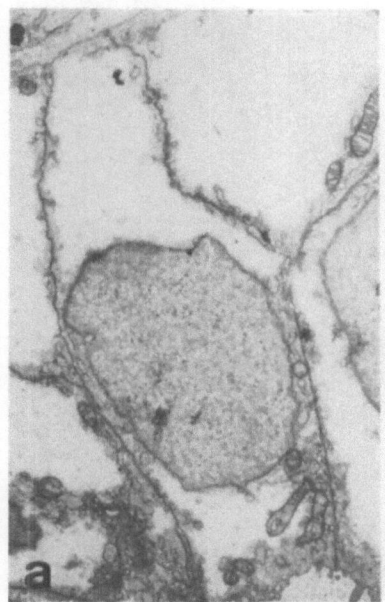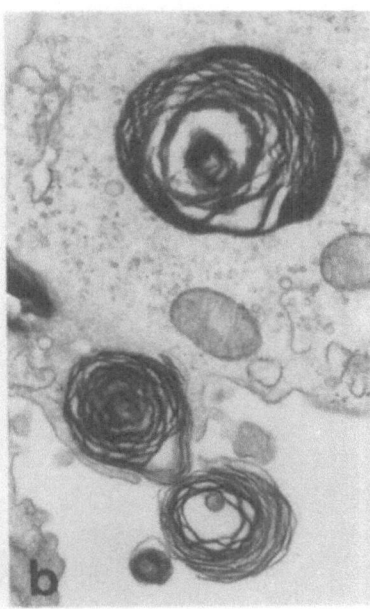

Figure 1.2 Rat lung primordia, originating from 13-day-old fetuses, grafted into 3.5-day-old chicken embryos: (**a**) after 7 days of grafting the epithelium is loaded with glycogen, and is still undifferentiated (× 4500); (**b**) after 13 days of grafting, normal lamellar bodies, specific for type II cells, have appeared, and are sometimes released in the lumina (× 1500)

are summarized here, we first explanted lung tissue from 16-day-old rat fetuses. These were either normal fetuses, or fetuses whose mothers had been adrenalectomized on day 10 of gestation. Lung tissue was maintained for 3 days on a gelified chemically defined medium (Waymouth's medium) without serum or hormones.

When explants were recovered, they were at a stage equivalent to 19 days of gestation. As shown by Fig. 1.5a, b normal type II cells had differentiated within the epithelium in the two series of cultures.

We then explanted lung primordia on day 13 of gestation, and kept them *in vitro* for 6 days, without serum or hormones. The survival was poor. But as long as explants did survive, lamellar bodies appeared in the epithelial cells (Fig. 1.6a). If serum was added to the medium the survival was better, and so was the differentiation (Fig. 1.6b). This remained true when charcoal-stripped serum was added to the medium, instead of normal calf serum (Fig. 1.7a), or when an antiglucocorticoid drug was used (Fig. 1.7b). So completely immature lung primordia gave rise to type II cells in the absence of hormones. Moreover, as had already been observed in other species[25-27], differentiation was accelerated, when compared to normal timing of development. As shown in Fig. 1.8a, normal lamellar bodies were found in explants after a 5-day culture period, after 4 days (Fig. 1.8b) and even after 3 days (Fig. 1.8c), i.e. at a stage equivalent to 16 days of gestation.

5

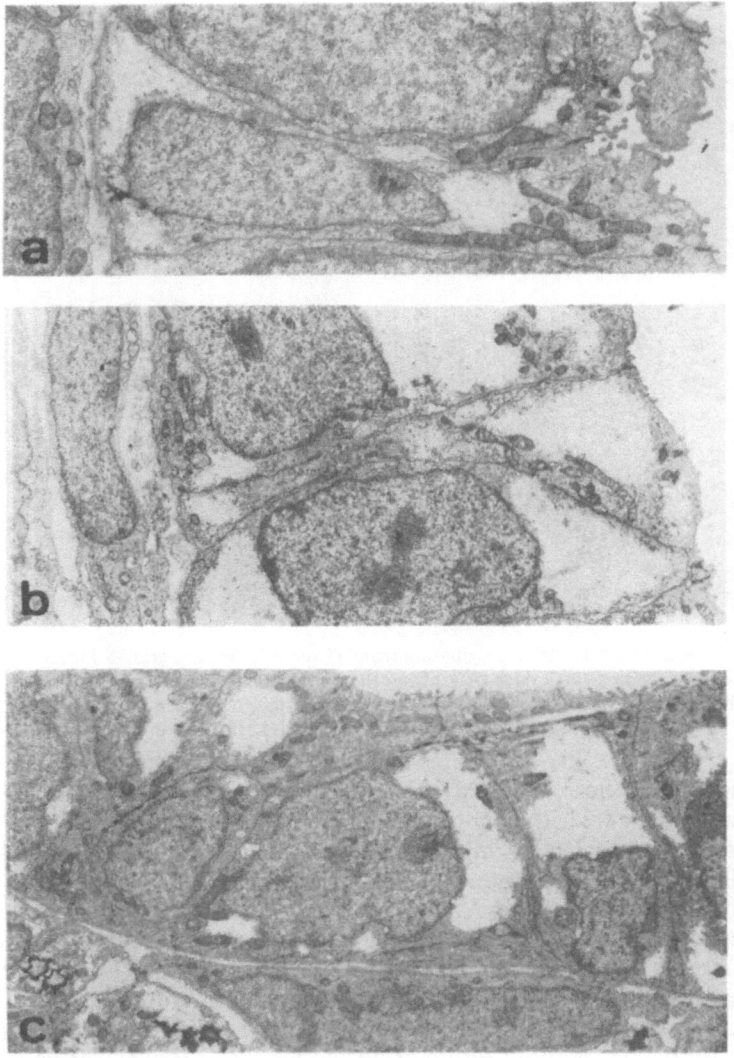

Figure 1.3 Fetal rat lung tissue grafted, in 3.5-day-old chicken embryos: **(a)** lung tissue originating from a 16-day-old rat fetus grafted for 3 days (× 3000); **(b)** lung tissue originating from a 17-day-old rat fetus, grafted for 2 days (× 4500); **(c)** lung tissue originating from an 18-day-old rat fetus, grafted for 1 day (× 3000). At this stage, which is equivalent to 19 days of gestation, the grafted epithelium is still undifferentiated

It is interesting to note that whereas differentiation is accelerated when fetal lung tissue is grown *in vitro*, it is delayed, and sometimes greatly delayed, when grafted in a living embryo. This may be due to the existence, in the latter, of some inhibiting factors, which are lacking *in vitro*, allowing the cultured cells to express morphological differentiation sooner

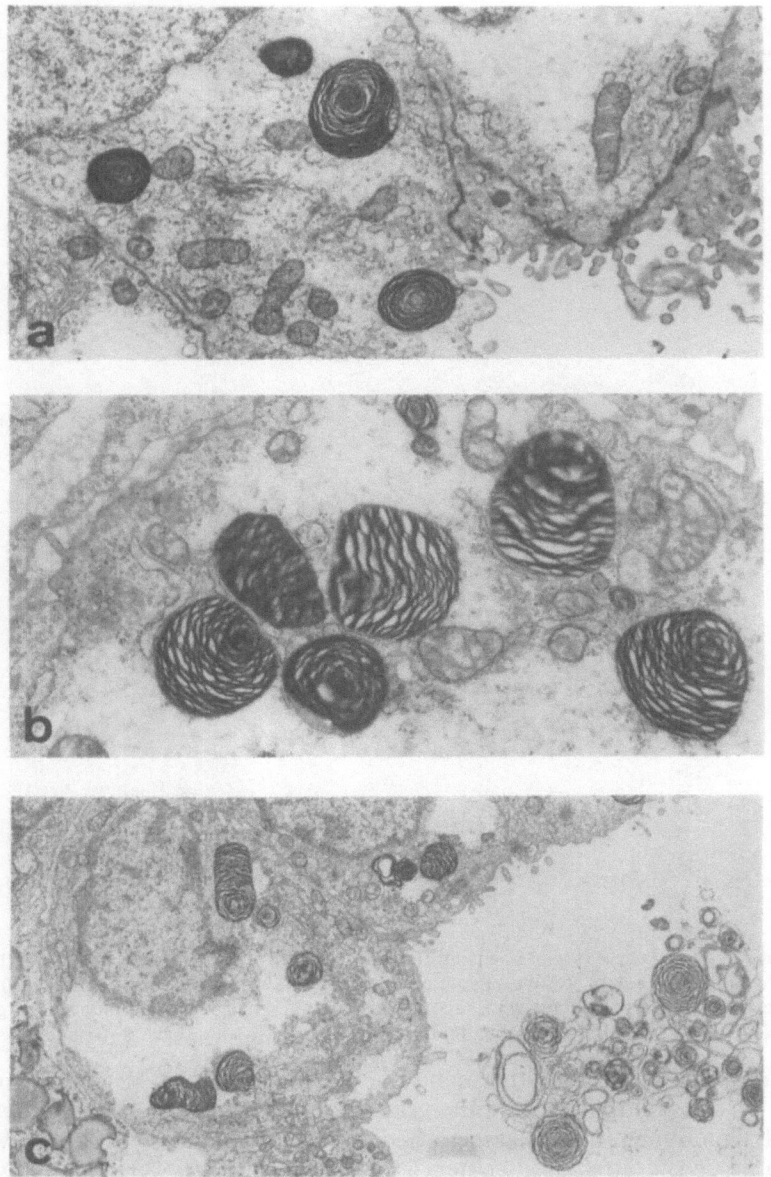

Figure 1.4 Fetal rat lung tissue grafted in 3.5-day-old chick embryos: **(a)** lung tissue originating from a 16-day-old rat fetus, which has been grafted for 5 days ($\times$ 7500); **(b)** lung tissue originating from a 17-day-old rat fetus, which has been grafted for 4 days ($\times$ 10500); **(c)** lung tissue originating from an 18-day-old rat fetus, which has been grafted for 3 days ($\times$ 4500). At this stage, which is equivalent to 21 days of gestation, type II cells have differentiated in the grafted tissue. Normal lamellar bodies have appeared, although the level of circulating hormones in the embryo is still very low

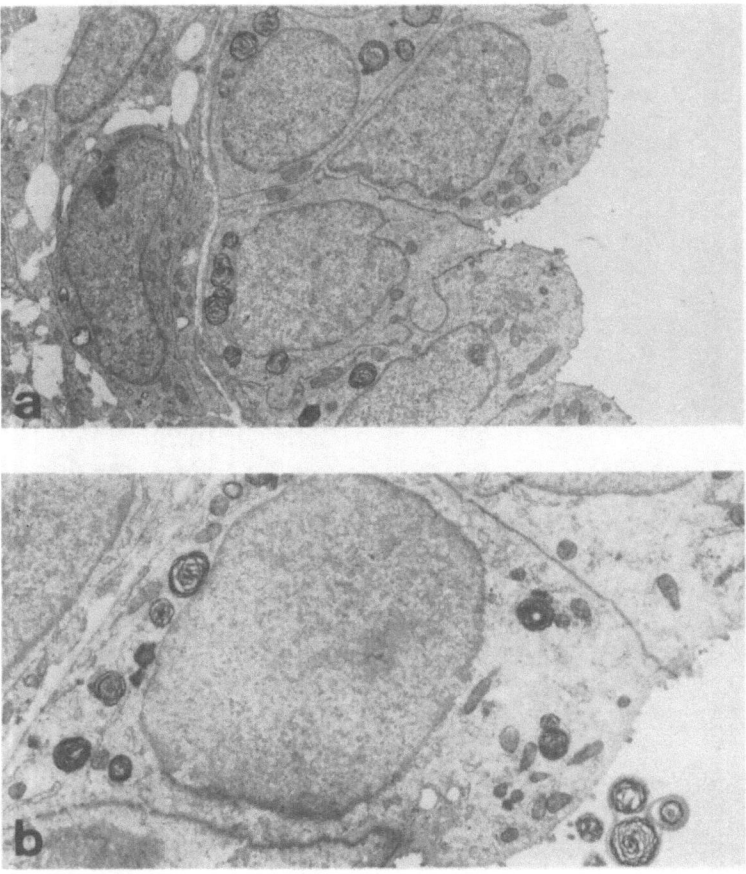

Figure 1.5 Lung tissue originating from 16-day-old rat fetuses, maintained *in vitro* for 3 days in Waymouth's medium: **(a)** lung tissue originating from a normal fetus (× 4500); **(b)** lung tissue originating from a fetus whose mother has been adrenalectomized on day 10 of gestation (× 3000). Type II cells, containing numerous lamellar bodies, have differentiated

than normally. On the other hand the phenomenon may be related to the rate of cell multiplication in the grafted or cultured tissues. Indeed, when 13-day-old lung primordia are grafted, their growth rate is very high. When lung tissue is grafted at later stages the growth rate is lower. Finally, when lung primordia, or fetal lung tissue, are transplanted *in vitro,* the growth rate remains very low.

In conclusion, our results suggest that hormones, which undoubtedly control lung maturation once it has started, might not be involved in the initiation of type II cell differentiation in the course of normal fetal development.

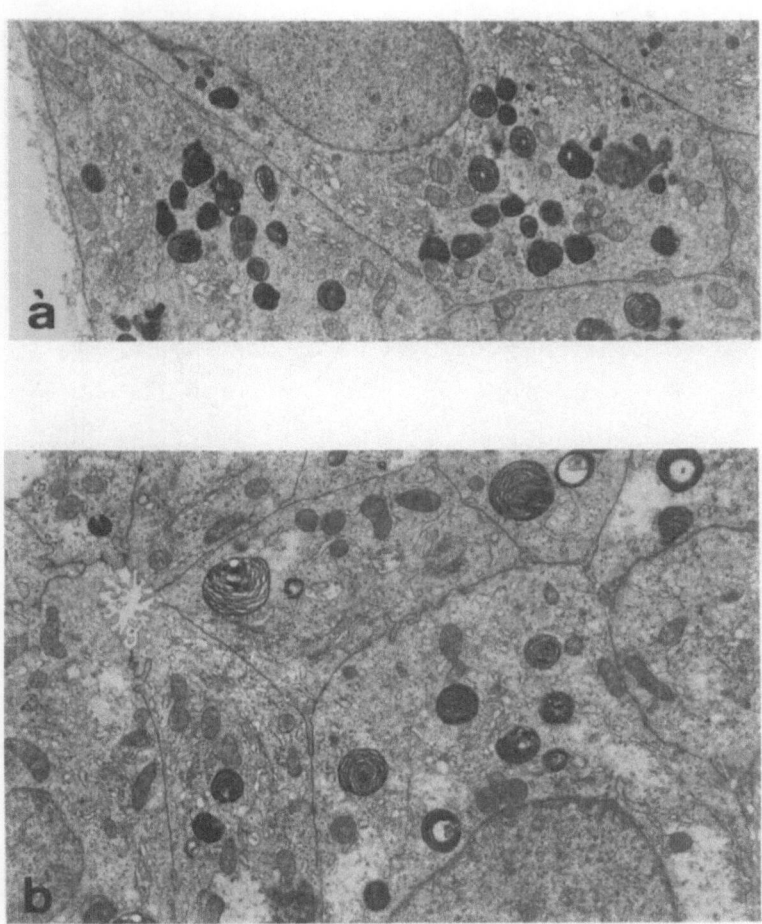

Figure 1.6 Lung tissue, originating from 13-day-old rat fetuses, which has been maintained *in vitro* for 6 days: **(a)** in Waymouth's medium, without serum or hormones ($\times$ 4500); **(b)** in Waymouth's medium, plus fetal calf serum ($\times$ 4500)

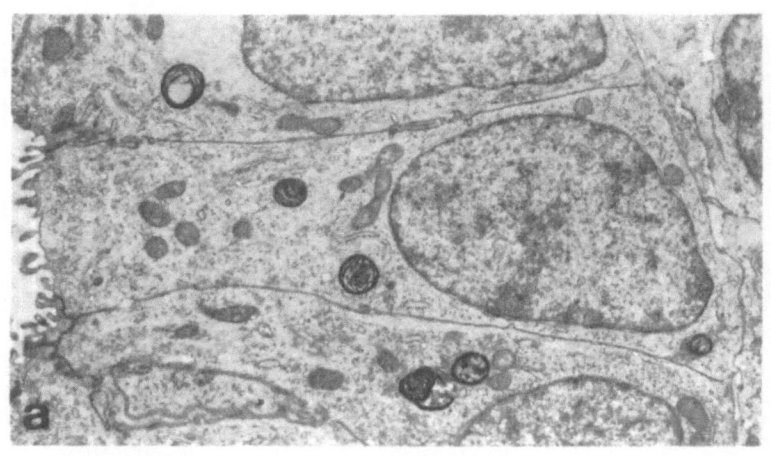

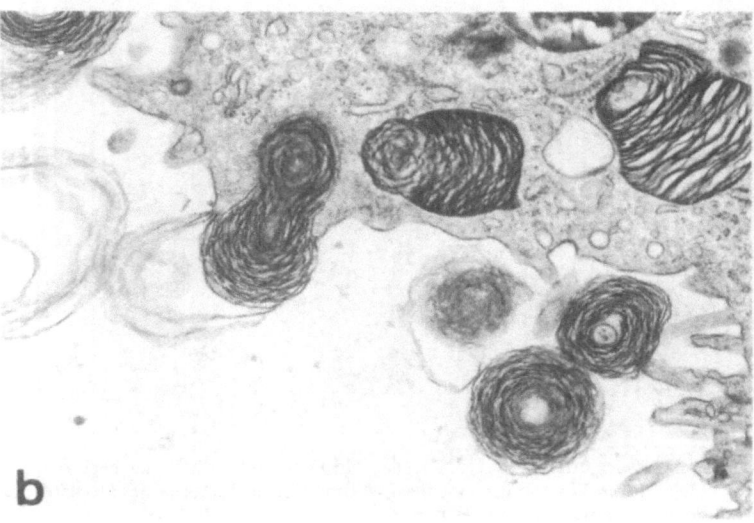

Figure 1.7 Same tissue as Fig. 1.6 maintained: **(a)** in Waymouth's medium plus charcoal-stripped calf serum (× 4500); **(b)** in Waymouth's medium, plus an antiglucocorticoid drug (× 15000)

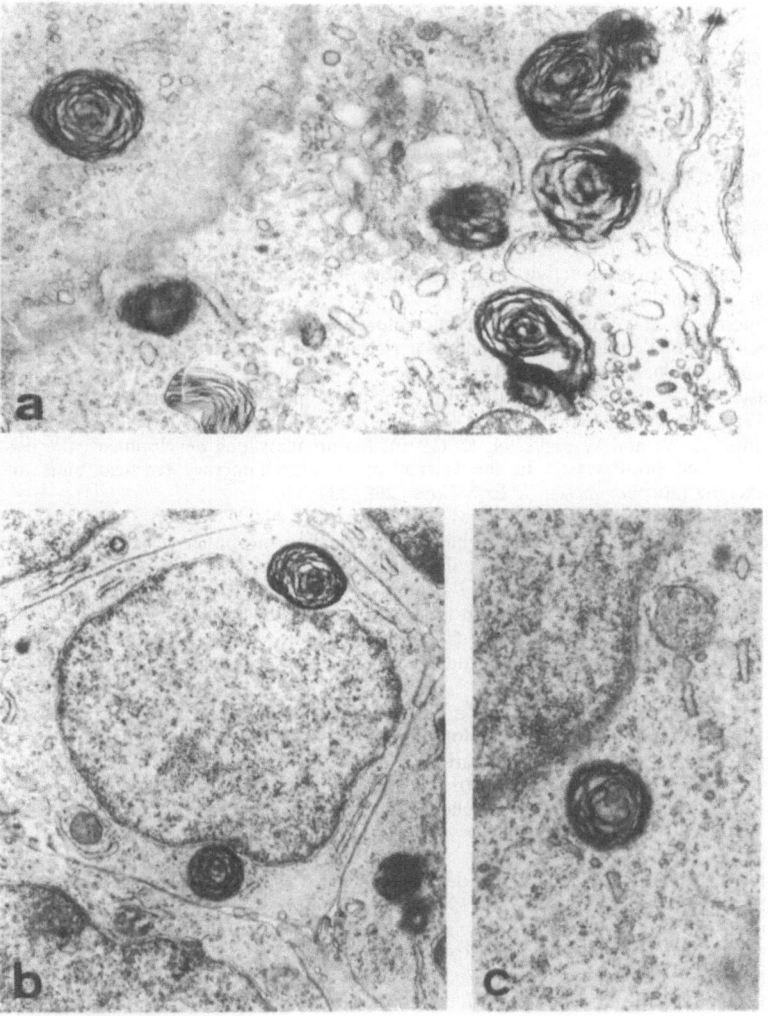

Figure 1.8 Lung tissue originating from 13-day-old rat fetuses, which has been maintained *in vitro* (a) for 5 days ($\times$ 15000); (b) for 4 days ($\times$ 7500); (c) for 3 days ($\times$ 15000). Normal lamellar bodies have appeared in epithelial cells. The timing of the differentiation has been accelerated, as compared to normal development (Figure 1.8b is reproduced with permission from *Cardiovascular and Respiratory Physiology in the Fetus and Neonate,* published by IN-SERM and John Libby and Company)

References

1. Avery, M. E. and Mead, J. (1959). Surface properties in relation to atelectasis and hyaline membrane disease. *Am. J. Dis. Child.*, **97**, 517
2. Farrell, P. M. and Avery, M. E. (1975). Hyaline membrane disease. *Am. Rev. Resp. Dis.*, **111**, 657–688
3. Rosenquist, G. C. (1970). The origin and movement of prelung cells in the chick embryo as determined by autoradiographic mapping. *J. Embryol. Exp. Morphol.*, **24**, 497–509
4. Alescio, T. and Cassini, A. (1962). Induction 'in vitro' of tracheal buds by pulmonary mesenchyme grafted on tracheal epithelium. *J. Exp. Zool.*, **150**, 83–94
5. Alescio, T. and Dani, A. M. (1971). The influence of mesenchyme on the epithelial glycogen and budding activity in mouse embryonic lung developing 'in vitro'. *J. Embryol. Exp. Morphol.*, **25**, 131–140
6. Dameron, F. (1968). Etude expérimentale de l'organogénèse du poumon: nature et spécificité de l'epithelium pulmonaire de l'embryon de poulet en culture 'in vitro'. *J. Embryol. Exp. Morphol.*, **20**, 151–157
7. Masters, J. R. W. (1976). Epithelial-mesenchymal interaction during lung development: the effect of mesenchymal mass. *Devel. Biol.*, **51**, 98–108
8. Goldin, G. V. and Wessells, N. K. (1979). Mammalian lung development: the possible role of cell proliferation in the formation of supernumerary tracheal buds and in branching morphogenesis. *J. Exp. Zool.*, **208**, 337–346
9. Goldin, G. V., Hindman, H. M. and Wessells, N. K. (1984). The role of cell proliferation and cellular shape change in branching morphogenesis of the embryonic mouse lung: analysis using aphidicolin and cytochalasins. *J. Exp. Zool.*, **232**, 287–296
10. Grant. M. M., Cutts, M. R. and Brody, J. S. (1983). Alterations in lung basement membrane during fetal growth and type 2 cell development. *Devel. Biol.*, **97**, 173–183
11. Jaskoll, T. F. and Slavkin, H. C. (1984). Ultrastructural and immunofluorescence studies of basal lamina alterations during mouse lung morphogenesis. *Differentiation*, **28**, 36–48
12. Ryan, U., Slawkin, H., Revel, J. P., Massaro, D. and Gail, D. (1984). Conference report: cell-to-cell interactions in the developing lung. *Tissue Cell*, **16**, 829–841
13. Smith, B. T. (1979). Lung maturation in the fetal rat: acceleration by the injection of fibroblast pneumocyte factor. *Science*, **204**, 1094–1095
14. Marin, L., Dameron, F. L. and Relier, J. P. (1982). Changes in the cellular environment of differentiating type II pneumocytes. A quantitative study in the perinatal rat lung. *Biol. Neonate*, **41**, 171–182
15. Hitchcock, K. R. (1980). Lung development and the pulmonary surfactant system: hormonal influences. *Anat. Rec.*, **198**, 13–34
16. Smith, B. T. (1984). Pulmonary surfactant during fetal development and neonatal adaptation: hormonal control. In Robertson, B., Van Golde, L. M. G. and Batenburg, G. G. (eds.) *Pulmonary Surfactant*, pp. 357–381. (Amsterdam: Elsevier)
17. Gross, I. (1984). Regulation of fetal lung maturation: initiation and modulation. In Raivio, Hallman, Kouvalainen and Valimaki (eds.) *Respiratory Distress Syndrome*, pp. 51–64. (New York: Academic Press)
18. Gross, I. and Wilson, C. (1983). Fetal rat lung maturation: initiation and modulation. *J. Appl. Physiol. Resp. Environ.*, **55**, 1725–1732
19. Marin, L., Dameron, F. L. and Relier, J. P. (1981). Le surfactant pulmonaire au cours du développement foetal et néonatal. Rôle des facteurs humoraux foetaux. In Minkowski, A. (ed.) *Biologie du Dévelopement*, pp. 27–57. (Paris: Flammarion)
20. Gaspard, K. J., Klitgaard, H. M. and Wondergem, R. (1981). Somatomedin and thyroid hormones in the developing chick embryo. *Proc. Soc. Exp. Biol. Med.*, **166**, 24–27
21. Hilfer, S. R. and Searls, R. L. (1980). Differentiation of the thyroid in the hypophy-sectomized chick embryo. *Devel. Biol.*, **79**, 107–118
22. Kalliecharan, R., and Hall, B. K. (1974). A developmental study of the levels of progesterone, corticosterone, cortisol and cortisone circulating in plasma of chick embryos. *Gen. Comp. Endocrinol.*, **24**, 364–372
23. Roth, J., Hernandez, E. and Pruss, R. M. (1982). Insulin is present in chicken eggs and early chick embryos. *Endocrinology*, **111**, 1909–1916

24. Thommes, R. C., Vieth, R. L. and Levasseur, S. (1977). The effects of hypophysectomy by means of surgical decapitation on thyroid function in the developing chick embryo. I. Plasma thyroxin. *Gen. Comp. Endocrinol.*, **31**, 29–36
25. Funckhouser, J. D. and Hughes, E. R. (1978). Differentiation of the pulmonary surfactant system. Disaturated phosphatidylcholine accumulation in fetal rat lung in vivo and in vitro. *Biochim. Biophys. Acta,* **530**, 9–16
26. Mendelson, C. R., Johnston, J. M., McDonald, P. and Snyder, J. M. (1981). Multihormonal regulation of surfactant synthesis by human fetal lung in vitro. *J. Clin. Endocrinol. Metabol.*, **53**, 307–317
27. Snyder, J. M., Mendelson, C. R. and Johnston, J. M. (1981). The effect of cortisol on rabbit fetal lung maturation in vitro. *Devel. Biol.,* **85**, 129–140

Discussion

Dr B. Smith	Your observations with the cultured lung and the antiglucocorticoid are very beautiful. However Dr John Torday has made opposite observations using biochemical techniques in our laboratory. Do you think it absolutely necessary that the morphology and biochemistry of the fetal lung progress in parallel?
Dr L. Marin	We did not make any biochemical assays on these explants, firstly because of having insufficient tissue and secondly because biochemical assays may not be sensitive enough to detect relevant changes. The lack of any detectable difference at the biochemical level does not always mean that there is none.
Smith	I would agree that hormones may have more influence on the final stages of maturation than in the initiation of development. They are probably modulators and timers rather than initiators.
Dr J. S. Wigglesworth	Your observations, Dr Marin, certainly fit in with findings in the human fetus. There appears to be a dissociation between endocrine function and lung development as the lungs in the anencephalic fetus may be normal even though there is gross disturbance of endocrine development. Looking at your slides, the alveolar spaces seemed to be very small in your cultured lung tissues, particularly in those transplanted into the chick embryo. Could you say whether there is any evidence of liquid accumulation within the air spaces?
Marin	This aspect is not constant from one explant to another. Some were expanded with liquid and others not; I can't tell why.
Dr L. B. Strang	Dr Wigglesworth, are you really justified in saying that the anencephalic fetus is necessarily inadequate in endocrine development? Is there not considerable variation in the damage to the hypothalamic region in these fetuses.
Wigglesworth	Most of them do not have normally formed posterior pituitaries or normal formation of the hypothalamus. In the 'true' anencephalic these structures are replaced by disorganized tissue although the anterior pituitary appears normal.
Strang	Are the adrenal glands present and of normal size?
Wigglesworth	The adrenal glands are always present but severely hypoplastic. Usually the two glands from an anencephalic fetus weigh well under 1.0 g at term, whereas the normal adrenals weigh about 8 g. There is almost total absence of the fetal cortex although the definitive cortex is present.
Smith	While I don't believe that individual case reports carry a lot of weight, on the question of anencephaly there are two reports which seem to be very important. One was from the US, where a group[1] followed a fetus, known by ultrasound to be anencephalic, with weekly amniocenteses for L/S ratios. The L/S ratio remained immature well past normal term – in fact until 45 weeks – when it became mature. Approximately 1 week later the infant was delivered after spontaneous labour. A second case, which we reported some years ago from Canada[2], concerned a set of twins born at 35 weeks. One was normal with normal corticosteroid

14

Smith   levels in cord blood and mature lungs, whereas the second, an anencephalic, had low corticosteroid levels and immature lungs. These two case reports tell me that in the appropriate time frame, hormones are important. I would add my opinion – and this is in agreement with Dr Marin's work – that hormones are not necessary for the lungs to mature, provided they are allowed enough time.

References

1. Weiss, R. R., Macri, J. N., Tejani, N., Tillitt, R. and Mann, L. I. (1974). Antenatal diagnosis and lung maturation in anencephaly. *Obstet. Gynecol.*, **44**, 368–372
2. Smith, D. T. and Worthington, D. (1976). Discordant lung maturation and corticosteroid levels in twins. *Pediatr. Res.*, **10**, 468 (Abstr.)

2
Differentiation of the Pulmonary Epithelium

B. T. SMITH, M. POST AND J. FLOROS

SUMMARY

1. Respiratory distress syndrome (RDS) reflects birth prior to the ability to synthesize adequate amounts of the pulmonary surfactant.
2. Exogenous glucocorticoids precociously stimulate surfactant production and thus reduce the incidence of RDS when administered to mothers in premature labour.
3. A major limitation to prevention of RDS by this means is the time required for demonstrable benefit: at least 24 hours must elapse between administration and delivery.
4. Belatedly, it has been recognized that this effect is modelled on the normal role of endogenous fetal glucocorticoids in timing and stimulating fetal lung maturation.
5. This effect is indirect: glucocorticoids act on the fetal lung fibroblast to induce production of fibroblast-pneumonocyte factor (FPF) which in turn stimulates surfactant synthesis by the alveolar type II cell.
6. In the fibroblast, glucocorticoid induction of FPF production is a pretranslational event and, hence, relatively slow.
7. At the level of the type II cell, FPF stimulates the rate-limiting enzyme in surfactant-associated phospholipid synthesis, and this effect is maximal within 60 minutes of incubation.

INTRODUCTION

The prenatal developmental repertoire of the pulmonary epithelium includes budding and branching activity to define the future airspaces; serving as a temporary prenatal site of glycogen storage; perhaps participating in the control of perinatal regression of interstitial tissue; achieving closer proximity to capillary endothelium and itself attenuating the physical barrier to postnatal gas exchange; and the subspecialization of a subpopulation of cells in the terminal airspaces for the synthesis and secretion of a highly specialized material, the pulmonary surfactant. This material, required to stabilize airspaces once air-breathing commences, is produced by the alveolar type II cells or 'pneumonocytes'. The recognition by Avery and Mead[1] that neonatal respiratory distress syndrome (RDS or hyaline membrane disease) is due to a deficiency in the pulmonary surfactant has led to a major revolution in our understanding of this important public health problem[2] and, indeed, to diagnostic[3], therapeutic[4,5], and even preventive[6,7] approaches. Most of these gains have been brought about by studies carried out at the organismic or organ level. The purpose of the present communication is to share more recent studies of the regulation of lung maturation at the cellular and molecular level, and to speculate upon possible future clinical implications of such new knowledge.

REGULATION OF FETAL LUNG MATURATION

In the context of this communication we shall equate regulation of lung maturation with regulation of the quantitative and temporal ability to elaborate components which serve as markers for the pulmonary surfactant. Most often utilized as a marker is the synthesis or content of saturated phosphatidylcholine, the major surface-active component of the surfactant. Phosphatidylglycerol also serves as a useful marker. A large number of agents, both hormones (glucocorticoids, thyroid hormones, thyrotropin releasing hormone, prolactin (?)) and exogenous agents (ambroxol, heroin, methylxanthines) can stimulate the production of surfactant by the fetal lung. The greatest experience has been with the glucocorticoids, and this is the only class of agents for which there is sufficient clinical experience to recommend routine clinical use for the prevention of RDS in fetuses at risk of premature delivery.

CLINICAL EXPERIENCE WITH GLUCOCORTICOIDS

After Liggins noted[8], quite by accident, that infusion of glucocorticoid into one of twin sheep fetuses resulted in better postnatal pulmonary aeration than in the untreated twins, a clinical trial was undertaken[6]. As compared to premature infants whose mothers, under double-blind conditions, received placebo, such infants born after *in utero* exposure to betamethasone had a significantly reduced incidence of RDS[6]. This benefit was restricted to infants born more than 24 h, but less than 7 days, after treatment was commenced. The requirements for at least 24 h of exposure to the hormone prior to birth now appears to be in keeping with our current understanding of the mechanism of action (see following) and represents a major limitation of such a preventive approach. The lack of statistically significant benefit if delivery occurred more than 7 days after therapy, however, may not represent so much the biology of the hormone effect as the fact that in this circumstance both the treatment and placebo groups had gained at least another week of maturation *in utero* ; thus the incidence of RDS was quite low in both of these sub-groups.

Several other studies have confirmed these findings, the most convincing being a large multicentred double-blind study carried out in North America[7]. Amongst 696 enrolled mothers, the incidence of RDS in the offspring was overall reduced from 18.1% to 12.7%, a statistically significant finding. Note, however, that the incidence of disease remains perturbingly high (albeit lowered) in the treatment group. Treatment failures were related to certain identified subgroups, including males and, again, those infants delivered within 24 h of treatment initiation. It was reported that 18.2% of the treated group (and 16.7% of the placebo group) delivered within this 24 h period. It must be noted, however, that this represents 16.7–18.2% of *enrolled* patients. Expected delivery within 24 h was the major criterion for exclusion of prospective candidates from this study. Indeed, out of 7893 mothers in premature labour screened for admission into the study, only 696 were enrolled[7], a figure of only 9%! Thus the relatively slow action of antenatal glucocorticoids is, in our view, the major limitation in their impact on the incidence of RDS.

PHYSIOLOGICAL ACTION OF GLUCOCORTICOIDS ON THE FETAL LUNG

It is interesting to note that the clinical and basic science of glucocorticoid regulation of lung maturation has been developed backwards. This is to say that the effect was demonstrated by serendipity[8], followed by clinical application[6,7], and only belatedly by recognizing that the clinical use of glucocorticoids is but an attempt to mimic a physiological process[9] – probably an imperfect attempt. Given preceding clinical application, is it valid to expend resources on elucidating underlying physiology? We shall leave the reader to reach his own conclusion.

There is now extensive evidence that the normal course of fetal lung maturation is temporally and quantitatively controlled by a complex panoply of hormonal regulators (reviewed in ref. 10), central among which are the glucocorticoids. The evidence for a physiological role of glucocorticoids in lung maturation has been previously reviewed[9,10], and includes studies and observations along classic endocrinological lines: (a) fetal plasma glucocorticoids rise just prior to the prenatal increase in surfactant production[11]; (b) administration of exogenous glucocorticoid increases and accelerates lung maturation in experimental animals (reviewed in ref. 10) and, as noted above, in proto-man; (c) ablation of the fetal pituitary[12,13] or of fetal adrenal function[14,15] delays lung maturation; and (d) the fetal lung contains specific glucocorticoid receptors[16–18] and a local metabolic apparatus for maintaining local glucocorticoid levels at relatively high levels[19].

CELLULAR MECHANISM OF GLUCOCORTICOID ACTION

As noted above, the surfactant is produced by the alveolar type II cell (or pneumonocyte). Since glucocorticoids stimulate surfactant production in organ cultures or mixed cell cultures (which contain multiple cell types) isolated from the fetal lung, it seemed reasonable to expect that this represented a direct effect on this epithelial cell type, especially since it is known to possess glucocorticoid receptors[20]. Surprisingly, this is not the case: the steroid acts on the fetal lung fibroblast to induce production of a small protein, fibroblast-pneumonocyte factor (FPF) which, in turn, stimulates surfactant production by the fetal alveolar type II cell[21]. Although first identified under tissue culture conditions, this protein appears to be physiologically relevant, since *in vivo* its injection accelerates lung maturation[22] and, conversely, injection of monoclonal antibodies against FPF delays the normal course of lung maturation[23]. It is present in human amniotic fluid near term[24]. Although relatively unexplored as yet, the multiple hormonal interactions known to be involved in the regulation of lung maturation[10] may also involve variations on this theme[25,26].

SUBCELLULAR MECHANISM OF GLUCOCORTICOID ACTION

As noted in the preceding section, glucocorticoid action on fetal lung maturation appears to involve a mesenchymal-epithelial action mediated by FPF. Only by consideration of the participation of the two cell types involved can a fuller picture emerge.

Production of FPF in the fetal lung fibroblast

As noted previously, this is regulated by glucocorticoids, The process is organ-specific[27], but not species-specific[28]. Recent evidence[29] suggests that FPF production is blocked by inhibitors of both protein and RNA synthesis, implying pretranslational regulation by the glucocorticoid. This is indeed confirmed by the observation that the glucocorticoid induces the appearance of messenger RNA which codes for FPF[29]. Interestingly, the primary translation product is biologically active[29]. As might be expected from the pretranslational nature of this effect, it is a relatively slow event: FPF mRNA is not detected for at least 7 h after glucocorticoid exposure, and the protein is not secreted by the cells in detectable amounts for at least 10 h (unpublished observations).

Action of FPF on the alveolar type II cell

This protein stimulates surfactant synthesis by isolated alveolar type II cells[21,30] as reflected by the biosynthesis of saturated phosphatidylcholine. Since the enzyme cholinephosphate cytidylyltransferase is rate-regulatory in phosphatidylcholine biosynthesis by this cell type[31], it was logical to speculate that this enzyme might be affected by FPF. Indeed, more recent studies suggest that this is indeed the case[32]. Most strikingly, stimulation of the activity of this enzyme is maximal within 60 min of incubation of the cells with FPF.

Taken together, the above observations suggest that the relatively delayed clinical effect of glucocorticoids in preventing RDS is more related to the time required for production of FPF within the fetal lung fibroblast than to the time required for it to act upon the alveolar type II cell. Thus, future availability of this protein could considerably increase the success of our attempts to prevent RDS in infants threatened with premature delivery.

Acknowledgements

The diphthongs herein result from appreciation for Professor Strang's excellent contribution to the organization of this meeting and from the senior author's British Commonwealth heritage. Supported by grants from the US National Institutes of Health (P50 HL-27372, RO1 HL-33069, and R23 HL-31956).

References

1. Avery, M. E. and Mead, J. (1959). Surface properties in relation to atelectasis and hyaline membrane disease. *Am. J. Dis. Child.*, **97**, 517–23
2. Farrell, P. H. M. and Wood, R. E. (1976). Epidemiology of hyaline membrane disease in the United States: analysis of national mortality statistics. *Pediatrics*, **58**, 167–76
3. Torday, J. S., Carson, L. and Lawson, E. E. (1979). Saturated phosphatidylcholine in amniotic fluid and prediction of the respiratory-distress syndrome. *N. Engl. J. Med.*, **301**, 1013–18
4. Gregory, G. A., Kitterman, J. A., Phibbs, R. A., Tooley, W. H. and Hamilton, W. K. (1971). Treatment of the idiopathic respiratory-distress syndrome with continuous positive airway pressure. *N. Engl. J. Med.*, **284**, 1333–40
5. Taeusch, H. W., Clements, J. A. and Benson, B. (1983). Exogenous surfactant for human lung disease. *Am. Rev. Resp. Dis.*, **128**, 791–4
6. Liggins, G. C. and Howie, R. N. (1972). A controlled trial of antepartum glucocorticoid treatment for prevention of the respiratory distress syndrome in premature infants. *Pediatrics*, **50**, 515–25
7. Collaborative Group on Antenatal Steroid Therapy (1981). Effect of antenatal dexamethasone administration on the prevention of respiratory distress syndrome. *Am. J. Obstet. Gynecol.*, **141**, 276–87
8. Liggins, G. C. (1969) Premature delivery of fetal lambs infused with glucocorticoids. *J. Endocrinol.*, **45**, 515–23
9. Smith, B. T. (1979). Prevention of hyaline membrane disease: an attempt to mimic a physiological process. In Moss, A. J. (ed.) *Pediatrics Update.* pp. 151–167. (New York: Elsevier)
10. Smith, B. T. (1984). Pulmonary surfactant during fetal development and neonatal adaptation: hormonal control. In Robertson, B., Van Golde, L. M. G. and Batenburg, J. J. (eds.) *Pulmonary Surfactants.* pp. 357–381. (Amsterdam: Elsevier)
11. Mulay, S., Giannopoulos, G. and Soloman, S. (1973). Corticosteroid levels in the mother and fetus of the rabbit during gestation. *Endocrinology*, **93**, 1342–8
12. Blackburn, W. R., Kelly, J. S., Dickman, P. S., Travers, H., Lopata, M. A. and Rhoades, R. A. (1973). The role of the pituitary-adrenal-thyroid axes in lung differentiation. II. Biochemical studies of developing lung in anencephalic fetal rats. *Lab. Invest.*, **28**, 352–60
13. DeLemos, R. A., Diserens, W. and Halki, J. (1971). Lung development after hypophysectomy in the goat fetus. *Comb. Abstr. Am. Ped. Soc., Soc. Ped. Res.* (Abstr.)
14. Kling, O. R. and Kotas, R. V. (1975). Endocrine influences on pulmonary maturation and the lecithin/sphingomyelin ratio in the fetal baboon. *Am. J. Obstet. Gynecol.*, **121**, 664–8

15. Vidyasagar, D. and Chernick, V. (1975). Effect of metopirone on the synthesis of lung surfactant in does and fetal rabbits. *Biol. Neonate*, **27**, 1–16
16. Ballard, P. L. and Ballard, R. A. (1974). Cytoplasmic receptor for glucocorticoids in lung of the human fetus and neonate. *J. Clin. Invest.*, **53**, 477–86
17. Giannopoulos, G. (1973). Glucocorticoid receptors in lung. I. Specific binding of glucocorticoids to cytoplasmic components of rabbit fetal lung. *J. Biol. Chem.*, **248**, 3876–83
18. Giannopoulos, G., Mulay, S. and Soloman, S. (1973). Glucocorticoid receptors in lung. II. Specific binding of glucocorticoids to nuclear components of rabbit fetal lung. *J. Biol. Chem.*, **248**, 5016–23
19. Torday, J. S., Post, M. and Smith, B. T. (1985). Compartmentalization of 11-oxidoreductase within fetal lung alveolus. *Am. J. Physiol.: Cell Physiol.*, **249**, C173–C176
20. Ballard, P. L., Mason, J. R. and Douglas, W. J. H. (1978). Glucocorticoid binding by isolated lung cells. *Endocrinology*, **102**, 1570–5
21. Smith, B. T. (1978). Fibroblast-pneumonocyte factor: intercellular mediator of glucocorticoid effect on fetal lung. In Stem, L. (ed.) *Neonatal Intensive Care*. pp. 25–32. (New York: Mason)
22. Smith, B. T. (1979). Lung maturation in the fetal rat: acceleration by injection of fibroblast-pneumonocyte factor. *Science*, **204**, 1094–5
23. Post, M., Floros, J. and Smith, B. T. (1984). Inhibition of lung maturation by monoclonal antibodies against fibroblast-pneumonocyte factor. *Nature*, **308**, 284–6
24. Seybold, W. D. and Smith, B. T. (1980). Human amniotic fluid contains fibroblast-pneumonocyte factor. *Early Hum. Devel.*, **4**, 337–45
25. Smith, B. T. and Sabry, K. (1983). Glucocorticoid-thyroid synergism in lung maturation: a mechanism involving epithelial-mesenchymal interaction. *Proc. Natl. Acad. Sci. USA*, **80**, 1951–4
26. Carlson, K. S., Smith, B. T. and Post, M. (1984). Insulin acts on the fibroblast to inhibit glucocorticoid stimulation of lung maturation. *J. Appl. Physiol.: Resp. Environ. Exercise Physiol.*, **57**, 1577–9
27. Smith, B. T. and Giroud, C. J. P. (1975). Effects of cortisol on serially propogated fibroblast cell cultures derived from the rabbit fetal lung and skin. *Canad. J. Physiol. Pharmacol.*, **53**, 1037–41
28. Smith, B. T. (1981). Lack of species-specificity in production of fibroblast pneumonocyte factor by perinatal lung fibroblasts. In Monset Couchard, M. and Minkowski, A. (eds.) *The Physiological and Biochemical Basis for Perinatal Medicine*. pp. 54–58. (Basel: Karger)
29. Floros, J., Post, M. and Smith, B. T. (1985). Glucocorticoids affect the synthesis of pulmonary fibroblast-pneumonocyte factor at a pretranslational level. *J. Biol. Chem.*, **260**, 2265–7
30. Post, M. and Smith, B. T. (1984). Effect of fibroblast-pneumonocyte factor on the synthesis of surfactant phospholipids in type II cells from fetal rat lung. *Biochim. Biophys. Acta*, **793**, 297–9
31. Post, M., Batenburg, J. J., Van Golde, L. M. G. and Smith, B. T. (1984). The rate-limiting reaction in phosphatidylcholine synthesis by alveolar type II cells isolated from fetal rat lung. *Biochim. Biophys. Acta*, **795**, 558–63
32. Post, M. and Smith, B. T. (1984). Fibroblast-pneumonocyte factor purified with the aid of monoclonal antibodies stimulates cholinephosphate cytidylyltransferase activity in fetal type II cells. *Pediatr. Res.*, **18**, 401A (Abstr.)

Discussion

Dr L. M. G. Van Golde	Although cholinephosphate cytidylyltransferase is a rate-limiting enzyme in the conversion of choline to phosphatidylcholine, another rate-limiting step in phosphatidylcholine synthesis may be between glycerol phosphate and diacylglycerols. Did you look to see whether FPF also affects other enzymes – let's say glycerol phosphate acyltransferase – or is the effect limited to cytidylyltransferase?
Dr B. Smith	I would be very surprised if it were limited to cholinephosphate cytidylyltransferase. The data relate to the only part of the pathway that we have examined as yet. It would be interesting to see whether the remodelling from unsaturated to saturated molecules of phosphatidylcholine might be affected by FPF. In some of the *in vivo* studies the major effect of FPF is on the percentage saturated phosphatidylcholine.
Van Golde	Did you look to see whether the activation of cholinephosphate cytidylyltransferase is accomplished by a translocation between cytosol and microsomes?
Smith	I can say that Dr Post is attempting these studies at the moment, but I don't think he has evidence for that yet.
Dr M. Hallman	You showed that glucocorticoid induces the synthesis of FPF. Do you think that if there were no glucocorticoid present you would still see differentiation?
Smith	Totally without data, my bias is that given sufficient time neither glucocorticoids nor FPF should be necessary for lung maturation. One of our interests in the future will be to look for genetic anomalies which might be expressed in the infant born very close to term who nonetheless develops respiratory distress syndrome.
Dr L. B. Strang	Would that view imply then that these mechanisms may be absent in the adult?
Smith	Yes, we have done studies in which we cannot detect production of FPF in postnatal lung fibroblasts. Both Dr Van Golde's group and Bob Mason's group have shown that FPF does not act on adult type II cells (personal communicatons).
Strang	Can you reassure us that fibroblasts from tissues other than the lung don't produce FPF?
Smith	It is exceedingly tissue specific.
Dr P. H. Burri	I would be interested to know more about the morphology of your culture system. You call it organotypic, but does it have anything like airspaces in it? Secondly, can you comment on the two types of fibroblasts, labelled and unlabelled?
Smith	In reply to the first question one of the systems which we use is organotypic; it is a three-dimensional system in which mixed fetal lung cells are placed on a sponge of gelfoam. In that system they reconstitute themselves three-dimensionally and there appear to be airspaces – i.e. spheres are formed. As to the second question, yes we believe there are multiple subpopulations of these fibroblasts, although this conclusion is based on some very preliminary evidence on differences in staining at the terminal parts of the differentiating lung buds. As you know, Dr Cunha's group[1] in San Francisco has looked at glucocorticoid receptors

	within lung mesenchyme and shown that they also show subanatomical localization adjacent to the epithelium.
Dr C. J. Morley	You imply that if you could get enough FPF you might be able to give it to women in premature labour, and that it would act faster than cortisol. Have you any idea what it does to tissue other than lung?
Smith	We have not as yet done toxicology studies which will be necessary before moving in the direction you suggest.
Dr E. A. Egan	With reference to the US collaborative study on the effects of corticosteroids on the incidence of RDS, you indicated that time lag is part of the reason for failure of treatment; but there is still a substantial failure rate after 24 h on steroids. How does this square with your view that a more rapidly acting agent would solve the problem?
Smith	There are, as you know, several subgroups that appear to be non-responsive to corticosteroids. In particular the male infant is less responsive than the female. Dr Torday in our group has found that the main difference in response between the sexes is at the level of the mesenchyme. The male lung fibroblast is less able to produce FPF than the female fibroblast, whereas the male type II cell responds to it as well as does the female cell. It has also been shown by Dr Kathleen Carlson in our group[2] that insulin inhibits production of FPF.
Dr C. L. Gaultier	What is the mechanism of action of T_3 and T_4 in lung maturation?
Smith	Apparently the thyroid hormones do not act on FPF or on the fibroblast, but rather on the type II cell making it more responsive to FPF.
Dr J. S. Wigglesworth	Is there any evidence on the need for maturation of the fibroblast itself before it is capable of producing FPF.
Smith	This protein is produced in small amounts at approximately 15 days gestation in the lung fibroblast of the fetal rat. It peaks at day 19–20, then falls off and is gone by the second or third postnatal day. One of our interests will be to learn how this gene is regulated in terms of its temporal expression during development.
Dr C. A. R. Boyd	Is there any homology of FPF with any of the known mesenchymal growth factors?
Smith	We do not yet have any sequence data, and hence we cannot synthesize oligonucleotide probes. With regard to functional similarity to other known mesenchymal factors, we have studied all those available and find that none share its pneumocyte-stimulating properties.

References

1. Sees, D. G., Cunha, G. R. and Malkinson, A. M. (1983). Autoradiographic demonstration of the specific binding and nuclear localisation of ³H-dexamethasone in adult mouse lung. *Lab. Invest.*, **49**, 725–34
2. Carlson, K. S., Smith, B. T. and Post, M. (1984). Insulin acts on the fibroblast to inhibit glucocorticoid stimulation of lung maturation. *J. Appl. Physiol. Resp. Environ. Exercise Physiol.*, **57**, 1577–9

3
Factors Affecting Fetal Lung Growth

J. S. WIGGLESWORTH

INTRODUCTION – THE CLINICOPATHOLOGICAL PROBLEM

The control of organ growth in quantitative terms is a subject of sufficient complexity to deter most developmental biologists, and particularly physiologists, surgeons and pathologists from too close an enquiry. However, it has become recognized that fetal lung growth is extraordinarily susceptible to adverse influences[1]. The most frequent effect of adverse influences on the human fetal lung is to retard growth so that the lungs at birth are hypoplastic and extrauterine respiration may not be established[2-5]. The human fetal lungs normally represent about 2–3% of body weight in the third trimester with a gradual fall in weight of the lungs relative to that of the body towards term[6]. Pathologists have regarded lungs representing 1.2% or less of body weight as unduly small[7,8]. We found that 14% of fresh stillbirths and early neonatal deaths at Hammersmith Hospital had hypoplastic lungs as indicated by a low lung/body weight ratio, and a frequency above 10% has been recognized by other pathologists[1,9]. Large lungs are far less frequent than small ones, and in my experience are invariably associated with congenital laryngeal atresia.

A very large number of conditions are associated with congenital lung hypoplasia. These may be grouped as shown in Table 3.1. One of the conditions most frequently seen in association with lung hypoplasia is oligohydramnios. Thomas and Smith[10] pointed out some years ago that both the hypoplastic lungs and the external anomalies seen in conditions with oligohydramnios are purely secondary to the lack of amniotic fluid. In rare cases where an infant with renal agenesis forms one of a monoamniotic twin pair the lungs grow normally and the infant may survive until renal failure supervenes[11,12]. In contrast an infant with normal renal tract but lack of amniotic fluid due to rupture of the membranes early in the second trimester, and subsequent leakage of amniotic fluid, may show the external features and hypoplastic lungs typically seen with renal agenesis[13-15].

Table 3.1 Conditions associated with lung hypoplasia

Prolonged oligohydramnios	Renal agenesis
	Severe renal cystic dysplasia
	Obstruction of lower urinary tract, prune belly syndrome
	Prolonged rupture of membranes
Skeletal dysplasias affecting integrity of thoracic wall	Thanatophoric dwarfism
	Asphyxiating thoracic dysplasia
	Osteogenesis imperfecta (lethal variant)
Anomalies affecting development of diaphragm	Congenital diaphragmatic hernia
	Congenital muscular dystrophy
	Congenital amyoplasia of diaphragm
Anomalies or damage to CNS	Anencephaly
	Iniencephaly
	Anoxic ischaemic lesions
	Meckel–Gruber syndrome
Miscellaneous conditions	Exomphalos
	Severe rhesus isoimmunization
	Extralobar sequestration of lung with pleural effusion.
	Other forms of non-immunologic hydrops (including some inborn errors of metabolism)

Congenital abnormalities associated with reduction of the intrathoracic volume are not unnaturally associated also with hypoplastic lungs. The most frequent of these is congenital diaphragmatic aplasia[16]; others include thoracic dysplasias such as thanatophoric dwarfism and asphyxiating thoracic dystrophy[9]. Anomalies or injury affecting the central nervous system may be associated with lung hypoplasia. Such conditions include some instances of anencephaly, intrauterine anoxic–ischaemic damage involving the brain stem and cord[4], and some cases of Werdnig–Hoffman disease with prenatal onset[17]. Many of the conditions that are associated with congenitally hypoplastic lungs of themselves suggest patterns of functional failure or of mechanical impairment to fetal lung growth rather than a primary organogenetic defect. Lack of space for lung growth or pressure from adjacent structures have long been assumed to account for many of these associations. However, this does not provide a satisfactory explanation for all cases. In cases of anencephaly in which the brainstem is preserved the lungs develop normally and the infant may survive for some hours or days after birth. In cases where the brainstem and upper spinal cord are involved in the anomaly there may be lung hypoplasia despite a normally developed thoracic cage and diaphragm. In such a situation, with increased amniotic fluid and no structural reason to account for lung hypoplasia, a functional basis for the condition seems likely. Similarly in several instances where undersized lungs were associated with anoxic–ischaemic damage to the CNS *in utero* it seemed likely that some functional impairment in lung growth had occurred[18].

KNOWLEDGE OF GROWTH CONTROL MECHANISMS IN THE MAMMALIAN FETAL LUNG

Embryologically, the lung develops as an outgrowth from the ventral aspect of the primitive foregut. In the human this occurs during the fourth week after conception when the embryo is 3–4 mm in length. The primitive epithelial tubule representing the trachea divides sequentially to form the major generations of bronchial branches. Initial epithelial branching is known to be under the control of the adjacent mesenchyme[19]. Indeed mesenchyme–epithelial reciprocal inductive processes may control a large proportion of basic pulmonary development[20]. Postembryonic structural lung development is subdivided into three classic separate stages: pseudoglandular, canalicular and terminal sac, as discussed elsewhere in this book. The close spatial relationship between epithelial tubules and the surrounding condensations of mesenchyme during the pseudoglandular phase (7–17 weeks in man) may reflect the interactions between these tissues. The main feature of the canalicular phase (17–24 weeks) is the thinning of the respiratory epithelium from a glandular to cuboidal pattern in association with transformation of the tubules into recognizable fluid-filled peripheral airways. Differentiation of the respiratory epithelium into type 1 and type 2 pneumonocytes and progressive elaboration of the airspaces to form alveoli are the characteristic features of the terminal sac phase from 24 weeks to term.

The presence of liquid within the lung from the canalicular stage onwards was in the past misinterpreted as indicating that the fetus expanded the lungs by inhaling amniotic fluid, a reasonable assumption in view of the frequent presence of amniotic debris within the lungs of stillborn infants. It was widely believed that the inhalation and expansion of the lungs with amniotic fluid was an essential mechanism to ensure normal fetal lung growth[21]. However, the experiments of Jost and Policard[22], in which decapitation of the fetal rabbit *in utero* was shown to be followed by development of normal or even large lungs, eventually caused this idea to be abandoned. In the Jost and Policard experiment the trachea became occluded following operation and the fetal lungs filled with fluid which had evidently formed *in situ,* providing one of the first demonstrations of lung liquid secretion. It has since become clear that the fluid produced by the lung forms a powerful mechanical stimulus to fetal lung growth. Although some inward movement of fluid occurs during periods of fetal breathing

27

the net flow is outwards. The fluid flows out of the trachea at an average hourly rate of 4.5 ml/kg during the last third of gestation in the fetal sheep[23]. As the fetal lung in this species represents about 2.5% of body weight, it can be estimated that the lung secretes its own volume in fluid over a period of $5\frac{1}{2}$ h. Alcorn and colleagues[24] showed that chronic drainage of liquid from the trachea of the fetal lamb results in lung hypoplasia, while surgical obstruction to the trachea, preventing egress of fluid to the amniotic cavity, results in grossly dilated fluid-filled lungs, as seen in the human fetus with laryngeal atresia[24,25].

Studies of fetal breathing movements during the past 15 years have shown that they do not normally produce dramatic inflow of amniotic fluid. Fetal respiratory movements can be recognized as bursts of high-frequency low-amplitude activity in the diaphragm, and to a lesser extent the chest wall, occurring in the human from early in the second trimester[26,27]. In lambs the movements have been considered to cause little net flux of tracheal fluid although they are associated with significant transthoracic pressure gradients. The normal episodic irregular low-amplitude movements are associated with pressure swings of 3-5 torr, but there are less frequent (about 1 per min) pressure changes of up to 20-30 torr[28,29].

There seems little a priori reason to believe that fetal breathing movements of this type would be of any significance for lung growth. However, the observations on human fetuses with CNS lesions, and other situations where it seemed likely that fetal respiratory movements might be impaired, led us to investigate the possibility that abolition of respiratory movements in the fetus with an intact airway might impair lung growth. We started from the basis that a significant growth-promoting role for fetal breathing would readily be disproved if section of the respiratory pathways in a fetus with patent trachea was followed by normal lung growth. An operation such as phrenectomy would be expected to cause atrophy of the diaphragm and might impair lung growth purely by a process of mechanical compression in a similar way to diaphragmatic hernia. We therefore severed the neural pathways between the medulla and the phrenic nucleus in order to produce an upper motor neurone type of lesion in which preservation of the reflex arc would allow maintenance of muscle tone and normal muscle growth, while abolishing co-ordinated breathing movements. Our experimental approach was designed to prevent co-ordinated respiratory movements without impairing development of chest wall and diaphragm, so as to avoid the possibility that lung growth impairment might result from compression by adjacent structures. We compared the effects of transecting the cord between the medulla and phrenic nucleus, which should prevent all respiratory movement, with those of transecting the cord between phrenic nucleus and thoracic inlet, which should allow diaphragmatic movement but prevent movement of the thoracic wall (Fig. 3.1).

Our experiments were performed at 23-24 days gestation on the fetal rabbit when the lung is about to change from the pseudoglandular to the canalicular stage. Spinal cord transection had no influence on fetal growth

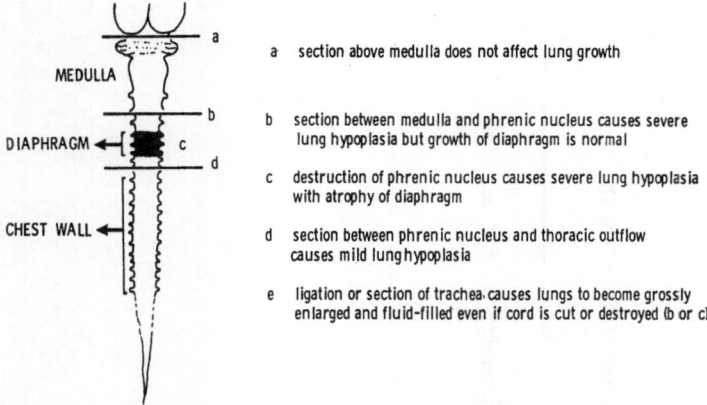

a   section above medulla does not affect lung growth

b   section between medulla and phrenic nucleus causes severe
     lung hypoplasia but growth of diaphragm is normal

c   destruction of phrenic nucleus causes severe lung hypoplasia
     with atrophy of diaphragm

d   section between phrenic nucleus and thoracic outflow
     causes mild lung hypoplasia

e   ligation or section of trachea causes lungs to become grossly
     enlarged and fluid-filled even if cord is cut or destroyed (b or c)

Figure 3.1 Summary of results of fetal surgery on lung growth in rabbits

in general, and did not impair growth of individual organs such as liver, kidney, heart or thymus. The growth of muscles, including the diaphragm, was also unaffected by the operation. There was, however, a consistent and marked effect on lung growth. Transection at C1–C3 between the medulla and the phrenic nucleus caused severe lung hypoplasia with a 70% reduction in lung growth over the period of the experiment, as measured by the increment of DNA[30]. Cord transection between the phrenic nucleus and the thoracic outflow (C6–C8), which would be expected to prevent thoracic movements but to allow normal diaphragmatic function, resulted in lungs of intermediate size between those of the high cord section group and those of control littermates. Destruction of the phrenic nucleus (C3–C5) caused complete atrophy of the diaphragm with an even more severe degree of lung hypoplasia than that associated with high cord section. Tracheal ligation at time of cord transection resulted in large fluid-filled lungs with a normal DNA content (Fig. 3.2). No consistent differences between the groups were demonstrated in respect of the concentration of phospholipid components such as lecithin palmitate, indicating a lack of difference in surfactant content.

The results were those to be expected if fetal respiratory movements play an important role in aiding fetal lung growth. The alternative explanation is that the effects were due to a non-specific loss of tone in chest wall and diaphragm associated with spinal shock. Spinal shock is analogous to a lower motor neurone injury and, if sufficiently long-lasting to cause impairment in lung growth, should also retard growth of the diaphragm. The normality of diaphragmatic growth in the high-section group suggests that spinal shock is not a significant factor.

The effects of high cord transection on fetal lung growth were confirmed by Liggins and colleagues using fetal lambs[31]. These workers also caused equally severe lung hypoplasia by inserting a flexible silastic membrane into the chest wall to abolish the pressure swings from fetal breathing while allowing it to continue[32]. Several groups have shown that section of the

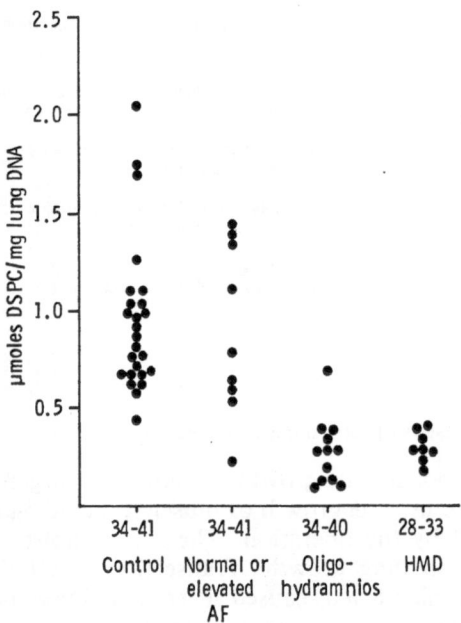

Figure 3.2 Concentration of disaturated phosphatidylcholine expressed per mg lung DNA in normally developed human fetal lungs as compared with hypoplastic lungs from infants with normal or elevated amniotic fluid volume, hypoplastic lungs from cases of oligohydramnios, and lungs from infants dying in the acute phase of hyaline membrane disease (HMD). Normal and hypoplastic lungs from gestations 34 weeks or more and HMD cases from 28 to 33 weeks. Figures for hypoplastic lungs with oligohydramnios significantly lower than 'controls' ($t = 5.725$, $p < 0.001$). No significant difference between control values and those for hypoplastic lungs from cases with normal or increased amniotic fluid

phrenic nerve causes fetal lung hypoplasia[33,34], but this procedure also causes atrophy of the diaphragm. Section of the vagus has no influence on fetal lung growth[33]. Dornan and colleagues[35] found that total absence of fetal breathing movements, or abnormal breathing movements in human fetuses with congenital abnormalities affecting the respiratory system, were associated with lung hypoplasia. Surfactant release but not surfactant synthesis were affected. Lung development was relatively normal in an anencephalic fetus with normal breathing movements[35]. There has been shown to be a reduced relative lung size in growth-retarded fetal sheep in which the incidence of fetal breathing movements is reduced[36].

Although none of these experiments individually provides conclusive proof of the role of fetal respiratory movements, it has become widely accepted as a result of these experiments, and human observations, that fetal breathing is important for lung growth in fetuses with normal airways.

The question arises as to how fetal respiratory movements might influence fetal lung growth. We originally suggested that fetal breathing must act by influencing lung volume. It seemed reasonable to assume that, even if the movements did not cause significant amniotic fluid inflow, they might well impose an increased resistance to fluid outflow. Studies by Murai and co-workers (quoted by Kitterman)[37] have shown an increase of lung liquid volume by 20% during periods of fetal breathing. The rate of lung liquid flow out of the trachea in the fetal lamb does not differ irrespective of whether breathing movements are abolished by phrenic section or increased by administration of inhibitors of prostaglandin synthesis[38]. Kitterman[37] believes that this indicates that there is, after all, an inflow of amniotic fluid during fetal breathing.

The effect of tracheal pressure has been investigated in the fetal lamb. In the absence of breathing movements tracheal pressure is about 3 torr above amniotic pressure, probably due to resistance to fluid outflow[39,40]. Abolition of tracheal pressure in one of twin lambs led to a decrease in lung growth[41]. Fewell and Johnson[40] have claimed that there is obstruction to inflow of fluid during fetal breathing by laryngeal adduction, but Harding[42] found electrical activity in laryngeal abductor muscles apparently opening the laryngeal orifice during the inspiratory phase of fetal breathing. It currently seems uncertain whether any increase of lung volume during fetal breathing can be ascribed to decreased outflow or to significant inflow. To answer the question will need measurement of both magnitude and direction of tracheal flows, as well as changes in lung volume during periods of fetal breathing.

Endocrine factors which are of importance in control of general body growth do not have any specific effect on growth of the fetal lung. Thus pituitary and thyroid hormones are without specific effect on quantitative fetal lung growth despite their known influences on pulmonary epithelial maturation[37]. Human infants with pituitary or thyroid aplasia are not typically born with hypoplastic lungs. Other growth factors such as EGF may also have an influence on maturation, but have not been shown to have an effect on gross lung growth, although EGF may stimulate growth and budding of the embryonic lung[43,44].

MECHANISMS OF HUMAN FETAL LUNG HYPOPLASIA

The relationships postulated among fetal breathing, fetal lung volume control, and fetal lung growth may help to explain some forms of human fetal lung hypoplasia such as those associated with abnormalities or intrauterine damage to the CNS or disorders of neuromuscular function. They do not provide any obvious explanation for lung hypoplasia in oligohydramnios.

The most popular theory relates lung hypoplasia to a decreased space for lung growth. There is some experimental evidence in support of this mechanism in that experimental surgical procedures causing reduction in intrathoracic space result in lung hypoplasia[45].

Nakayama and colleagues[46] produced oligohydramnios in the rabbit by obstructing the bladder neck, and attempted to prevent lung hypoplasia by creating an abdominal hernia. As an alternative the fluid was replaced by a continuous saline infusion. Partial reversal was obtained by such means.

31

However, the reduction in alveolar number at term following a single removal of amniotic fluid in the monkey experiments of Hislop and co-workers[47] is against a simple compressive mechanism.

A superficially attractive hypothesis related lung hypoplasia in renal agenesis to lack of the normal proline production by the fetal kidney[48]. However the similarity of lung hypoplasia in oligohydramnios of any cause, irrespective of the presence or absence of normal fetal renal tissue, renders this hypothesis untenable. We have found a relatively high concentration of hydroxyproline in this group of hypoplastic lungs, suggesting that proline availability is unlikely to be a limiting factor in their growth (Wigglesworth and Desai, in preparation).

An effect on fetal breathing is worth considering. Nathanielz et al.[49] noted tonic focal contractions of both sheep and monkey uterus, which they call contractures, and which cause deformation of the fetal thorax and may abolish fetal breathing. The effects of such uterine contractions on the fetus may be more severe in the absence of amniotic fluid. Amniocentesis in human pregnancy causes a decrease in fetal breathing movements for up to 2 days[50]; but breathing movements do occur in infants with oligohydramnios[51]. It is also of interest that spinal cord transection has been shown to accentuate lung hypoplasia in experimental oligohydramnios[52].

This leaves consideration of reduced fluid content in airways and airspaces. The most striking feature of these lungs at a histological level is the small size of the acini and a characteristic form of impaired epithelial maturation[4]. This can be seen irrespective of whether the cause of oligohydramnios is renal agenesis or prolonged rupture of the membranes. If such infants survive for some hours they develop HMD. This is in marked contrast to the lungs of infants with lung hypoplasia associated with normal or increased amniotic fluid, which have a normally developed structure for the gestation.

We have found that disaturated phosphatidylcholine concentration in the lungs of the oligohydramnios group at 34 weeks or more is as low as in infants who die in the acute stage of HMD at an earlier gestation, in comparison with the normal levels seen in the equally hypoplastic lungs of infants with normal or increased amniotic fluid (Fig 3.2). The narrow airways and small airspaces of the lungs in oligohydramnios, in addition to impaired epithelial maturation, seem likely effects of lack of liquid retention. Experimentally one might wish to see the effect of obstructing lung liquid outflow at laryngeal level on lung growth in oligohydramnios. The combination of renal agenesis and laryngeal atresia does indeed occur in some infants with the synophthalmos (Fraser) syndrome. In a recent case of this condition we found that the lungs were large and oedematous, and both structural and biochemical indices of lung size and alveolar number were within normal limits. We have previously observed cases with this combination of anomalies in which the lungs were large rather than hypoplastic[1].

IMPLICATIONS OF FUNCTIONAL CONTROL OF FETAL LUNG GROWTH

The recognition that normal fetal lung growth is highly dependent on both secretion of lung liquid and its retention by neuromuscular activity involving fetal breathing movements carries important implications for perinatal medicine. Both types of function are readily interfered with by stresses to which the fetus is subject. Lung liquid secretion can be abolished in fetal lambs by infusion of catecholamines or β_2 adrenergic agents[53]. Thus it may be expected that any acute stress affecting the fetus may temporarily depress the secretion of lung liquid or lead to its resorption, with consequent impairment in lung growth. Fetal respiratory movements are readily depressed by a wide variety of influences including hypoxia, maternal hypoglycaemia, smoking or the maternal ingestion of CNS depressant drugs such as alcohol or barbiturates[27,54,55].

Thus on theoretical grounds it might be expected that infants subject to recurrent episodes of intrauterine asphyxia would have smaller lungs than those not exposed to such stress. We have recently shown that normally formed infants who die during or soon after birth near term have smaller lungs related to body weight than those who die earlier in gestation or those who present as unexpected death at 2 weeks age or later (Table 3.2). This group of normally grown and normally formed mature infants are mainly cases of intrapartum asphyxia, many of whom show subtle signs of preceding intrauterine stress on pathological examination[56]. A small group of such normally formed infants with borderline or frank lung hypoplasia was recognized by Page and Stocker[9], and the occurrence has been reported as 'primary lung hypoplasia'[5]. These findings give support to the hypothesis that the common forms of prenatal asphyxial stress do indeed retard fetal lung growth.

Table 3.2 Comparison of lung weight and DNA content relative to body weight at different ages in infants without conditions known to be associated with lung hypoplasia

Age	n	Lung weight as percentage of body weight (Mean ± SD)	Lung DNA in mg per kg body weight (Mean ± SD)
28–36 weeks	24	2.1 ± 0.4	156 ± 10.6
		$p < 0.01$	$p < 0.01$
37–42 weeks	20	1.7 ± 0.4	120.5 ± 6.7
		$p < 0.001$	$p < 0.01$
Infant 2 weeks–8 months	19	2.1 ± 0.3	151 ± 32.9

Infants in 37–42 weeks group mainly cases of intrapartum asphyxia. Statistical comparisons by *t* test

Lung size is likely to become limiting for neonatal survival only at the extreme limits, as yet undefined. It must be assumed that many infants with mild or moderate impairment in lung growth will survive the perinatal period. It is interesting to speculate whether compensatory growth of the lung can occur postnatally in such cases or whether the low respiratory reserve will have a limiting influence on tissue oxygenation, and thus on bodily growth in general. Additional point is given to this question by recent observations on alveolar development in the fetal and infant lung, which indicate that a significant proportion of the adult alveolar number develops within the last third of gestation, rather than after birth[57,58]. Our studies on the lungs of prematurely born infants dying at (corrected) postnatal ages up to 9 months after prolonged mechanical ventilation for respiratory distress syndrome show generalized persistent emphysema with severe impairment in alveolar development long after the stage at which the original damage to lung structure has been remodelled (Hislop, Wigglesworth and Desai, in preparation). Although the mechanisms of lung growth impairment after preterm birth in these infants may differ from those retarding lung growth *in utero* the study supports the hypothesis that the lung may have strict limitation to its powers of compensatory growth after birth.

The latter half of gestation may well prove to be a critical period for growth of the peripheral portion of the lung lobule in the way that the first half of gestation is critical for development of the branches of the bronchial tree[59].

References

1. Wigglesworth, J. S. and Desai, R. (1982). Is respiratory function a major determinant of perinatal survival? *Lancet*, 1, 264–7
2. Perlman, M. and Levin, M. (1974). Fetal pulmonary hypoplasia, anuria and oligohydramnios: clinicopathologic observations and review of the literature. *Am. J. Obstet. Gynecol.*, 18, 1119–23
3. Wigglesworth, J. S. (1976). The effects of placental insufficiency on the fetal lung. *J. Clin. Pathol.*, 29, (suppl. 10), 27–30
4. Wigglesworth, J. S., Desai, R. and Guerrini, P. (1981). Fetal lung hypoplasia: biochemical and structural variations. *Arch. Dis. Child.*, 56, 606–15
5. Swischuk, L. E., Richardson, C. J., Nichols, M. M. and Ingman, M. J. (1979). Primary pulmonary hypoplasia in the neonate. *J. Pediatr.* 95, 573–7
6. Wigglesworth, J. S. and Desai, R. (1981). Use of DNA estimation for growth assessment in normal and hypoplastic fetal lungs. *Arch. Dis. Child.*, 56, 601–5
7. Reale, F. R. and Esterly, J. R. (1973). Pulmonary hypoplasia: a morphometric study of the lungs of infants with diaphragmatic hernia, anencephaly, and renal malformation. *Pediatrics*, 51, 91–6
8. Askenazi, S. S. and Perlman, M. (1979). Pulmonary hypoplasia: lung weight and radial alveolar count as criteria of diagnosis. *Arch. Dis. Child.*, 54, 614–18
9. Page, D. V. and Stocker, J. J. (1982). Anomalies associated with pulmonary hypoplasia. *Am. Rev. Respir. Dis.*, 125, 216–21
10. Thomas, I. T. and Smith, D. W. (1974). Oligohydramnios, cause of the non-renal features of Potter's syndrome, including pulmonary hypoplasia. *J. Pediatr.*, 84, 811–14
11. Kohler, H. (1972). An unusual case of sirenomelia. *Teratology*, 6, 295–301
12. Mauer, S. M., Dobrin, R. S. and Vernier, R. L. (1974). Unilateral and bilateral renal agenesis in monoamniotic twins. *J. Pediatr.*, 84, 236–8

13. Perlman, M., Williams, J. and Hirsch, M. (1976). Neonatal pulmonary hypoplasia after prolonged leakage of amniotic fluid. *Arch. Dis. Child.*, **51**, 349-53
14. Fliegner, J. R., Fortune, D. W. and Egger, T. R. (1981). Premature rupture of the membranes, oligohydramnios and pulmonary hypoplasia. *Aust. N.Z. J. Obstet. Gynaecol.*, **21**, 77-81
15. Nimrod, C., Varela-Gittings, F., Machin, G., Campbell, D. and Wesenberg, R. (1984). The effect of very prolonged membrane rupture on fetal development. *Am. J. Obstet. Gynecol.*, **148**, 540-3
16. Butler, N. and Claireaux, A. E. (1962). Congenital diaphragmatic hernia as a cause of perinatal mortality. *Lancet*, **1**, 659-63
17. Cunningham, M. and Stocks, J. (1978). Werdnig–Hoffman disease. The effects of intrauterine onset on lung growth. *Arch. Dis. Child.*, **53**, 921-5
18. Wigglesworth, J. S. (1984). *Perinatal Pathology.* pp. 114-15. (Philadelphia: W. B. Saunders)
19. Wessells, N. K. (1970). Mammalian lung development; interactions in formation and morphogenesis of tracheal buds. *J. Exp. Zool.*, **175**, 455-66
20. Franzblau, C., Hayes, J. A. and Snider, G. L. (1977). Biochemical insights into the development of connective tissue. In Hodson, W. A. (ed.) *Development of the Lung.* pp. 367-399. (New York: Marcel Dekker)
21. Snyder, F. F. (1961). Pulmonary hyaline membrane disease. *Obstet. Gynaecol.*, **18**, 677-94
22. Jost, A. and Policard, A. (1948). Contribution experimentale a l'étude du développement prenatal du poumon chez le lapin. *Arch. Anat. Micr. Morph. Exp.*, **37**, 323-32
23. Mescher, E. J., Platzker, A. C. G., Ballard, P. L., Kitterman, J. A., Clements, J. A. and Tooley, W. H. (1975). Ontogeny of tracheal fluid, pulmonary surfactant and plasma corticoids in the fetal lamb. *J. Appl. Physiol.*, **39**, 1017-21
24. Alcorn, D., Adamson, T. M., Lambert, T. F., Maloney, J. E., Ritchie, B. C. and Robinson, P. M. (1977). Effects of chronic tracheal ligation and drainage in the fetal lamb lung. *J. Anat.*, **123**, 649-60
25. Carmel, J. A., Friedman, F. and Adams, F. H. (1965). Fetal tracheal ligation and lung development. *Am. J. Dis. Child.*, **109**, 452-6
26. Dawes, G. S., Kox, H. E., Leduc, B. M., Liggins, C. G. and Richards, J. S. (1972). Respiratory movements and rapid eye movement sleep in the foetal lamb. *J. Physiol.*, **220**, 119-43
27. Boddy, K. and Dawes, G. S. (1975). Fetal breathing. *Br. Med. Bull.*, **31**, 3-7
28. Maloney, J. E., Adamson, T. M., Brodecky, V., Cranage, S., Lambert, T. F. and Ritchie, B. C. (1975). Diaphragmatic activity and lung liquid flow in the unanaesthetised fetal sheep. *J. Appl. Physiol.*, **39**, 423-8
29. Dawes, G. S. (1984). The central control of fetal breathing and skeletal muscle movements. *J. Physiol.*, **346**, 1-8
30. Wigglesworth, J. S. and Desai, R. (1979). Effects on lung growth of cervical cord section in the rabbit fetus. *Early Hum. Devel.*, **3**, 51-65
31. Liggins, G. C., Vilos, G. A., Campos, G. A., Kitterman, J. A. and Lee, C. H. (1981). The effect of spinal cord transection on lung development in fetal sheep. *J. Devel. Physiol.*, **3**, 267-74
32. Liggins, G. C., Vilos, G. A., Campos, G. A., Kitterman, J. A. and Lee, C. H. (1981). The effect of bilateral thoracoplasty on lung development in fetal sheep. *J. Develop. Physiol.*, **3**, 275-82
33. Alcorn, D., Adamson, T. M., Maloney, J. E. and Robinson, P. M. (1980). Morphological effects of chronic bilateral phrenectomy or vagotomy in the fetal lamb lung. *J. Anat.*, **130**, 683-95
34. Fewell, J. E., Lee, C. and Kitterman, J. A. (1981). Effects of phrenic nerve section on the respiratory system of fetal lambs. *J. Appl. Physiol.*, **51**, 293-7
35. Dornan, J. C., Ritchie, J. W. K. and Meban, C. (1984). Fetal breathing movements and lung maturation in the congenitally abnormal human fetus. *J. Devel. Physiol.*, **6**, 367-75
36. Maloney, J. E., Bowes, G., Brodecky, V., Dennett, X., Wilkinson, M. and Walker, A. (1982). Function in the future respiratory system in the growth retarded fetal sheep. *J. Devel. Physiol.*, **4**, 279-97
37. Kitterman, J. H. (1984). Fetal lung development. *J. Devel. Physiol.*, **6**, 67-82

38. Kitterman, J. A., Liggins, G. C., Clements, J. A. and Tooley, W. H. (1979). Stimulation of breathing movements in fetal sheep by inhibition of prostaglandin synthesis. *J. Devel. Physiol.*, **1**, 453-66
39. Vilos, G. A. and Liggins, G. C. (1982). Intra-thoracic pressures in fetal sheep. *J. Devel. Physiol.*, **4**, 247-56
40. Fewell, J. E. and Johnson, P. (1983). Upper airway dynamics during breathing and during apnea in fetal lamb. *J. Physiol.*, **339**, 495-504
41. Fewell, J. E., Hislop, A., Kitterman, J. A. and Johnson, P. (1983). Effect of tracheostomy on lung development in fetal lambs. *J. Appl. Physiol.*, **55**, 1103-8
42. Harding, R. (1980). State related and developmental changes in laryngeal function. *Sleep, 3*, 307-22
43. Sundell, H. W., Gray, M. E., Serenius, F. S., Escobedo, M. B. and Stahlman, M. T. (1980). Effects of epidermal growth factor on lung maturation in fetal lambs. *Am. J. Pathol.*, **100**, 707-26
44. Carpenter, G. and Cohen, S. (1979). Epidermal growth factor. *Ann. Rev. Biochem.*, **48**, 193-216
45. Harrison, M. F., Jester, J. A. and Ross, N. A. (1980). Correction of congenital diaphragmatic hernia in utero. I. The model: intrathoracic balloon produces fatal pulmonary hypoplasia. *Surgery*, **88**, 174-82
46. Nakayama, D. K., Glick, P. L., Harrison, M. R., Villa, R. L. and Noall, R. (1983). Experimental pulmonary hypoplasia due to oligohydramnios and its reversal by relieving thoracic compression. *J. Pediatr. Surg.*, **18**, 347-53
47. Hislop, A., Fairweather, D. V. I. Blackwell, R. J. and Howard, S. (1984). The effect of amniocentesis and drainage of amniotic fluid on lung development in *Macaca fascicularis*. *Br. J. Obstet. Gynaecol.*, **91**, 835-42
48. Hislop, A., Hey, E. and Reid, L. (1979). The lungs in congenital bilateral renal agenesis and dysplasia. *Arch. Dis. Child.*, **54**, 32-8
49. Nathanielz, P. W., Jansen, C. A. M., Lowe, C. K. and Buster, J. E. (1981). Changing patterns of steroid production in the fetus and placenta and their effects on development. In: *The Fetus and Independent Life*, **86**, pp. 66-88. Ciba Foundation Symposium. (London: Pitman)
50. Manning, F. A., Platt, L. D. and Lemay, K. (1977). Effect of amniocentesis on fetal breathing movements. *Br. Med. J.*, **2**, 1582-3
51. McFadyen, I. R., Wigglesworth, J. S. and Dillon, M. J. (1983). Fetal urinary tract obstruction: is active intervention before delivery indicated? *Br. J. Obstet. Gynaecol.*, **90**,342-9
52. Adzick, N. S., Harrison, M. R., Glick, P. L., Villa, R. L. and Finkbeiner, W. (1984). Experimental pulmonary hypoplasia and oligohydramnios: relative contributions of lung fluid and fetal breathing movements. *J. Pediatr. Surg.*, **19**, 658-63
53. Walters, D. V. and Olver, R. E. (1978). The role of catecholamines in lung liquid absorption at birth. *Pediat. Res.*, **12**, 239-42
54. Manning, F. A. and Feyerabend, C. (1976). Cigarette smoking and fetal breathing movements. *Br. J. Obstet. Gynaecol.*, **83**, 262-70
55. Fox, H. E., Steinbrecher, M., Pessel, D., Inglis, J., Medvid, L. and Angel, E. (1978). Maternal ethanol ingestion and the occurrence of human fetal breathing movements. *Am. J. Obstet. Gynecol.*, **132**, 354-8
56. Wigglesworth, J. S. (1984). *Perinatal Pathology*. pp. 104-109, (Philadelphia: W. B. Saunders)
57. Langston, C., Kida, K., Reed, M. and Thurlbeck, W. M. (1984). Human lung growth in late gestation and in the neonate. *Am. Rev. Respir. Dis.*, **129**, 607-13
58. Hislop, A. A., Wigglesworth, J. S. and Desai, R. (1986). Alveolar development in the human fetus and infant. *Early Hum. Devel.* **13**, 1-11
59. Chamberlain, D., Hislop, A., Hey, E. and Reid, L. (1977). Pulmonary hypoplasia in babies with severe rhesus isoimmunisation: a quantitative study. *J. Pathol.*, **122**, 43-52

Discussion

Dr L. B. Strang	I wonder if you have considered sufficiently the effect of muscle action on thoracic wall compliance?
Dr J. S. Wigglesworth	In the Liggins and Kitterman experiments referred to in my presentation in which a 'window' was inserted into the chest wall, an attempt was made to answer that question. After recovery from the operation, the muscle tone in these lambs should have been relatively normal. They certainly carried on making normal respiratory movements. If tone was really critical over a long period of time, then I would expect it to be important for growth of the thorax in general. But in our experiments you get normal growth of the thorax and the same occurs in the anencephalic fetus. There is adequate volume within the thoracic cage but the diaphragm is very high up within it. I don't see how tone could be critical for lung growth without being critical also for growth of the whole thoracic chamber.
Dr A. C. Bryan	A contracting muscle is a stiffer muscle, there's no doubt; but I don't think that's where the issue lies. It is rather with the thyroaryteroid muscles. As in the newborn so in the fetus, the upper airway muscles have a crucial function in maintaining FRC. It is not so much the rate of ingress or egress of liquid but the magnitude of the respiratory resistance that determines lung volume.
Dr J. P. Mortola	I think, as Dr Bryan does, that the upper airways must contribute to the maintenance of lung volume in the fetus; this could also explain your finding of a positivity of tracheal pressure with respect to amniotic pressure.
Dr B. Robertson	Is there any experimental or other evidence that there is indeed increased drainage of fetal lung liquid in fetal lung hypoplasia due to prolonged rupture of the membranes?
Dr E. A. Egan	I'm not aware that anyone has actually measured the output of lung liquid in these circumstances. However, in experiments in which all the liquid was drained from the trachea, the lungs didn't grow (see Alcorn et al[1]).
Wigglesworth	Premature rupture of the membranes also produces accelerated maturation of the lung, probably because this tends to be associated with infection which induces stress.
Dr G. Enhorning	My impression as an obstetrician is that with premature rupture of the membranes present for some time, there is accelerated maturation of the lung and reduced risk of RDS. When the rupture of the membrane is longstanding, and no infection develops, the result is likely to be hypoplasia.

Reference

1. Alcorn, D., Adamson, T. M., Lambert, T. F., Maloney, J. E., Ritchie, B. C. and Robinson, P. M. (1977). Morphological effects of chronic tracheal ligation and drainage in the fetal lamb lung. *J. Anat. London,* **123**, 649–60

4
Postnatal Lung Development and Modulation of Lung Growth

P. H. BURRI

INTRODUCTION

The human lung at birth is not simply a miniaturized version of the adult one. A newborn lung has to undergo very marked structural changes in order to match adult morphology. We know that between 17 and 50 million alveoli are present at birth, whereas the lung of a man of 75 kg body weight contains around 300 million alveoli. Furthermore, the pulmonary microvasculature is completely restructured in the early postnatal period. Although this process markedly transforms septal morphology, very little is known about it. The late E. A. Boyden, an expert in structural pulmonary development, whose careful three-dimensional reconstructions of the developing lung represented pioneering work, seriously argued that the 'alveoli' counted at birth were saccules[1]. Therefore the alveolar stage of lung development has been placed after birth (Fig. 4.1). Recently Langston and co-workers[2] have published a study on 42 fetal lungs showing that shallow alveoli were present sometimes as early as the 32nd or 34th week. At birth they counted on average 50 million alveoli, a finding which renewed the discussion about the degree of alveolization of the newborn human lung. Practically, this would mean that the human lung could be born in a more mature state than assumed so far. Nevertheless, these new data do not overthrow the fact that the bulk of alveoli develop after birth. Indeed, on average only 15–20% of their final number is present in the first days of postnatal life.

In order to give an insight into the process of alveolar formation and postnatal lung maturation, the general principles of the structural and ultrastructural transformation will be discussed on the basis of findings obtained in the postnatal rat lung. After familiarization with the mechanisms,

39

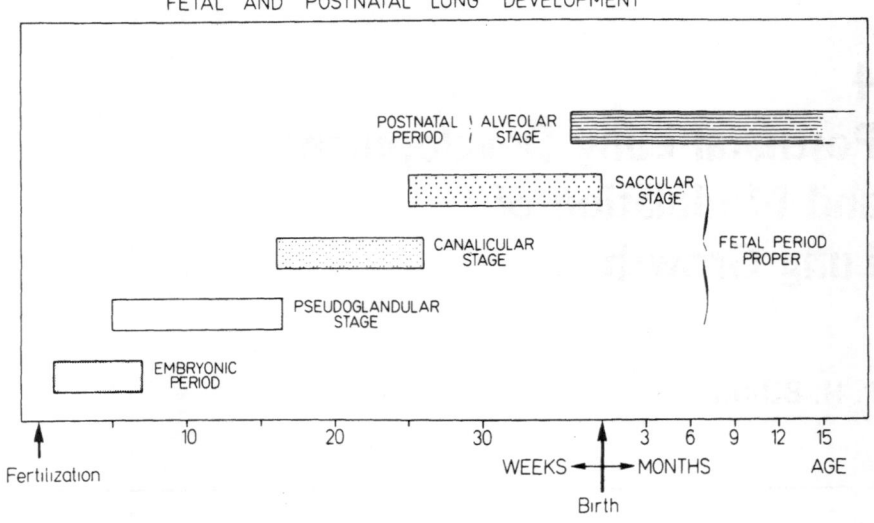

Figure 4.1 Stages and timing of human lung development. Dating is based on the time point of ovulation. Reproduced with permission from Ref. 31

comparisons will be made to the situation in man, as we were able to observe it recently in babies.

POSTNATAL LUNG DEVELOPMENT

At birth the rat lung is devoid of alveoli. The pulmonary parenchyma is formed by smooth-walled channels, which divide and end in a small saccules which have often been interpreted as alveoli (Fig. 4.2a). We called the septa present at birth primary septa[3]. They are straight, relatively thick and show a capillary network on either side of a connective tissue sheet (Figs. 4.2a, 4.3, 4.5a). In contrast, the gas exchange region in animals after weaning (i.e. older than 3 weeks), has tremendously increased in complexity. Within a few days the saccules have been transformed into alveolar sacs and the smooth-walled channels into alveolar ducts by the outgrowth of new, so-called secondary septa, which represent the prospective interalveolar walls (Fig. 4.2b). The morphometric findings reflect these dramatic alterations. Figure 4.6 shows a double logarithmic plot of alveolar and capillary surface areas (Sa and Sc) versus lung volume (VL). The curve shows a triphasic growth pattern with a very steep slope between days 4 and 21. If one assumes airspaces to grow by simple expansion, airspace surface area would increase with lung volume to the power of $\frac{2}{3}$. The much higher regression coefficient of 1.6 signifies that the rapid increase in surface area is achieved by a change in airspace shape. As Fig. 4.2b shows, the secondary septa increase the internal surface complexity of the lung.

40

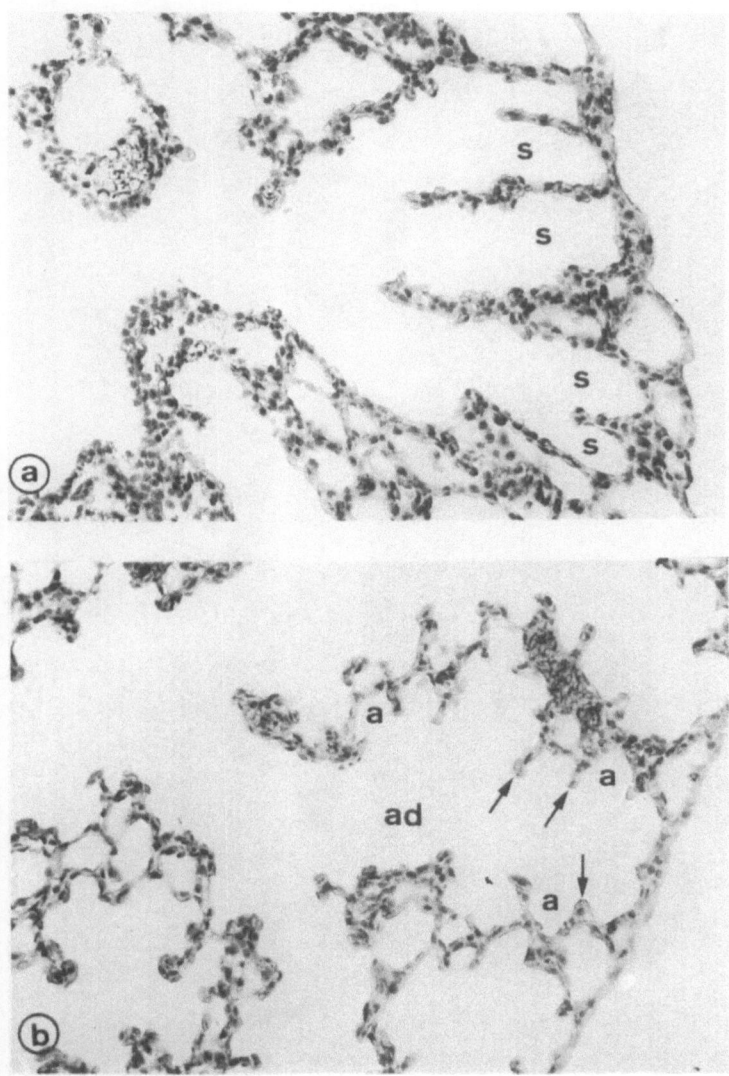

Figure 4.2 Comparison of light micrographs from rat lungs aged 1 day (**a**) and 21 days (**b**) at the same magnification. On day 1 lung parenchyma contains smooth-walled channels and saccules (s) with no alveoli. On day 21 secondary septa have been formed (arrows) and the saccules have been transformed into alveolar ducts (ad) with alveoli (a). (× 230)

We can imagine a secondary septum to be formed by a folding up of capillary loops from the primary septum. Therefore all septa present during alveolar formation have two capillary layers; i.e. they are all of the immature, primitive type (Fig. 4.5a). During the third postnatal week, along

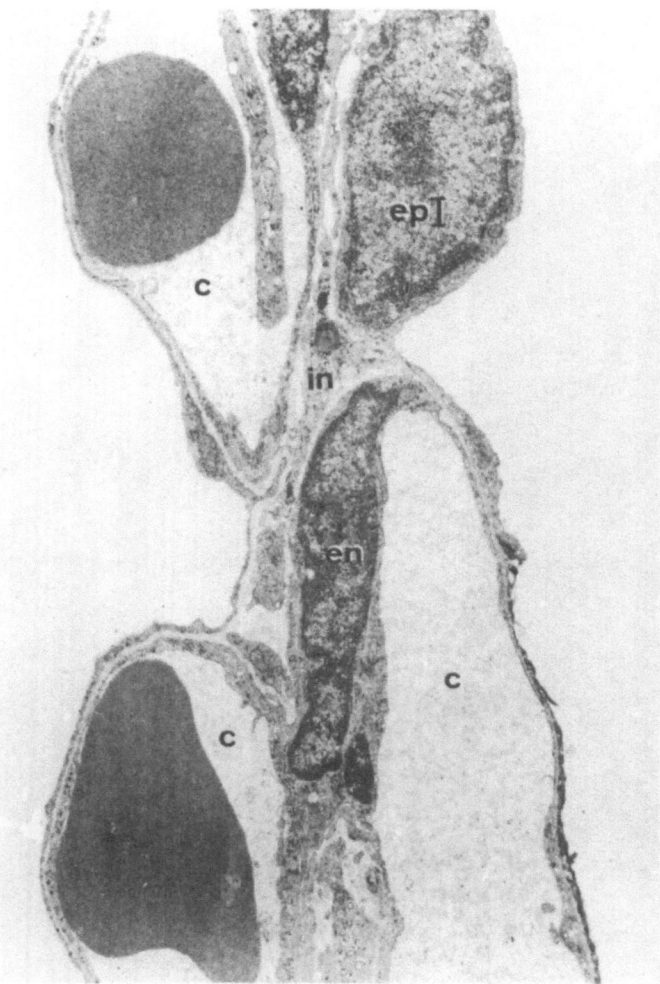

Figure 4.3 Transmission electron micrograph from rat lung aged 4 days. The septum is thick and presents a central layer of interstitium (in) with a capillary network (c) on both sides; en = endothelial cell; epI = epithelial cell nucleus of type I. (× 8000)

with a marked decrease in septal interstitial volume[4] the structure of the capillary bed is dramatically altered, so that at 21 days and later a large part of the parenchyma is made of mature septa (Fig. 4.5b). Transections show the typical adult structure with a central capillary forming a gas-exchange barrier on both its sides (Fig. 4.4). Based on a recent scanning electron microscopic investigation of Mercox casts of the pulmonary vasculature we proposed the hypothesis that the transformation of the septal capillary

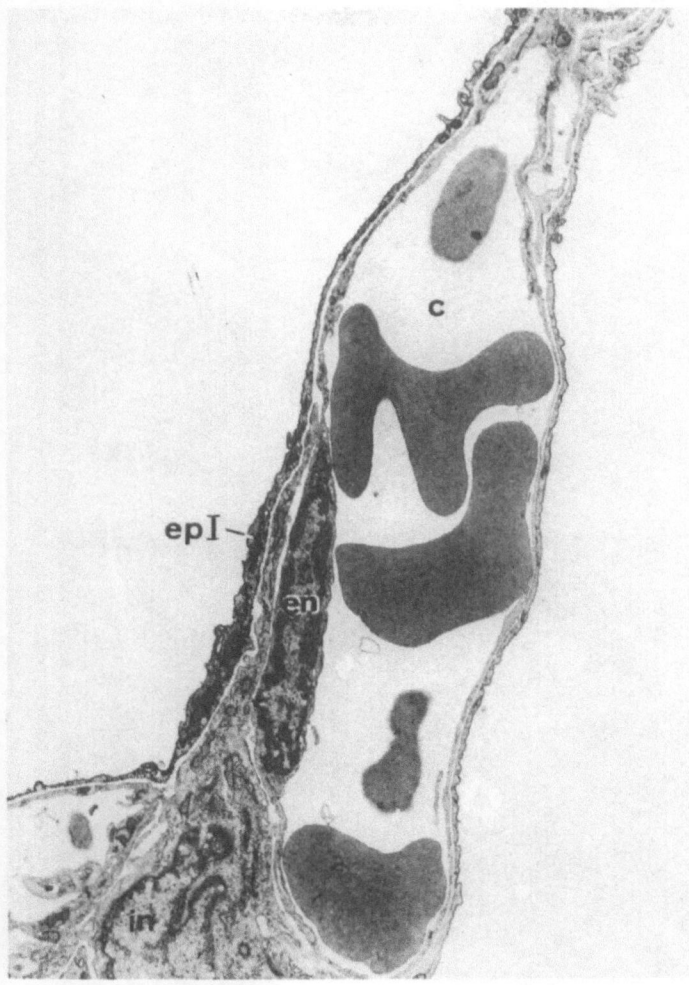

Figure 4.4 Transmission electron micrograph of a mature interalveolar septum of an adult rat lung. The septum is slender, the capillary (c) occupies the central axis of the septum; en = endothelial cell; epI = epithelial cell of type I. (× 6300)

system occurred by two additive processes: a patchwise fusion of the two capillary layers combined with subsequent preferential growth[5]. It is clear, however, that direct proof of such dynamic processes cannot be definitively provided by static pictures. Nonetheless the scanning pictures demonstrated a narrowing of the intervening interstitial space and an approximation of the two capillary layers, which strongly supports the fusion process in transformation of the septal capillaries.

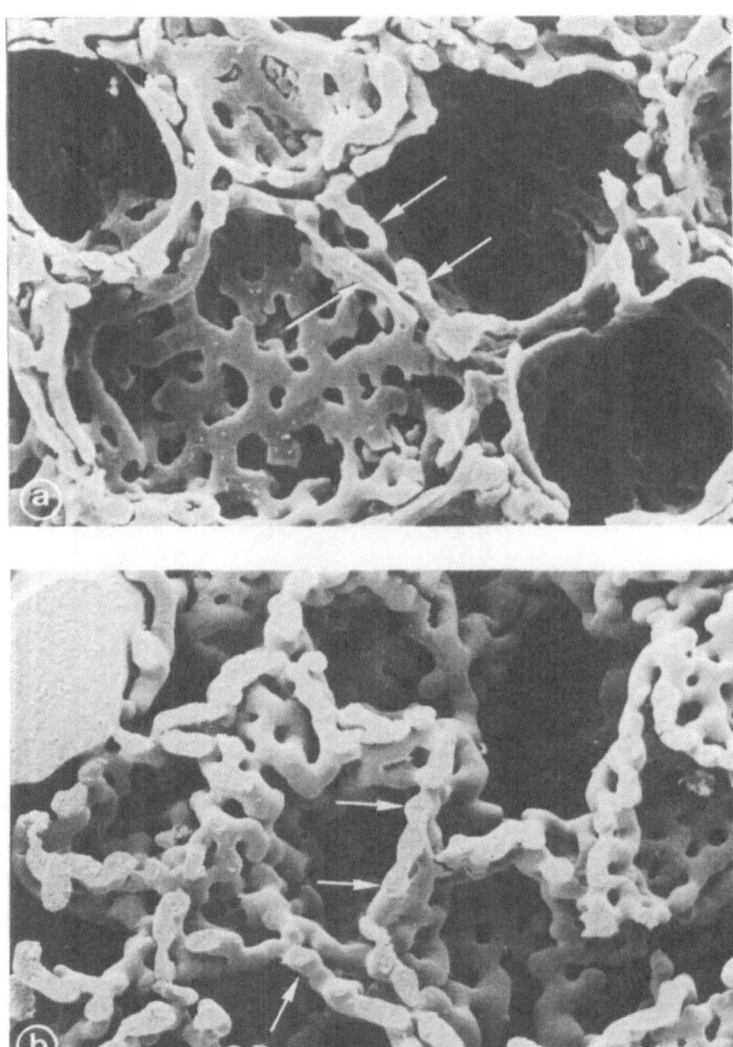

Figure 4.5 Scanning electron micrographs showing casts of the microvasculature of rat lungs aged **(a)** 4 days and **(b)** 139 days at same magnification of × 500. Immature status of parenchymal septa with two capillary networks (arrows) in **(a)** and mature parenchymal microvasculature with a single capillary network per septum (arrows) in **(b)**

As a follow-up to pulmonary vascular development the occurrence of capillary fusions appears highly plausible. Figure 4.7 illustrates that there is a continuous process of capillary approximation during the fetal period. In the pseudoglandular stage of development the capillaries form a loose

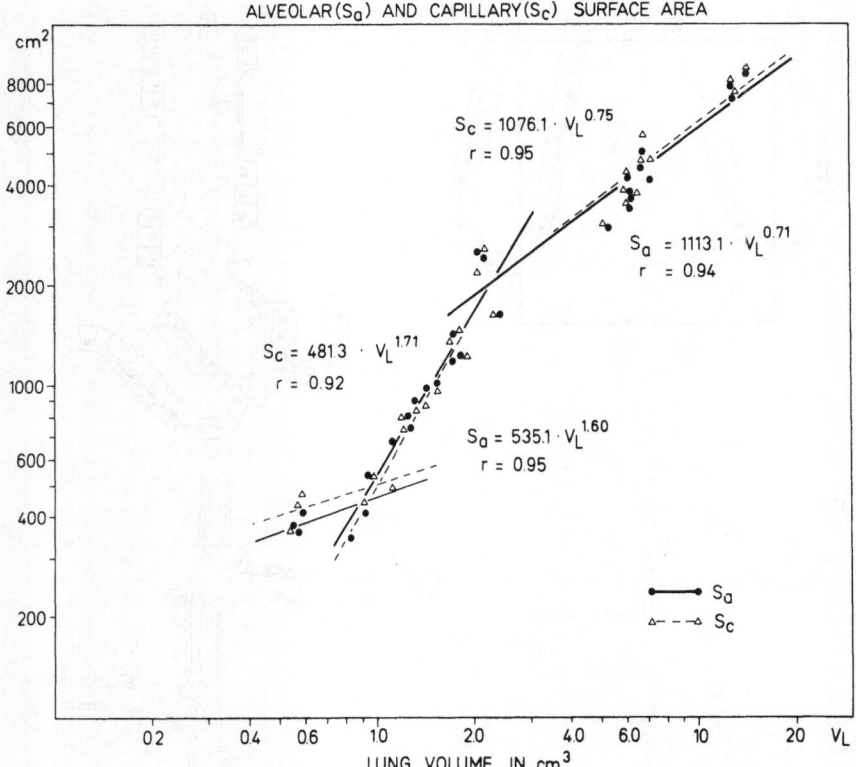

ALVEOLAR (S$_a$) AND CAPILLARY (S$_c$) SURFACE AREA

$$S_c = 1076.1 \cdot V_L^{0.75}$$
$$r = 0.95$$

$$S_a = 1113.1 \cdot V_L^{0.71}$$
$$r = 0.94$$

$$S_c = 481.3 \cdot V_L^{1.71}$$
$$r = 0.92$$

$$S_a = 535.1 \cdot V_L^{1.60}$$
$$r = 0.95$$

LUNG VOLUME IN cm^3

Figure 4.6 Double logarithmic plot of alveolar (S$_a$) and capillary (S$_c$) surface areas against lung volume (VL) in growing rat lung. Intense increase of surface area between days 4 and 21 corresponds to phase of alveolar formation and septal transformation. Data from Ref. 4

three-dimensional network in the pulmonary mesenchyme. The tubular sprouts derived from the entoderm grow into the mesenchyme and give the organ the appearance of a gland. In the canalicular stage the airways enlarge, and at some places the capillaries come into close contact with the cuboidal airway epithelium. Where 'contact' is made the epithelium flattens and a thin air–blood barrier is established. Through the dilatation and growth of the peripheral airways the relative proportion of intervening mesenchymal mass is greatly reduced and the capillaries are rearranged around the airspaces. This leads to a situation in which every airspace is surrounded by its own capillary system. During the saccular stage of development the prospective peripheral airspaces increase in size and further thin out the inter-airspace septa. Inevitably, the capillary networks of two neighbouring airways come to lie close to each other. At this stage, which corresponds to the situation at birth, the two networks show many inter-

45

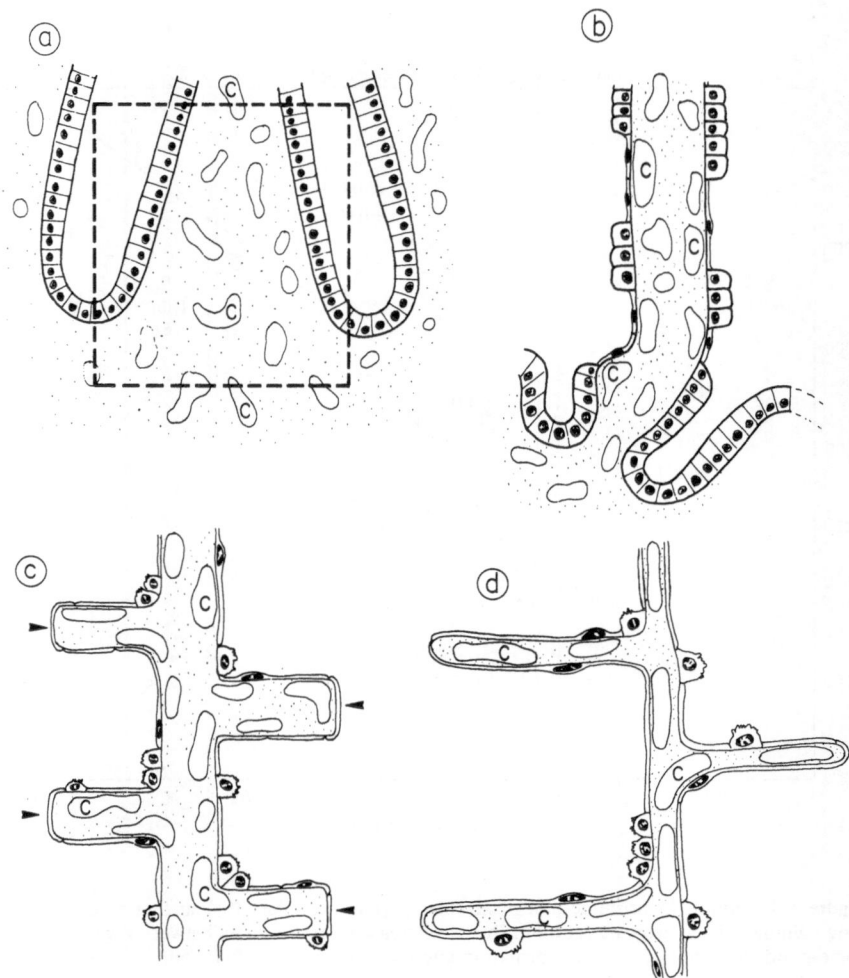

Figure 4.7 Follow-up of the capillary arrangement in the developing lung. **(a)** Pseudoglandular stage: the mesenchyme contains a three-dimensional capillary network (c). **(b)** Canalicular stage: epithelial tubes of figure **(a)** have enlarged; epithelium differentiates into type I and type II cells. Capillaries are rearranged around the tubes, the mass of intervening mesenchyme is reduced, so that ultimately the capillaries between the tubes are forming a double interconnected network. **(c)** Secondary septa (arrowheads) are formed perinatally by lifting off one capillary layer from the primary septa. Both types of septa are immature and contain two capillary networks. **(d)** Mature interalveolar septa with a single capillary network meandering through the interstitium. Reproduced with permission from Ref. 31

connections because they originate from a three-dimensional network. It is highly plausible that, following alveolar formation through the outgrowth of secondary septa, a further reduction of the interstitium ends up in fusion of the capillaries (Fig. 4.7). If, as has been proposed, the secondary septa form by a lifting off of one of the two capillary layers, the formation

46

of alveoli is structurally linked to the presence of immature septa. It would appear, therefore, that new alveoli can only be formed as long as parts of the lung parenchyma still contain immature septa.

It is not known at what age alveolar formation is completed in the rat lung. The spurt in alveolar formation occurs in the first two postnatal weeks in the rat lung and the process appears to be open-ended. Figure 4.6 shows that alveolar surface area increases as the power of 0.71 of lung volume after the age of 21 days, which is not significantly different from that expected with proportional lung growth (0.67). These results suggest that alveolar formation is complete around 21 days. Even a significantly higher rate of increase would not prove further alveolar formation, however, because surface area can be added simply by increasing the height or the complexity of the existing septa. Thus, the presently available quantitative information does not allow us to determine whether alveolar formation continues at a slow pace after the third postnatal week, nor at what age it finally stops. However, our results support proportional lung growth rather than alveolar formation after 21 days.

What is the situation in man? Recently, we had the opportunity to investigate the lungs of seven children dying from non-respiratory causes aged between $3\frac{1}{2}$ weeks and 6 years. Figure 4.8 compares a 1-month-old child's lung with a 1-week-old rat lung. The pictures demonstrate clearly that the parenchymal structures are absolutely identical except for the obvious size differences in airspace dimensions. It is remarkable that both human and rat lung parenchyma show thick primary septa from which the secondary septa arise, project into the airspaces and partition the latter into a number of shallow alveoli. The septal ultrastructure presents the immature aspect with two capillary systems. At 17–18 months of age, however, a child's lung is practically mature. Even at 5 months, large parts of the lung parenchyma display the adult pattern, as is shown by Fig. 4.9. From a morphological point of view, it appears therefore very unlikely that the process of alveolization should last to an appreciable extent up to the age of 8 or even 20 years, as postulated by Dunnill[6] or Emery and Wilcock[7], respectively. The data of Thurlbeck[8] on alveolar counts performed in 36 boys' and 20 girls' lungs in the age range of 6 weeks to 14 years are much more in line with our findings. Despite a large scatter of the data, he was able to conclude that only limited or no alveolar formation occurred after 2 years of age.

MODULATION OF LUNG GROWTH

The second part of this contribution will address the question whether the phase of isomorphic growth following the alveolization is genetically fixed or whether it can be influenced by various conditions, like exposure to altered pO_2 or increased O_2 consumption due to training or cold exposure. Alternatively, the equilibrium between size of the gas exchange apparatus on the one hand, and oxygen requirements of the organism on the other hand, can be altered by resection of lung tissue. Such experiments, performed over the past 15 years, were based on the general hypothesis that

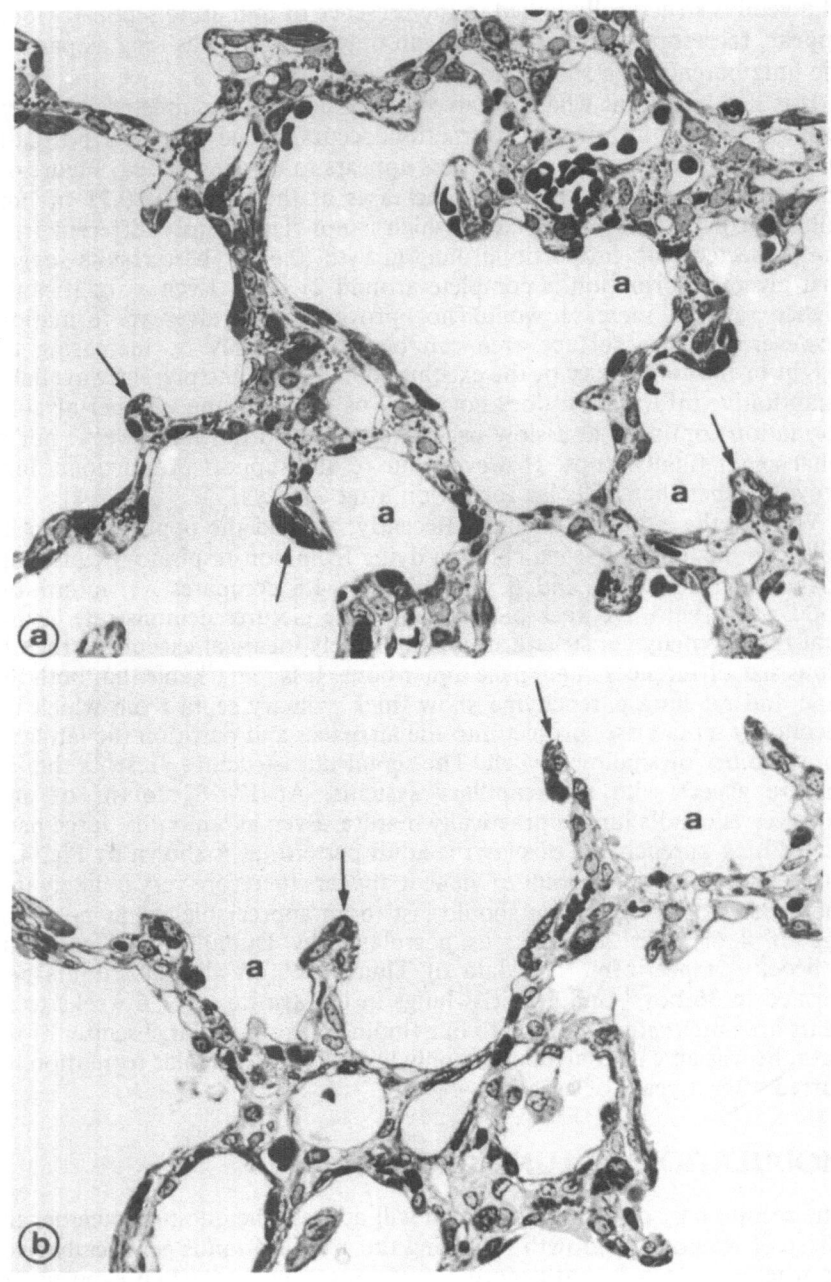

Figure 4.8 Comparison of alveolar formation in rat lung and human lung. **(a)** Rat lung, aged 1 week. Alveoli are formed by outgrowth of secondary septa (arrows) which subdivide airspaces into alveoli (a). (Light micrograph, × 540) **(b)** Human lung, aged about 1 month. Same structural features as in rat lung can be identified. Airspace dimensions are larger than in rat lung. (Light micrograph, × 400)

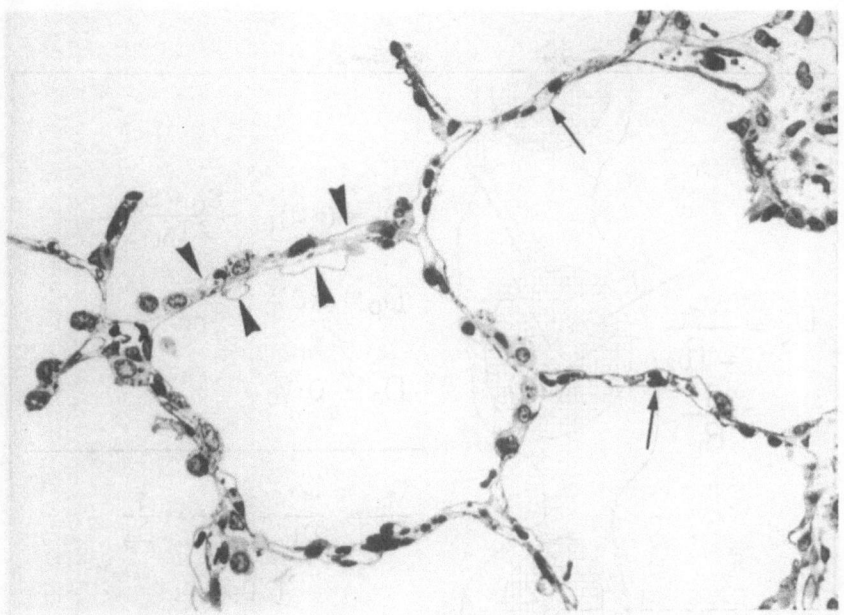

Figure 4.9 Light micrograph of human lung parenchyma at age 5 months. Most septa are already mature (arrows); at places primitive septa are still present (arrowheads) (× 400). Reproduced with permission from Ref. 32

lung structure was quantitatively balanced to meet the oxygen requirements of the organism. Clearly the answer to such questions can only be found by exact quantitation of the pulmonary structures. Advanced morphometric techniques, introduced into histology during the past 20 years, permit reliable measurement of the parameters that determine the gas exchange function of the lung. These parameters are the airspace and capillary surface areas, the capillary volume and the barrier thicknesses of tissue and plasma intervening between air and the erythrocytes. Figure 4.10 illustrates how these parameters have been assembled into a model that permits estimation of the pulmonary diffusion capacity on the basis of the structural dimensions of the gas exchange apparatus[9].

Effect of environmental pO_2 alteration on the growing lung

Why people living at high altitude are fairly well able to cope with hypoxia has always interested physiologists. The physiological mechanisms involved in adaptation to hypoxia have received considerable attention. Little effort was made, however, to answer the question as to what kind of structural adaptations were responsible for the relatively large chests[10] and larger lungs[11] of high-altitude natives compared with lowlanders. After the publication of the findings that growing rats and dogs exposed to hyperoxia showed a deficient growth in alveolar surface area[12,13] the question seemed worthy of experimental investigation. To test the hypothesis of whether

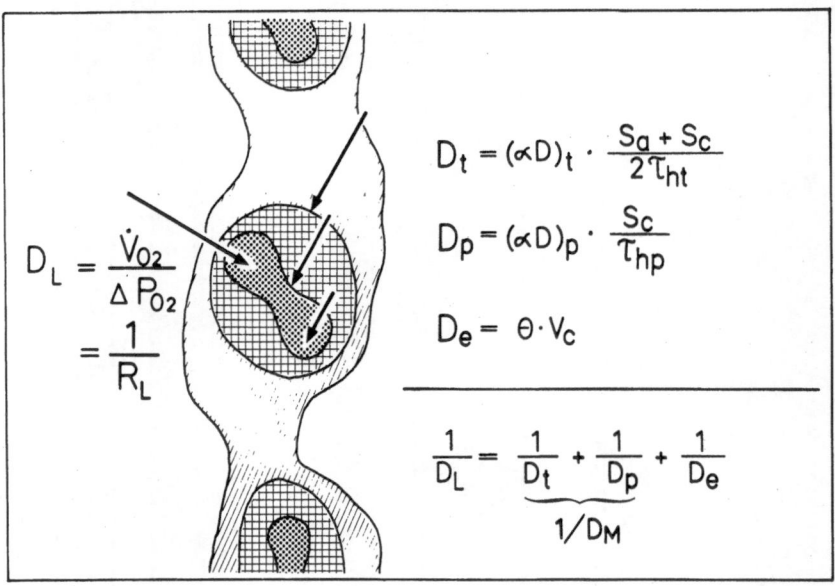

Figure 4.10 Weibel's model for calculation of the morphometric pulmonary diffusion capacity D_L. The relevant morphometric parameters are alveolar (S_a) and capillary (S_c) surface areas, capillary volume (V_c) and the harmonic mean thicknesses of the tissue (τht) and plasma barrier (τhp). For explanation of the model, see Ref. 9. Reproduced with permission from Ref. 33

environmental pO_2 could influence lung growth, rats aged 23 days were exposed to hypoxia at high altitude (pO_2 = 100 mmHg), to hyperoxia in an O_2 chamber (pO_2 = 290 mmHg), and to room air (pO_2 = 150 mmHg) for a period of 3 weeks. In these experiments the rats grown under hyperoxia had significantly smaller lungs with a compartmental volume distribution of airspaces, tissue and blood corresponding to that of control animals. This unchanged relative distribution resulted in smaller absolute volumes of every compartment and in diminished gas exchange surface areas. The hypoxic rats showed just the opposite findings. With a slightly larger average lung volume despite a body mass 11% smaller than in controls, all the lung parameters were significantly reduced when compared to rats raised in normoxia[14]. Finally, the morphometric diffusing capacity expressed per 100 g body weight was increased by 20% in hypoxic and decreased by 15% in hyperoxic animals. Subsequently, this type of adaptive response to a hypoxic environment was confirmed by other authors in a number of animal species exposed to both experimental[15] and natural hypoxic environments[16].

The single morphometric study performed in man seems to indicate that high-altitude people have more and larger alveoli with a larger alveolar surface than a comparable sea-level population[17].

Effect of increased O_2 consumption on the growing lung

Decades ago, it was postulated that physical exercise was able to enlarge the lungs and to increase the number of alveoli[18,19]. In 1971 Geelhaar and Weibel[20] investigated the gas exchange tissue of Japanese Waltzing Mice (JWM), animals suffering from a genetic defect of the vestibulo-cochlear system. Within a few weeks after birth, these mice develop a hyperkinetic syndrome showing choreo-athetotic movements and the typical high-speed waltz of up to three turns per second. The morphometric diffusion capacity of these animals was found to be increased in proportion to their heavily augmented $\dot{V}O_2$ when compared with normal white laboratory mice. Although the authors interpreted the findings as functional adaptation, it was shown later by Bartlett and Areson[21] that these lung parameters were genetically determined, as were the defects of the inner ear.

In a further attempt to test the hypothesis that increased oxygen demand could stimulate lung growth, the lungs of IDPN-mice were quantitatively analysed. IDPN stands for the drug imino-$\beta'\beta$-dipropionitrile, which induces (after three single injections) a waltzing syndrome in normal white mice quite similar to the one observed in JWM[22]. Three and a half months after the induction of the waltzing syndrome, the morphometric pulmonary D_LO_2 per gram body weight was increased by 45% over the control values of litter mates and matched closely the elevated O_2 consumption[23]. In a third experiment with increased $\dot{V}O_2$, growing rats were exposed for 3 weeks to a temperature of 11^0C. The cold exposure augmented $\dot{V}O_2$ by 64% when compared with rats[24] raised at 24^0C. Concomitantly, lung volume was enlarged by 24%, the gas exchange surface areas by 18% and the morphometrically derived D_LO_2 by 20% over control values. In the aforementioned experiments the results had to be normalized to body weight for intergroup comparisons, because the experimental animals showed a smaller body mass than the controls. In the last experiment, however, the body masses of the cold-exposed rats were identical to those of the control group, so that the full extent of the adaptive response could be attributed to changes in lung parameters.

In a similar experiment performed in hamsters exposed to an ambient temperature of only 5^0C, Thompson[25] found the 26% higher $\dot{V}O_2$ compared with controls was matched by a proportionally increased alveolar surface area.

Consequences of lung tissue resection in the growing lung

It may appear problematic to put the 'regenerative' response occurring after lung tissue resection on a par with the adaptive response following exposure to hypoxia, exercise or cold. The resection of lung lobes disturbs the natural balance between the oxygen needs of the organism and the dimensions of the gas exchange apparatus, but the observed responses to resection may rely more on the grounds of tissue homeostasis than on physiological adaptation mechanisms. The results of resection experiments, however, are well suited to document the enormous plasticity of the pulmonary tissues. Having shown in a first set of experiments that 6½ weeks after the resection of lung tissue in growing rats, the size of the gas exchange apparatus was back to normal[26], we investigated the time course and structural features of the recovery in a second set of experiments[27,28]. Rats aged 23 days were subjected to the resection of the upper and middle lobes which comprised 25% of the total lung volume. On days 1, 4, 6, 9, 12, 18 and 30 after surgery, their lungs were fixed under controlled conditions processed for light, transmission (TEM) and scanning electron microscopy, and quantitatively investigated by means of stereological techniques. From this combined morphological and morphometric approach it was possible to extract the following essentials of the 'regenerative' response.

After surgery the remaining lung increased so rapidly in volume that even on the first postoperative day the mean lung volume of the operated group was no longer significantly smaller than that of the sham-operated group or of the control group. In scanning electron micrographs, widening of the airspaces was apparent on day 1 in the alveolar ducts in particular, and 3 days later also in the alveoli. On day 6, and even more so on day 9, no morphological differences could be detected between groups, and the airspaces appeared normal in size[28]. The morphometric results revealed that the initial volume gain of the lung was due solely to a dilatation of the parenchymal airspaces and that tissue mass increased to the preoperative value with a short delay between days 4 and 6. It is known from other investigations that RNA- and DNA-synthesis reached maximal rates on days 4 to 6 after surgery[29], and that collagen synthesis was elevated during this phase of intense cellular reaction in rabbits[30]. These results permitted establishment of the following sequence of events in the remaining lung after lung tissue resection. An initial phase of overinflation of the remaining lung parenchyma is followed by a proliferative response in pulmonary tissues which restores the original tissue mass within a few days. In less than 10 days the remnants of the original lung restored the tissue surgically lost in a highly ordered fashion, so that the dimensions of every single parenchymal component equalled the preoperative values. The 'recovery' of lung function is best reflected by the morphometric diffusion capacity, which from the sixth postoperative day onward is not significantly different from the values of non-operated animals (Fig. 4.11). These studies, however, also indicate that parenchymal structures seem to have a greater adaptive potential than non-parenchymal structures. 'Regenerated' rat lungs had smaller volume densities in the conductive airway and in the blood vessel fraction than control lungs[26]. Reduction of non-respiratory tissue could lead to such functional problems as ventilation/perfusion inequalities in regenerated lungs. However, such potential problems escape our analysis because our type of approach quantifies only respiratory tissues.

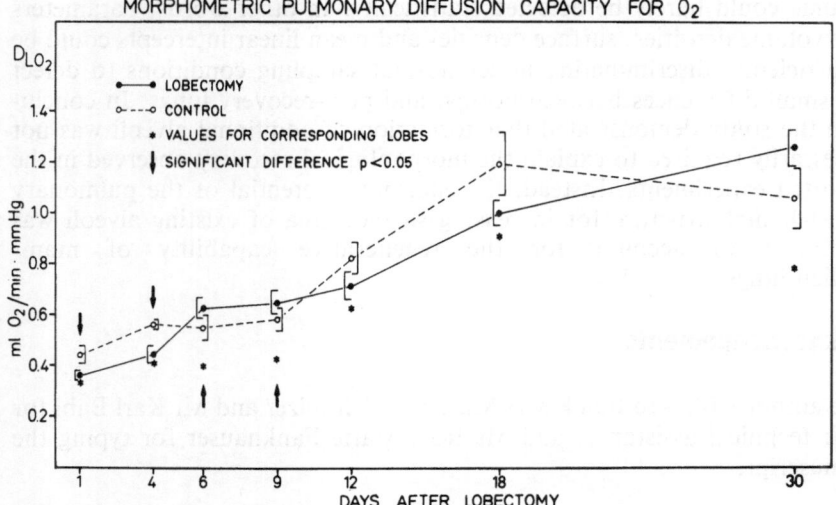

Figure 4.11 The morphometrically determined pulmonary diffusion capacity summarizes adequately the results on the timing of the 'regenerative' response following resection of the right upper and medium lobes (= 25% of total lung volume) of rat lungs. The diagram shows that from postoperative day 6 onwards the operated lungs have completely restored the lost tissue. Arrows indicate significant differences between controls and lobectomized animals. Asterisks give values for corresponding lobes of controls (i.e. for total lung minus right upper and medium lobes). Data from Ref. 27

MORPHOLOGY OF THE ADAPTIVE RESPONSE

A final problem is the question of the structural mechanism of the adaptive increase in the number of airspace units, the alveoli, called hyperplasia. (Both these terms, hypertrophy and hyperplasia, are in fact misnomers. It would be preferable to use instead airspace dilatation and alveolar formation, respectively.) Despite the use of morphometric techniques in recent publications this controversy is still alive.

Given the mode of alveolar formation described in the first part of this paper, it is unlikely that alveolar formation to any great extent can occur in a lung made of mature interalveolar septa, because as we have seen, formation of secondary septa is based on the presence of a double capillary network. If, however, focally distributed areas with immature septal structure were present in the lung of older animals, a limited number of new alveoli could be produced at these sites.

In our scanning electron microscopic study we found no clues for the formation of new alveoli. On the other hand, the pictures of operated and non-operated lungs 9 days after bilobectomy appeared to be identical. As explanation for these paradoxical findings we proposed that the initial dilatation of the airspaces could subsequently be masked to the observer's eye by an increase in height of the interalveolar septa. To support this notion, we developed a two-dimensional model which illustrates this possibility[28]. By means of measurements performed on the model, we could show that the small changes in linear dimensions needed to restore the lost volume could barely be detected statistically. In other words, parameters like volume densities, surface densities and mean linear intercepts could be insufficiently discriminating under normal sampling conditions to detect the small differences between normal and post-recovery lungs. In conclusion the study demonstrated that formation of additional alveoli was not necessarily required to explain the morphological recovery observed in the reported experiments. Instead, the enormous potential of the pulmonary parenchymal structure for increasing surface area of existing alveoli was sufficient to account for the regenerative capability of mammalian lungs.

Acknowledgements

The author wishes to thank Mrs Marianne Schweizer and Mr Karl Babl for their technical assistance, and Ms Rose-Marie Fankhauser for typing the manuscript.

References

1. Boyden, E. A. (1977). Development and growth of the airways. In Hodson, W. A. (ed.) *Lung Biology in Health and Disease. Development of the Lung.* Vol. 6, pp. 3–35. (New York: Dekker)
2. Langston, C., Kida, K., Reed, M. and Thurlbeck, W. M. (1984). Human lung growth in late gestation and in the neonate. *Am. Rev. Respir. Dis.,* **129,** 607–13
3. Burri, P. H. (1974). The postnatal growth of the rat lung. III. Morphology. *Anat. Rec.,* **180,** 77–98
4. Burri, P. H., Dbaly, J. and Weibel, E. R. (1974). The postnatal growth of the rat lung. I. Morphometry. *Anat. Rec.,* **178,** 711–30
5. Caduff, J. H., Fischer, L. C. and Burri, P. H. (1986). Scanning electron microscopic study of the developing microvasculature in the postnatal rat lung. *Anat. Rec.,* (in press)
6. Dunnill, M. S. (1962). Postnatal growth of the lung. *Thorax,* **17,** 329–33
7. Emery, J. L. and Wilcock, P. F. (1966). The postnatal development of the lung. *Acta Anat.,* **65,** 10–29
8. Thurlbeck, W. M. (1982). Postnatal human lung growth. *Thorax,* **37,** 564–71
9. Weibel, E. R. (1970/71). Morphometric estimation of pulmonary diffusion capacity. I. Model and method. *Respir. Physiol.,* **11,** 54–75
10. Frisancho, R. A. (1969). Human growth and pulmonary function of high altitude Peruvian Quechua population. *Hum. Biol.,* **41,** 366–79
11. Brody, J., Lahiri, S., Simpser, M., Motoyama, E. and Velasquez, T. (1977). Lung elasticity and airway dynamics in Peruvian natives to high altitude. *J. Appl. Physiol.,* **42,** 245–51
12. Kistler, G. S., Caldwell, P. R. B. and Weibel, E. R. (1966). Pulmonary pathology of oxygen toxicity. II. Electron microscopic and morphometric study of rat lungs exposed to 97% O_2 at 258 torr (27 000 feet). *Aerosp. Med.,* 1–14
13. Schwinger, G., Weibel, E. R. and Kaplan, H. P. (1967). Pulmonary pathology of oxygen toxicity. III. Electron microscopic and morphometric study of dog and monkey lungs exposed to 98% O_2 at 258 torr for 7 months and followed by 1 month recovery in room air. Aerospace Med. Res. Lab. AMRL, Interim Scientific Report, January
14. Burri, P. H. and Weibel, E. R. (1971). Morphometric estimation of pulmonary diffusion capacity. II. Effect of PO_2 on the growing lung. Adaptation of the growing rat lung to hypoxia and hyperoxia. *Respir. Physiol.,* **11,** 247–64
15. Bartlett, D. Jr. and Remmers, J. E. (1971). Effects of high altitude exposure on the lungs of young rats. *Respir. Physiol.,* **13,** 116–25
16. Pearson, O. P. and Pearson, A. K. (1976). A stereological analysis of the ultrastructure of the lungs of wild mice living at low and high altitude. *J. Morphol.,* **150,** 359–68

7. Saldaña, M. and Garcia-Oyola, E. (1970). Morphometry of the high altitude lung. *Lab. Invest.*, **22**, 509

8. Tiemann, F. (1936). Wachstum und Hypertrophie der Lunge von Mensch und Tier. *Verh. Dtsch. Ges. Inn. Med.*, **48**, 217–43

9. Gehrig, H. (1951). Ueber tierexperimentelle Einwirkung von körperlicher Ueberanstrengung und sportlichem Training (Schwimmen) auf die Lungenmorphologie. Würzburg, West Germany: Universität Würzburg. Inaugural dissertation

20. Geelhaar, A. and Weibel, E. R. (1971). Morphometric estimation of pulmonary diffusion capacity. III. The effect of increased oxygen consumption in Japanese waltzing mice. *Respir. Physiol.*, **11**, 354–66

21. Bartlett, D. Jr. and Areson, J. G. (1978). Quantitative lung morphology in Japanese waltzing mice. *J. Appl. Physiol.*, **44**, 446–9

22. Burri, P. H., Gehr, P., Müller, K. and Weibel, E. R. (1976). Adaptation of the growing lung of increased $\dot{V}O_2$. I. IDPN as inducer of hyperactivity. *Respir. Physiol.*, **28**, 129–40

23. Hugonnaud, C., Gehr, P., Weibel, E. R. and Burri, P. H. (1977). Adaptation of the growing lung to increased oxygen consumption. II. Morphometric analysis. *Respir. Physiol.*, **29**, 1–10

24. Gehr, P., Hugonnaud, C., Burri, P. H., Bachofen, H. and Weibel, E. R. (1978). Adaptation of the growing lung to increased $\dot{V}O_2$: III. The effect of exposure to cold environment in rats. *Respir. Physiol.*, **32**, 345–53

25. Thompson, M. E. (1980). Lung growth in response to altered metabolic demand in hamsters: influence of thyroid function and cold exposure. *Respir. Physiol.*, **40**, 335–47

26. Burri, P. H. and Sehovic, S. (1979). The adaptive response of the rat lung after bilobectomy. *Am. Rev. Respir. Dis.*, **119**, 769–77

27. Berger, L. C. and Burri, P. H. (1985). Timing of the quantitative recovery in the regenerating rat lung. *Am. Rev. Respir. Dis.*, **132**, 777–83

28. Burri, P. H., Pfrunder, B. and Berger, L. C. (1982). Reactive changes in pulmonary parenchyma after bilobectomy: a scanning electron microscopic investigation. *Exp. Lung Res.*, **4**, 11–28

29. Brody, J. S., Bürki, R. and Kaplan, N. (1978). Deoxyribonucleic acid synthesis in lung cells during compensatory lung growth after pneumonectomy. *Am. Rev. Respir. Dis.*, **117**, 307–16

30. Cowan, M. J. and Crystal, R. G. (1975). Lung growth after unilateral pneumonectomy: Quantitation of collagen synthesis and content. *Am. Rev. Respir. Dis.*, **111**, 267–77

31. Burri, P. H. (1984). Fetal and postnatal development of the lung. *Ann. Rev. Physiol.*, **46**, 617–28

32. Burri, P. H. (1986). Pulmonary development and lung regeneration. In Fishman, A. P. (ed.) *Pulmonary Diseases and Disorders*, 2nd edn. chapter 19. (New York: McGraw-Hill) (In press)

33. Burri, P. H., Gil, J. and Weibel, E. R. (1983). The ultrastructure and morphometry of the human lung. In Shields, Th. W. (ed.) *General Thoracic Surgery*, 2nd edition. pp. 18–42. (Philadelphia: Lea and Febiger)

Discussion

Dr L. B. Strang	Am I right in believing that hyperventilation induced by carbon dioxide does not cause increased lung growth?
Dr P. H. Burri	Bartlett[1] reported experiments on hyperventilating animals with CO_2 and found no adaptive response. I think one has to differentiate between this kind of mechanical pulmonary stress and the stress experienced by residual lung after removal of part of it. I believe, despite Bartlett's negative results, that mechanical stress plays a role in adaptive response, as is illustrated by pneumonectomy experiments.
Strang	To follow up that idea, it would seem that the internal volume of either the fetal or the postnatal lung – the stretch applied to lung tissue – is an important determinant of growth. If one lobe is removed, is there any difference between the adaptive growth in the remaining lung on that side and the opposite lung? With a mobile mediastinum there should not be much difference in the transpulmonary pressure on the two sides.
Burri	The response to lobectomy seems to depend on the age of the animal. In experiments in which the right upper and middle lobes were removed from young rats aged 23 days and from adult rats of 250 g, we found in the young animals that both lung sides contributed exactly the same percentage of their own remaining volume to full recovery[2], whereas in adult rats the right lung (on the side of the lobectomy) contributed more[3]. In the old rats the mediastinum is presumably less compliant – hence the stretch on the right side is greater than the stretch on the left side, whereas in the young rats the more compliant mediastinum would equalize pressures on the two sides. The effect of hypoxia in favouring an adaptive response could be due to an increase in end expiratory level, documented by Verzar[4].
Dr L. Marin	Can you comment on the effect of growth hormone?
Burri	It is an unsettled point. I think growth hormone has a certain influence, mainly in the sense of an overall growth stimulation[5,6]. Unfortunately some experiments on this topic, such as decapitation, are rather crude.
Dr B. Smith	In the regenerating kidney, somatomedin C in the regenerating tissue is elevated. In the hypophysectomized rat when there is no demonstrable growth hormone, a lower level of tissue and serum somatomedin C is seen. After nephrectomy there is still a small amount of regeneration and a small increase in tissue somatomedin C level. Thus although somatomedin C is primarily under the control of growth hormone, it is also influenced by local factors.
Strang	Does lung regeneration involve the formation of new alveoli?
Burri	I think new alveoli probably cannot be formed, in substantial number, because as we have seen this requires a pre-existing double capillary network. In the early stages of postnatal development you can lift off one capillary network and get a new wall in the airspace, but in a mature lung only few of these double networks are left. On the other hand, an increase in gas exchange surface area following lung resection can be produced in another way, i.e. by a lengthening of existing septa. We have tried to work out a model which is based on the fact that a volume gain of 33% after bilobectomy can be achieved by only a 9% increase in linear

56

dimensions. If the lung model is expanded without lengthening of the alveolar walls you can recognize dilated air spaces. But if the walls are lengthened by 10%, restoring the original proportions between alveolar depth and duct size, the distension of individual airspaces is no longer detectable. The changes in dimensions are even unlikely to be statistically significant on morphometry[7].

Dr A. C. Bryan
I think the chairman is driving us into a dangerously reductionist position, particularly in equating postnatal lung growth with antenatal growth. The most impressive finding of your group, Dr Burri, is that gas exchange and the surface area of the lung are matched to metabolic requirements over a wide variety of animal species. Hence lung growth in the postnatal period seems not to be determined solely by stretch (or available thoracic volume).

Strang
Although breathing a hypoxic mixture increases lung growth and breathing a hyperoxic mixture slows growth[9,8], the effect of an increase in oxygen consumption by the growing animal is not so clearly defined. Bartlett[10] showed no effect of increased O_2 uptake induced by treadmill exercise or L-thyroxine in rats. On the other hand, Japanese Waltzing Mice, whose O_2 consumption is well above normal, have a larger pulmonary exchange surface than normal mice[11].

Burri
That is a genetic factor. We have produced another model, the IDPN mouse, which becomes a waltzing mouse after three injections of the substance imino-$\beta'\beta$-dipropionitrile ($=$IDPN)[12,13]. This mouse does not turn as much as the Japanese Waltzing Mouse, but it increases oxygen consumption by about 50%. These animals show an increase in all lung parameters as compared with the untreated littermates. However, the increase has to be expressed with respect to body weight, as the mice (like the hypoxic animals) are smaller and have slightly larger lungs for body weight than the controls. A third type of experiment uses cold exposure to increase O_2 consumption. In these experiments the controls and the cold-exposed animals had similar body weights, yet the morphometric diffusion capacity was increased by about 20% in the cold-exposed[14]. The matter of adaptation remains controversial, however, as Lechner and Banchero[15], who exposed guinea pigs at altitude, claim that the effect was only to produce an acceleration of growth, and that the difference between experimental and control animals, seen after 3 or 4 weeks, became very small as the growth period came to an end.

Dr L. L. Gaultier
Do you feel that it is really feasible to compare adaptation in the rat, which is very immature at birth, and Lechner's work on the guinea pig, which is very mature at birth.

Burri
There is probably a difference. On the other hand, the quantitative structural recovery after lung resection in rats occurs not only in the neonatal period, but also at later stages when the lung seems to be mature. However, the rat may be a special case; it continues growing until it dies.

Dr J. P. Mortola
There are many examples in nature of excellent matching between structure and function of the lung, but I would interpret this as a process of evolutionary adaptation rather than a cause–effect relationship. Most of our structures, including the lung, are far more abundant than we actually need. Experimental removal of 25% of the lung certainly does not decrease the amount of oxygen available, or oxygen consumption, yet structural compensation takes place, suggesting that oxygen needs are not directly determining the structural development of the lung. I'm not saying that you have compensation because the animal doesn't get enough oxygen. There might be another mechanism related to tissue homeostasis, analogous to that which allows a full recovery of liver volume within 2 weeks after a two-thirds hepatectomy in rats.

Burri

Dr J. S. Wigglesworth	To what extent do alveoli actually develop *in utero* during the latter part of the pregnancy? All the older investigators were quite happy about there being lots of alveoli in the fetal lung, but in recent years it has been said there are none.
Burri	The results are controversial. In alveolar counting one uses a formula with a shape factor, but alveolar formation cannot take place without shape changes, which creates problems. Besides that, Hansen and Ampaya[16] have shown that, in sections, it is not possible to distinguish between alveoli and alveolar ducts. Large errors are revealed when the counts of alveoli in sections are compared with counts made in three-dimensional models reconstructed from these sections. Presently, alveolar counts at birth are in the range of 20–50 million. Since an adult lung has on average 300 million alveoli, it is still justified to state that alveolar formation occurs after birth.
Strang	I've never been sure of what is defined by the word alveolus. From to-day's discussion it appears to be a small airspace with a single capillary circulation. Up to now, we've always been told that alveoli appear at a certain stage, but to me these 'new' structures were just small airspaces not fundamentally different in kind from other small spaces. Now we learn that at birth these spaces have a double capillary network, and that in the course of postnatal development new airspaces are formed and that, furthermore, one of the capillary networks is lost. This I can understand to be a fundamental change justifying the term 'remodelling'. These postnatally developing airspaces seem to be of a new kind; call them alveoli or not as you wish.
Burri	It's not sensible to make such an important point of when alveoli appear. They start to appear probably in late fetal life. The important point is that we still have an immature lung at birth, and that, in addition to the formation of alveoli, a transformation of the capillary network takes place after birth, a kind of maturation of the microvasculature and of the interalveolar septa.
Wigglesworth	A tremendous change in lung structure is going on throughout late gestation as well as in the postnatal period. It is not a case of there being a saccular stage which remains unchanged between 30 weeks and term.
Burri	Important changes also take place later in life. The lung of a man aged 20 is not composed in the same way as that of a man aged 50. The volumetric composition – airspace volume, tissue volume and capillary volume – is continuously changing.

References

1. Bartlett, D. Jr. (1972). Postnatal development of the mammalian lung. In Goss, R. J. (ed.) *Regulation of Organ and Tissue Growth*, pp. 197–209. (New York: Academic Press)
2. Burri, P. H. and Sehovic, S. (1979). The adaptive response of the rat lung after bilobectomy. *Am. Rev. Respir. Dis.*, **119**, 769–77
3. Wandel, G., Berger, L. C. and Burri, P. H. (1983). Morphometric analysis of adult rat lung after bilobectomy. *Am. Rev. Respir. Dis.*, **128**, 968–72
4. Verzar, F. Die Regulation des Lungenvolumens. *Pflugers Arch.*, **232**, 322–41
5. Bartlett, D. Jr. (1971). Postnatal growth of the mammalian lung: influence of excess growth hormone. *Respir. Physiol.*, **12**, 297–304
6. Brody, J. S., Fisher, A. B., Gocmen, A. and DuBois, A. B. (1970). Acromegalic pneumonomegaly: lung growth in the adult. *J. Clin. Invest.*, **49**, 1051–60
7. Burri, P. H., Pfrunder, B. and Berger, L. C. (1982). Reactive changes in pulmonary parenchyma after bilobectomy: a scanning electron microscopic investigation. *Exp. Lung Res.*, **4**, 11–28

8. Burri, P. H. and Weibel, E. R. (1971). Morphometric estimation of pulmonary diffusion capacity. II. Effect of pO_2 on the growing lung. Adaptation of the growing rat lung to hypoxia and hyperoxia. *Respir. Physiol.,* **11,** 247-64

9. Bartlett, D. Jr. and Remmers, J. E. (1971). Effects of high altitude exposure on the lungs of young rats. *Respir. Physiol.,* **13,** 116-25

10. Bartlett, D. Jr. (1970). Postnatal growth of the mammalian lung: influence of exercise and thyroid activity *Respir. Physiol.,* **9,** 50-7

11. Geelhaar, A. and Weibel, E. R. (1971). Morphometric estimation of pulmonary diffusing capacity. III. The effect of increased oxygen consumption in Japanese Waltzing Mice. *Respir. Physiol.,* **11,** 354-66

12. Burri, P. H., Gehr, P., Muller, K. and Weibel, E. R. (1976). Adaptation of the growing lung to increased vO_2. I. IDPN as inducer of hyperactivity. *Respir. Physiol.,* **28,** 129-40

13. Hugonnaud, C., Gehr, P., Weibel, E. R. and Burri, P. H. (1977). Adaptation of the growing lung to increased oxygen consumption. II. Morphometric analysis. *Respir. Physiol.,* **29,** 1-10

14. Gehr, P., Hugonnaud, C., Burri, P. H., Bachofen, H. and Weibel, E. R. (1978). Adaptation of the growing lung to increased vO_2: III. The effect of exposure to cold environment in rats. *Respir. Physiol.,* **32,** 345-53

15. Lechner, A. J. and Banchero, N. (1980). Lung morphometry in guinea pigs acclimated to hypoxia during growth. *Respir. Physiol.,* **42,** 155-69

16. Hansen, J. E. and Ampaya, E. P. (1974). Lung morphometry: a fallacy in the use of the counting principle. *J. Physiol.,* **37,** 951-4

5
The Secretion and Absorption of Fetal Lung Liquid

D. V. WALTERS AND C. A. RAMSDEN

At the birth of a mammal dramatic changes must occur if the liquid-filled lungs of the fetus are to be transformed into an air-filled organ capable of supporting gas exchange. The aim of this paper is to examine some of the physiological mechanisms which bring about this metamorphosis, in particular those concerned with ion transport across the pulmonary epithelium.

FETAL LUNG LIQUID SECRETION

It has been known for at least 100 years that the lumen of the fetal lung is filled with liquid[1]. This liquid is a secretion of the lung and not, as once supposed, inhaled amniotic liquor. Experiments of nature in which occlusion of the airway during development produced distension of the lungs with liquid first suggested that the site of lung liquid production is the lung itself[2]. More direct evidence was presented by Jost and Policard[3] who, in experiments designed to study endocrine effects, ligated the neck of fetal rabbits and incidentally observed that after a few days the lungs became distended with a liquid which was under considerable pressure.

Adams, Moss and Fagan[4] were the first to examine the chemical composition of fetal lung liquid, but they were unable to decide whether it was an ultrafiltrate or a secretion. However, in more detailed studies, Adamson et al.[5] were able to demonstrate the fluid to be distinct from both plasma and amniotic liquor (Table 5.1). The high chloride and low bicarbonate concentrations led the authors to conclude that lung liquid must be a result of active ion transport by the lung; an hypothesis later confirmed by Olver and Strang[6].

For a secretory organ to be capable of generating a chemical gradient a barrier must be present to restrict molecular diffusion. Normand et al.[7] showed that in the fetal lung this barrier resides in the pulmonary epithelium. In their experiments the capillary endothelium of the fetal lung was found to present little barrier to molecular diffusion, whereas the pulmonary epithelium was relatively 'tight', completely restricting the movement of molecules larger than mannitol. Describing their results in terms of pore theory, the effective pore radius of the capillary endothelium was in excess of 11 nm, while that of the epithelium was only 0.6 nm. This may explain why lung liquid contains such a small concentration of protein (molecular radius of albumin is about 3.5 nm).

Table 5.1 Composition of lung liquid, plasma and amniotic liquid in mature fetal lambs (from Adamson et al[5]).

	Na^+	K^+	Cl^-	HCO_3^-	Protein
Plasma	150	4.8	107	24	4.09
Lung liquid	150	6.3	157	2.8	0.027
Amniotic liquid	113	7.6	87	19	0.10

Units are mmol/kg H_2O except for protein, which is g/100 ml

The mechanism of lung liquid secretion was investigated a few years later by Olver and Strang[6]. They measured unidirectional fluxes of various ions across the pulmonary epithelium, and compared the observed fluxes with those predicted for passive diffusion by the Ussing flux ratio equation. Agreement between the observed and predicted flux ratios for a particular ion suggests that it is distributed passively across the epithelium, whereas a significant discrepancy may be taken to indicate that the ion in question is actively transported. Olver and Strang demonstrated net movement of chloride ions (and of other halides) into the lumen of the fetal lung against an electrical and chemical gradient. They found not only that there was a discrepancy between observed and predicted fluxes, but also that the observed flux ratio was greater than 1, whereas the predicted ratio was less than 1. This observation provided strong evidence for the active transport of chloride into the lung lumen.

They also found evidence for active movement of potassium ions into the lumen and of hydrogen ions into (or bicarbonate ions out of) the lumen. The quantitative fluxes of these latter ions were small compared with that of the chloride ion, and Olver and Strang were able to conclude that active transport of chloride was the dominant force mediating lung liquid secretion. Sodium appeared to be distributed passively in these experiments. The permeability of the pulmonary epithelium to the chloride ion is lower than would be expected simply from the size of its hydrated shell. Olver and Strang suggested that this was because of a standing negative charge on the surface of the epithelium, a proposition supported by the relative permeabilities of the other halides they investigated.

The capacity of the pulmonary epithelium to actively transport chloride ions and to present a permeability barrier between the interstitium and alveolar space is established very early in gestation[8]. Lung liquid is certainly secreted before 70 days gestation in the fetal lamb and no change in permeability was detected in the lung between this gestation and term (147 days). In these experiments the number of strands comprising the tight junctions between epithelial cells was examined, and found to decrease with advancing gestation. This suggests that in the developing lung there is not a straightforward relationship between tight junction structure and permeability, unlike the observations of Claude and Goodenough[9].

The lungs of the mature fetal lamb contain about 30 ml of lung liquid/kg body weight, and secrete liquid at a rate of between 3 and 5 ml/h per kg body weight[6-8,10]. Thus a fetal lamb near term secretes a volume approaching $\frac{1}{2}$ litre every 24 hours. The liquid volume contained in the potential airspaces appears to have an important role in normal lung growth; interference with lung volume, either by artificially withdrawing liquid or by preventing its escape, profoundly alters lung histology and tissue weight[11-13] (see also Chapter 3 in this volume).

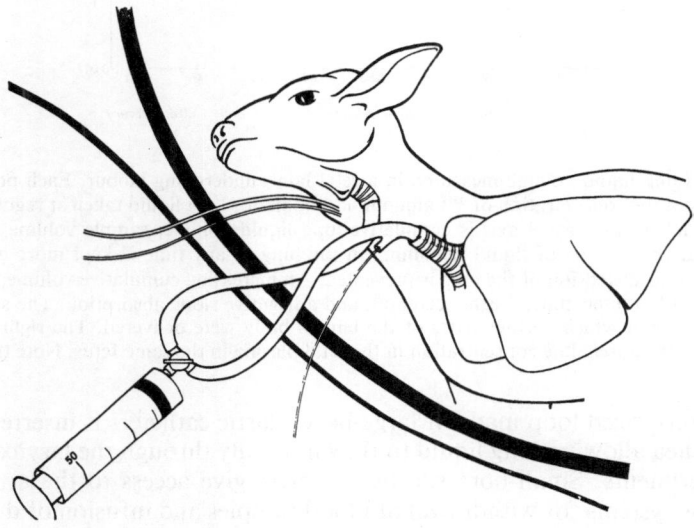

Figure 5.1 Pregnant ewes were operated on under sterile conditions, and catheters were inserted as shown. The large-bore silastic tracheal catheters produced a pressure drop of 0.22 cmH$_2$O along their combined lengths at a flow of 35 ml/h – a value well in excess of normal lung liquid secretion rates. In some preparations, in order to measure electrical p.d., a fine catheter filled with KCl agar was inserted through a watertight seal into the lung catheter and advanced so that its tip lay in the 8th to 10th bronchial generation. A circuit was completed using two calomel half-cells and a catheter connected to the vascular space to allow measurement of the vascular–lung lumen electrical p.d.

LABOUR, ADRENALINE AND FETAL LUNG LIQUID ABSORPTION

To investigate the effect of labour on lung liquid secretion, we have used the chronically catheterized fetal lamb model[14,15]. In our preparation (Fig.

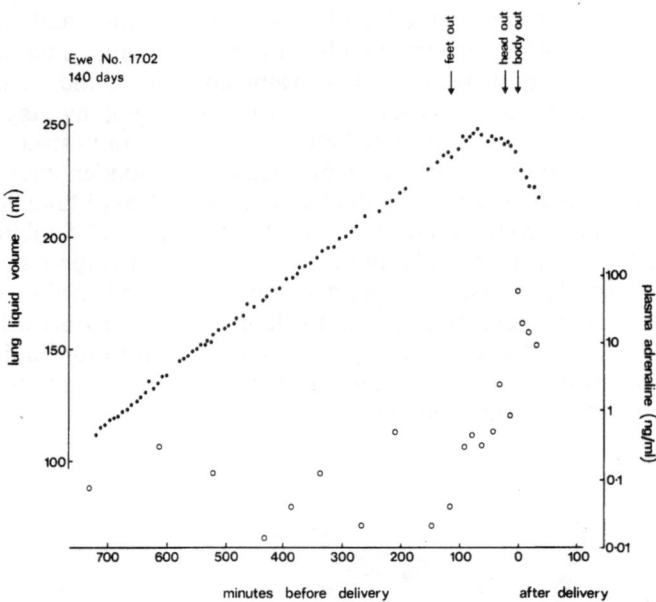

Figure 5.2 Lung liquid volume measured in a fetal lamb undergoing labour. Each point is calculated from the concentration of ^{125}I albumin in samples of lung liquid taken at regular intervals. The left-hand vertical axis is cumulative lung liquid volume; sample volume is adjusted so that the volume of liquid remaining in the lung at any time is kept more or less constant and thus distension of the lung is prevented. An increasing cumulative volume, i.e. a positive slope of volume/time, means secretion, and a negative slope absorption. The arrows indicate the time at which various parts of the lamb's body were delivered. The right-hand vertical axis is the adrenaline concentration in the fetal plasma in the same fetus. Note the log scale

5.1) an exteriorized loop made of large-bore silastic catheters is inserted into the trachea allowing lung liquid to flow normally through the larynx between experiments. Small-bore silastic catheters give access to the arterial and venous systems for withdrawal of blood samples and infusion of drugs. To perform an experiment the tracheal loop is interrupted and a syringe attached to the proximal catheter. About half the liquid volume can be gently withdrawn and put back into the lung. Frequent repetition of this action ensures thorough mixing of the liquid. By introducing a known amount of a volume marker (radiolabelled albumin) into the liquid, volume and thus secretion rate can be calculated from the concentration of albumin in serial samples. The labelled albumin is confined to the lung lumen because the pulmonary epithelium is completely impermeable to a molecule of this size. (The catheter to the larynx is closed off for the duration of the experiment.) Corrections are made for the amount of albumin removed in samples, and the sampling volume is adjusted so that the volume of lung liquid remaining in the enclosed system is as constant as possible. Figure 5.2 gives an example of an experiment in which lung liquid secretion rate was measured over several hours. In this experiment the ewe was in labour.

Lung liquid continued to be secreted early in labour, but as delivery of the fetus approached, secretion slowed, and absorption of lung liquid was observed when a presenting part (the forelimbs) appeared at the vaginal outlet. Similar results were obtained in other experiments and these are summarized in Table 5.2. The observations immediately following birth were made by restraining the ewe and allowing the fetus to lie quietly at the vaginal outlet. The placental circulation was maintained by applying warm saline packs around the exposed cord. Because of the characteristics of the sheep placenta, oxygenation of the fetus may be maintained for a substantial period after birth despite the fetus being unable to breathe.

Table 5.2 Pooled data from experiments in which lung liquid secretion rate was measured in fetal lambs undergoing labour and delivery (from Ref. 14)

	Time before delivery (min)			Time after delivery (min)
	900–150	150–50	50–0	0–50
J_V (ml/h)	+ 7.1	− 2.2	− 15.2	− 28.7
[A] (ng/ml)	0.087	0.524	6.86	7.17
[NA] (ng/ml)	1.7	3.8	12.1	9.1

J_V is secretion (+) or absorption rate (−); [A] and [NA] are fetal plasma adrenaline and noradrenaline concentrations. The number of animals contributing to any value was between three and seven; all values after delivery are the means from four animals. Note that adrenaline concentration increased almost 100-fold, whereas noradrenaline concentration increased only 5-fold

How then to explain the reversal of liquid flow across the pulmonary epithelium during labour? We had already observed and reported that adrenaline had profound effects on lung liquid secretion[15]. An example of the effect of intravenous infusion of adrenaline is shown in Fig. 5.3. This infusion rate (0.5 μg/min) produces a plasma adrenaline concentration similar to that observed in labour. The effect on secretion is related to gestational age: infusion of the same dose in young fetuses (about 120 days) has little effect, but the response increases as the fetus matures until after 130 days absorption is the rule, and by 140 days rapid absorption is generally observed (see Table 5.3).

The effect appears to be mediated by β-receptors since it is blocked by propranolol and large concentrations of noradrenaline have little effect, whereas isoprenaline is even more potent than adrenaline[15].

Can the absorption of lung liquid seen during labour be explained by the action of endogenously derived adrenaline released in response to the stress of delivery? To answer this question we constructed dose–response curves by infusing adrenaline at different rates into fetuses of various gestational ages[14]. The animals were grouped into 3-day gestational periods

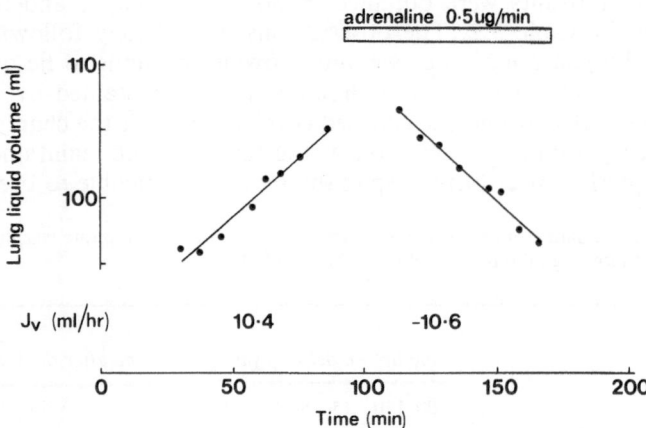

Figure 5.3 The effect of adrenaline infused intravenously on lung liquid secretion. In this fetus, at 132 days gestation, absorption of lung liquid was produced. The lines are the calculated regression lines and their slopes give J_V. A negative value for J_V indicates absorption

Table 5.3 Data demonstrating the maturation in the response of fetal lamb lungs to adrenaline in the last weeks of gestation. Term is 145 + days. (from Ref. 14)

Gestation period (days)	J_{vc} (ml/h)	J_{va} (ml/h)	ΔJ_v (ml/h)	ΔJ_v cAMP (ml/h)
120–124	11.7	6.5	5.2* ⎫	2.8
125–129	13.2	4.5	8.6* ⎭	
130–134	17.3	− 1.3	18.5*	6.0
135–139	17.0	− 9.2	26.1*	15.8
140 +	10.3	− 17.9	28.2†	48.4

* Indicates significance at $p<0.001$, and † = $p<0.02$
J_{vc} is the resting secretion rate, J_{va} the secretion or absorption rate during infusion of 0.5 µg/min of adrenaline, and J_v is ($J_{vc} - J_{va}$)
ΔJ_{vc}AMP is the response to dibutyryl cyclic AMP introduced into the lung liquid to give a final concentration of 10^{-4} mol/l, in a separate series of experiments
The values are means; n varied between 4 and 12 for each gestation period

and within each group we were able to correlate the rate of lung liquid secretion or absorption to the prevailing plasma adrenaline concentration.

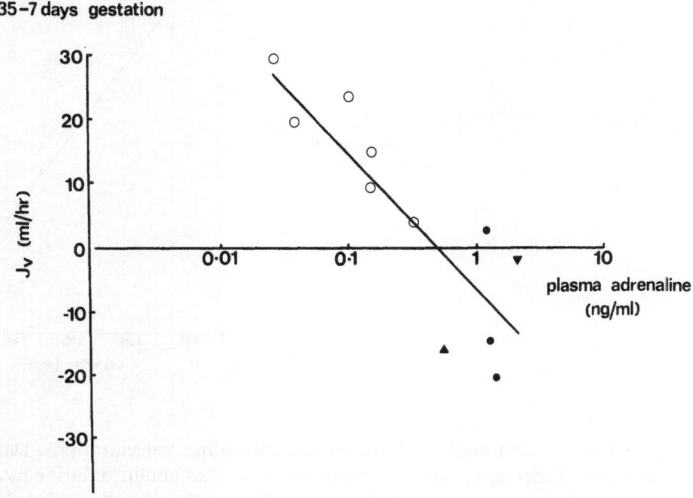

135-7 days gestation

Figure 5.4 The relationship between the secretion or absorption rate of lung liquid (J_V) and fetal plasma adrenaline concentration during control periods (open symbols) and infusions of adrenaline (closed symbols). Pooled data from five fetal lambs of gestational age 135–137 days. The regression line is shown ($r = 0.85$, $p < 0.01$) and this is line b in Fig. 5.5

An example of the results for a single group of animals is given in Fig. 5.4. A similar analysis was performed for fetuses undergoing labour, but in these experiments the adrenaline in fetal blood was the result of endogenous fetal catecholamine release. The relationship observed in labouring animals was closely similar to that obtained from fetuses of similar gestation into which adrenaline had been intravenously infused (Fig. 5.5a). More quantitatively, Fig. 5.5b demonstrates that all of the slowing of secretion and absorption of lung liquid observed during labour can be explained by the endogenous release of adrenaline by the fetus.

Other experiments in rabbits support this conclusion: β-adrenergic stimulation of rabbit fetuses near term can produce lungs which contain less water[16]; exposure to labour also produces drier lungs in fetal rabbits – an effect unaltered by subsequent route of delivery (by hysterotomy or normally by the vagina)[17]. Estimations of plasma catecholamines in fetal scalp blood samples from human infants followed for several hours *before* delivery show that adrenaline concentrations are high early in labour[18]. Indeed they are higher than would be required to produce very rapid absorption of lung liquid if the sensitivity of the human lung is similar to that of the lamb.

It is noteworthy that the concentrations of adrenaline required in the term lamb fetus to produce cessation of lung liquid secretion are extremely

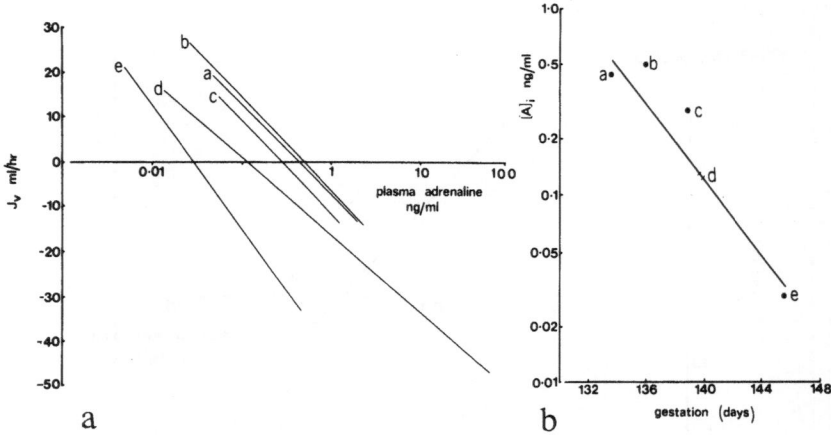

Figure 5.5 (a) The regression lines of J_v on plasma adrenaline concentrations. Data points are omitted for clarity. Lines *a, b, c* and *e* are derived from data obtained during i.v. adrenaline infusions in gestation groups *a:* 132–134, *b:* 135–137, *c:* 138–140 and *e:* >141 days. Line *d* is obtained from fetuses undergoing labour during which the elevated adrenaline concentrations are the result of endogenous secretion, not infusion: gestation range 134–144. (b) [A_i], the intercepts of the regression lines from (a) plotted against the mean gestation of each group. [A_i] is the concentration of adrenaline which stops secretion but does not cause absorption. The regression line is calculated from the adrenaline infusion data only (i.e. points *a, b, c* and *e*). Note, however, that point *d* lies on the line. This means that the changes in lung liquid secretion rate observed during delivery can be attributed to endogenous adrenaline release. No other mechanism needs to be postulated to explain the data

low. In fact, such low concentrations of adrenaline have not been reported in any postnatal mammal even under resting conditions[19]. This has important implications for the physiology of the postnatal lung; even if no further maturational changes take place after birth there appears to be always enough adrenaline in the circulation to produce continuous stimulation of absorption of lung liquid. In this respect it is relevant that the adult sheep pulmonary epithelium has been demonstrated to be capable of absorbing liquid against large oncotic pressure gradients[20] and sodium absorption has been reported in primate distal airway epithelium[21].

THE MECHANISM OF ABSORPTION

Absorption of fetal lung liquid could be the result of several very different mechanisms. For example, the large protein oncotic difference between lung liquid and the interstitium would be expected to produce passive absorption of liquid if the active transport of chloride into the luminal space were to be totally inhibited, or if the permeability of the epithelium, particularly to chloride ions, were to be increased sufficiently to allow little restriction to ions but not enough to allow unrestricted protein movement. (Indeed, a very temporary increase in epithelial permeability of this type,

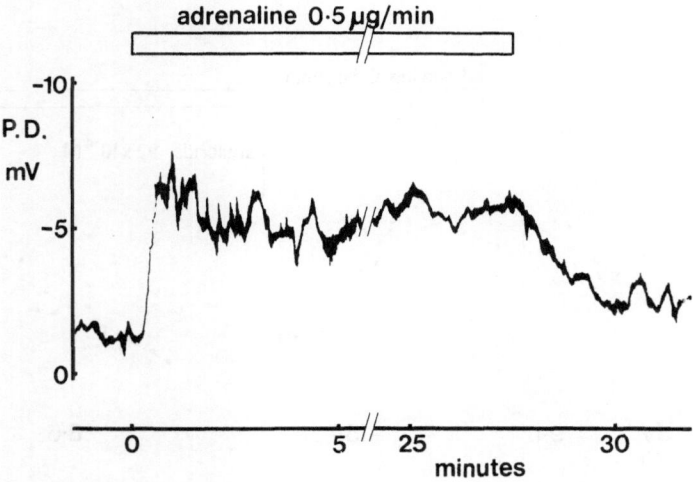

Figure 5.6 The effect of i.v. adrenaline infusion on the electrical p.d. measured between the fetal lung lumen and the vascular compartment. Note that the p.d. becomes more negative during adrenaline infusion

presumably due to stretching of the alveolar surface, has been described in the first few hours of spontaneous breathing in neonatal lambs[22]). It is possible that alterations in pulmonary blood flow could affect liquid movement across the pulmonary epithelium by an effect on the hydrostatic pressure gradient. However, Olver and Strang demonstrated that changes in pulmonary vascular pressure sufficient to double lung lymph flow had no effect on the rate of lung liquid secretion[6]. Furthermore, adrenaline can induce rapid absorption of lung liquid in a dose that has no measurable effect on pulmonary blood flow as detected by electromagnetic flow meters placed around the pulmonary artery (personal observations, Walters, D. V. and Cassin, S.). Also it is known that isoprenaline and adrenaline have opposite effects on the pulmonary vasculature but similar effects on lung liquid secretion[23].

Other possibilities are that adrenaline could reverse the direction of the chloride 'pump' or it could stimulate some other active transport system orientated towards the interstitium. The first evidence we obtained to support the latter hypothesis came from observations of the electrical potential difference across the pulmonary epithelium during adrenaline infusion[10]. An example experiment is shown in Fig. 5.6. The lung lumen, which is normally electrically negative with respect to blood, became even more negative during adrenaline infusion. This observation, whilst not compatible with reversal of active chloride transport, provides supporting evidence for the active transport of a positively charged ion (Na^+) in the direction lung lumen to plasma. Much more convincing evidence im-

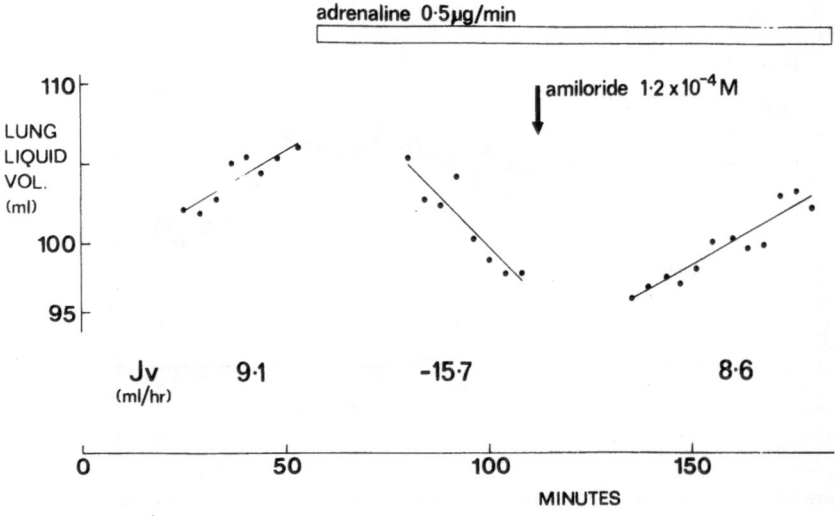

Figure 5.7 The effect of amiloride on adrenaline-induced lung liquid absorption. Amiloride was mixed into the lung liquid at the time indicated by the arrow to give a final concentration of 1.2×10^{-4} mol/l. It completely blocked the absorption produced by adrenaline

plicating active movement of sodium ions was obtained by examining the effect of amiloride, an agent known to block sodium channels on the apical membranes of some transporting epithelia. When amiloride is given into the lung liquid during resting secretion it has little effect but it completely prevents the absorption which is produced by adrenaline in a mature fetus (Fig. 5.7). The blocking effect of amiloride is invariable, and occurs whether it is given before or during an adrenaline infusion[10]. The concentration of amiloride required to produce half maximal inhibition of the effect of adrenaline, the K_I, is 4.3×10^{-6} mol/l, a figure in agreement with that reported for amiloride in other tissues studied *in vivo*[24].

Thus β-receptor stimulation of the fetal lung appears to stimulate sodium transport from lung lumen to plasma, an effect which is dependent on activation of sodium channels in the apical surface of the epithelial cells. This could be the result of configurational changes of pre-existing channels, or the insertion of preformed channels into the membrane. When an adrenaline infusion is stopped the effect on the lung wears off rapidly and the epithelium begins to secrete again within minutes. The capacity of the sodium channels of the fetal lung to be activated and deactivated so quickly is, as far as we know, unique to this tissue.

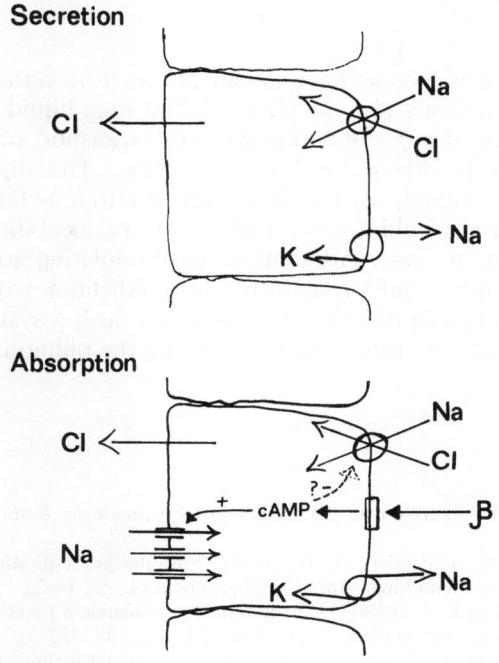

Figure 5.8 A model which may explain the fetal (secretory) and postnatal (absorptive) states of the lung. In this model Na^+ entry channels play a key role; when they are closed liquid is secreted and when they are open liquid is absorbed. β-Adrenergic stimulation, by modulating the sodium channel number or function, determines the direction of net fluid movement. *Secretion:* Na^+/K^+ ATPase generates a gradient for Na^+ which enters the intracellular space across the basolateral membrane linked to Cl^-, the latter ion being moved 'uphill' against its electrochemical gradient. Cl^- having entered the cell will pass into the lumen of the lung down the electrochemical gradient across the apical membrane (perhaps through specialized chloride channels) resulting in net transport of Cl^- from plasma to lung lumen. *Absorption:* During β-adrenergic stimulation Na^+ channels open in the apical membrane of the cell. Under these conditions Na^+ will preferentially enter the intracellular space across the apical membrane and be extruded across the basolateral membrane by Na^+/K^+ ATPase, resulting in net transport of Na^+ from the lumen to plasma. Entry of Na^+ across the apical membrane may dissipate the electrochemical gradient for linked Na^+ and Cl^- transport at the basolateral membrane, causing active Cl^- transport to decrease or even cease during β-adrenergic stimulation

MECHANISM OF MATURATION

A synthetic analogue of cyclic AMP, dibutyryl cyclic AMP, when mixed into lung liquid produces changes which are similar to those of adrenaline, i.e. an effect on secretion which is related to gestation (Table 5.3) and which can be inhibited by amiloride. Besides confirming that adrenaline is working via the adenylate cyclase system, it also suggests that the limiting step in the maturation of the response to adrenaline is 'downstream' from the β-receptor and the generation of intracellular cyclic AMP.

CONCLUSION

The experimental evidence we have to date allows us to postulate a cellular model for the secretion and absorption of fetal lung liquid which is summarized in Fig. 5.8. It is possible that the active transport of both chloride and sodium ions is driven by Na^+/K^+ATPase. The direction of net transport in such a model, whether it is chloride into lung liquid or sodium into the interstitium, would depend solely on the permeability of the apical membrane to sodium ions. Adrenaline, by modulating sodium channel function or number, could transform the epithelium from a state of chloride secretion to one of sodium absorption. Such a system may allow very fine control of the amount of liquid lining the pulmonary epithelium in postnatal lungs.

References

1. Preyer, W. (1885). In Fernam, L. (ed.) *Specielle Physiologie des Embryos*. (Leipzig: Th. Grieker's Verlag)
2. Potter, E. L. and Bohlender, G. P. (1941). Intrauterine respiration in relation to development of the foetal lung. *Am. J. Obstet. Gynecol., 42*, 14-22
3. Jost, A. and Policard, A. (1948). Contribution experimentale a l'etude du development prenatal du poumon chez le lapin. *Arch. Anat. Microsc., 37*, 323-32
4. Adams, F. H., Moss, A. J. and Fagan, L. (1963). The tracheal fluid of the foetal lamb. *Biol. Neonat., 5*, 151-8
5. Adamson, T. M., Boyd, R. D. H., Platt, H. S. and Strang, L. B. (1969). Composition of alveolar liquid in the foetal lamb. *J. Physiol., 204*, 159-68
6. Olver, R. E. and Strang, L. B. (1974). Ion fluxes across the pulmonary epithelium and the secretion of lung liquid in the foetal lamb. *J. Physiol., 241*, 327-57
7. Normand, I. C. S., Olver, R. E., Reynolds, E. O. R., Strang, L. B. and Welch, K. (1971). Permeability of lung capillaries and alveoli to non electrolytes in the foetal lamb. *J. Physiol., 219*, 303-30
8. Olver, R. E., Schneeberger, E. E. and Walters, D. V. (1981). Epithelial solute permeability, ion transport and tight junction morphology in the developing lung of the fetal lamb. *J. Physiol., 315*, 395-412
9. Claude, P. and Goodenough, D. A. (1973). Fracture faces of zonulae occludentes from 'tight' and 'leaky' epithelium. *J. Cell. Biol., 58*, 390-400
10. Olver, R. E., Ramsden, C. A., Strang, L. B. and Walters, D. V. (1986). The role of amiloride blockable sodium transport in adrenaline induced lung liquid reabsorption in the fetal lamb. *J. Physiol., 376*, 321-40
11. Alcorn, D., Adamson, T. M., Lambert, T. F., Maloney, J. E., Ritchie, B. C. and Robinson, P. M. (1977). Morphological effects of chronic tracheal ligation and drainage in the fetal lamb lung. *J. Anat. London, 123*, 649-60
12. Fewell, J. E., Hislop, A. A., Kitterman, J. A. and Johnson, P. (1983). Effect of tracheostomy on lung development in fetal lambs. *J. Appl. Physiol., 55*, 1103-8
13. Liggins, G. C., Campos, G. A., Vilos, G. A., Kitterman, J. A., Lee, C. C. and Clements, J. A. (1981). The effect of bilateral thoracoplasty on lung development in fetal sheep. *J. Dev. Physiol., 3*, 275-82
14. Brown, M. J., Olver, R. E., Ramsden, C. A., Strang, L. B. and Walters, D. V. (1983). Effects of adrenaline and of spontaneous labour on the secretion and absorption of lung liquid in the fetal lamb. *J. Physiol., 344*, 137-52
15. Walters, D. V. and Olver, R. E. (1978). The role of catecholamines in lung liquid absorption at birth. *Ped. Res., 12*, 239-42

16. Enhorning, G., Chamberlain, D., Contreras, C., Burgoyne, R. and Robertson, B. (1977). Isoxuprine-induced release of pulmonary surfactant in the rabbit fetus. *Am. J. Obstet. Gynecol.*, **129**, 197-202

17. Bland, R. D., McMillan, D. D. and Bressack, M. A. (1979). Labor decreases lung water content of newborn rabbits. *Am. J. Obstet. Gynecol.*, **134**, 364-7

18. Lagercrantz, H., Bistoletti, P. and Nylund, L. (1981). Sympathoadrenal activity in the foetus during delivery and at birth. In Stern, L. *et al.* (eds.) *Intensive Care of the Newborn.* pp. 1-12. (New York: Mason Press)

19. Buhler, H. V., Da Prada, M., Haefely, W. and Picotti, G. B. (1978). Plasma adrenaline, noradrenaline and dopamine in man and different animal species. *J. Physiol.*, **276**, 311-20

20. Matthay, M. A., Landolt, C. C. and Staub, N. C. (1982). Differential liquid and protein clearance from the alveoli of anesthetized sheep. *J. Appl. Physiol.*, **53**, 96-104

21. Legris, G. J., Will, P. C. and Hopfer, V. (1982). Human and baboon bronchial sodium absorption: implications for airway fluid movement and the mucociliary clearance mechanism. *Chest,* **81**, (Suppl.), 9S-11S

22. Egan, E. A., Olver, R. E. and Strang, L. B. (1975). Changes in non-electrolyte permeability of alveoli and the absorption of lung liquid at the start of breathing in the lamb. *J. Physiol.*, **244**, 161-79

23. Cassin, S., Dawes, G. S. and Ross, B. B. (1964). Pulmonary blood flow and vascular resistance in immature foetal lambs. *J. Physiol.*, **171**, 80-9

24. Edmonds, C. J. (1981). Amiloride sensitivity of the trans-epithelial electrical potential of sodium and potassium transport in the rat distal colon, in vivo. *J. Physiol.*, **313**, 547-59

Discussion

Dr J. T. Gatzy	Can the developmental change in apparent sensitivity to adrenaline be traced to differences in receptor affinity, stimulus effectiveness, or perhaps to the presence of other effectors in the system?
Dr D. V. Walters	We haven't looked at β-receptor number or affinity. The resting levels of adrenaline early in gestation are slightly higher than later in gestation, but we haven't taken it any further. The fact that the response to dibutyryl cAMP is also gestation-dependent suggests that maturation is 'downstream' from the β-receptor.
Gatzy	Are there other factors which seem to tune this sytem for adrenaline?
Walters	We have somewhat inconclusive evidence that neither corticosteroids nor thyroid hormones are involved.
Dr B. Robertson	It is interesting that tight junctions are already so tight on the 70th day of gestation. Is there any morphological difference between mature and immature junctions?
Walters	My answer comes from the work we did with Dr Schneeberger[1]. We looked at tight junction morphology by the freeze–fracture method and found that there are fewer strands in the mature fetus than in the immature one; yet in terms of pore theory their permeability is absolutely identical. Thus we must ask whether the junctional strands have anything to do with permeability. The claims that strand number and permeability are related are based on comparisons between different types of epithelia[2], which is perhaps less valid than our comparison of the same epithelium at different stages of development.
Dr E. A. Egan	As the fetus delivered was there substantial expulsion of fluid into the syringe from the thorax, which might be expected if chest squeeze is important in clearing lung liquid?
Walters	No, there wasn't.
Dr C. A. R. Boyd	In your final model you didn't mention a number of the ions that were studied in the earlier paper on the composition of lung liquid[3], in particular potassium ions and protons.
Walters	We haven't given detailed consideration to the role of other ions in the proposed model.
Dr J. A. Clements	May I ask a question about the stoichiometry between volume of water removed and the number of chloride ions removed and whether or not the ratio between sodium and potassium is the same during lung liquid secretion and absorption?
Walters	It seems to be an isotonic absorption. Bicarbonate, chloride and sodium concentrations in lung liquid do not alter during reabsorption. There is a small rise in potassium.
Clements	The lung liquid Na level is 150 mmol/l, the K 5–6 mmol/l and the Na/K exchange 3/2 at the Na/K ATPase. I'm having trouble balancing the books.
Walters	There are several membranes between the lung lumen and interstitial space. We know the Na/K ATPase works at a 3/2 ratio but we would be wrong to expect the same ratio across the whole epithelium as the K is free to leak out of the basolateral membrane of the cell down the electrochemical gradient established by the pump. Indeed the plasma membrane is usually permeable to K^+ and behaves as a K^+ electrode.

Dr G. Enhorning	Is it known what happens when infusion of a β-adrenergic agonist is used in an attempt to arrest labour? Is there a rebound increase in secretion when the β-agonist is stopped?
Walters	We have never seen a rebound – the resting secretion rate seems to be very stable.
Dr J. P. Mortola	Several aspects of the breathing pattern and respiratory mechanics after birth do not seem to be strikingly different between babies born naturally and those born by Caesarean section[4,5]. In a baby delivered artificially before labour begins, would the absorption rate of the fetal pulmonary fluid be much slower than in the naturally born infant?
Walters	Adrenaline is released in the fetus in response to the stress of labour. The adrenaline concentration is high in the cord blood of babies whether delivered normally or by Caesarean section, but in the infant born by elective Caesarean section we can assume that the adrenaline level must have been high for only a very short time. The increased incidence of transient tachypneoa of the newborn (TTN) in Caesarean babies may be due to lack of adrenaline stimulation over a sufficient period.
Gatzy	Have you tried to change the composition of the liquid to see if the absorption is dependent on both Na^+ and K^+?
Dr C. A. Ramsden	We attempted to remove Na^+ from the liquid but we presumed that a concentration below 20 mmol/l – if not below 10 mmol/l – would be required to have an effect on transport. That is difficult or impossible to achieve in our preparation due to backflux of Na^+ from plasma to lung liquid.

References

1. Olver, R. E., Schneeburger, E. E. and Walters, D. V. (1981). Epithelial solute permeability, ion transport and tight junction morphology in the developing lung of the lamb. *J. Physiol.* **315**, 395–412
2. Claude, P. and Goodenough, D. A. (1973). Fracture faces of zonulae occludentes from 'tight' and 'leaky' epithelium. *J. Cell Biol.,* **58**, 390–400
3. Adamson, T. M., Boyd, R. D. H., Platt, H. S. and Strang, L. B. (1969). Composition of alveolar liquid in the foetal lamb. *J. Physiol.,* **204**, 159–68
4. Mortola, J. P., Fisher, J. T., Smith, J. B., Fox, G. S., Weeks, S. and Willis, D. (1982). Onset of respiration in infants delivered by caesarean section. *J. Appl. Physiol.,* **52**, 716–24
5. Fisher, J. T., Mortola, J. P., Smith, J. B., Fox, G. S. and Weeks, S. (1982). Respiration in newborns. Development of the control of breathing. *Am. Rev. Resp. Dis.,* **125**, 650–7

6
Development of Epithelial Ion Transport in Fetal and Neonatal Airways

J. T. GATZY, C. U. COTTON, R. C. BOUCHER,
M. R. KNOWLES AND C. W. GOWEN, JR.

ABSTRACT

The mode of secretion of lung liquid by the pulmonary epithelium of the sheep during late gestation and reabsorption of this liquid around the time of birth has been elucidated, but the role of different regions of the epithelium in these processes has not been examined. We studied bioelectric properties and ion flows across upper airway epithelia excised from fetal sheep and fetal and neonatal dogs. Transepithelial nasal p.d. values of human neonates were also assessed *in vivo*. The tracheal epithelium of fetal sheep (143 days gestation) secreted Cl^- (1.4 μEq cm^{-2} h^{-1} hour). Na^+ movement (1.8 μEq cm^{-2} h^{-1}) was passive. Transepithelial p.d. (12 mV, lumen negative), short-circuit current (1.6 μEq cm^{-2} h^{-1}) and Cl^- secretion were stimulated by isoproterenol but were not affected by amiloride. Tracheal and 4th to 6th generation bronchial epithelia of maternal sheep absorbed Na^+; Cl^- movement was passive. Amiloride inhibited p.d., short-circuit current and Na^+ transport, but isoproterenol had no effect. Canine fetal and neonatal (up to about 1 month) tracheas exhibited patterns of bioelectric properties, ion flow and drug response similar to those of fetal sheep trachea. Whereas the dominant ion transport deduced from drug responses of canine fetal bronchi resembled those processes of fetal and neonatal trachea, bronchi from 1 month neonates absorbed Na^+ and responded to amiloride. Although these results suggest that Na^+ absorption by upper airway epithelia matures after birth and proceeds from distal to proximal regions, the transepithelial p.d. values of the nasal turbinate of term and preterm infants were close to the mature value (-30 mV, lumen negative) at birth. Moreover, amiloride induced a similar inhibition of p.d. (40%) of turbinates of infants and adults. This departure from the pattern predicted from the canine studies could reflect species and/or regional differences in airway epithelial function.

INTRODUCTION

Because of the efforts of Drs Walters, Olver, Strang and their co-workers[1-3], we know a good deal about the maturation of ion transport and permeability of the fetal pulmonary epithelium of the sheep around the time of birth. Production of lung liquid by the fetus appears to be driven by the secretion of Cl^-. This flow slows as term approaches and is supplanted by an absorption of Na^+ (Cl^-) and liquid that can be inhibited by amiloride. The changeover is induced by interaction of β-adrenergic receptors with the rising concentration of circulating catecholamines which accompanies the last days of gestation. Recent studies by Bland and co-workers[4] demonstrated that labour stimulates $Na^+ - Rb^+$ exchange by disaggregated granular pneumocytes. These results imply that Na^+ pumps, as well as amiloride-inhibitable Na^+ channels, are activated around the time of birth.

However, there is little direct evidence about the role of the different regions of the pulmonary epithelium in the fetus or neonate, although the alveolar epithelium, with its enormous surface area, is usually assumed to dominate any measurements of epithelial function. McAteer and co-worker's studies of alveolar buds from fetal rat lung in subculture[5] indicate that the primitive alveolar epithelium is capable of producing a liquid, but, for the most part, direct studies of this region are, if you will pardon the pun, 'in their infancy'. Moreover, there is no direct information about solute transport and permeability of small airways even though there is reason to believe that the aqueous phase which bathes the cilia of distal airway cells is produced by the epithelium[6]. Consequently, this paper will be limited to a description of the behaviour of a more accessible region – namely, the large airways of fetal and neonatal sheep, dog, and man.

IN VITRO METHODS

Our approach to the study of developing airways of sheep and dogs drew on traditional flux chamber techniques. Tracheas or large bronchi were excised from anesthetized fetal, neonatal or adult animals and were mounted as sheets between half chambers that were filled with mammalian Ringer solution. Potential difference was measured between Ringer–agar bridges that were connected by calomel half-cells to a high impedance voltmeter. Direct current was passed through a second pair of bridges and half cells. Transepithelial conductance was taken as the ratio of the current required to clamp the p.d. to zero (short-circuit) to the open circuit p.d. Unidirectional fluxes of radiolabelled solutes were estimated from the steady-state rate of appearance of tracer that was added to the solution bathing one surface of the tissue (source) in the other bath (sink).

Table 6.1 Bioelectric properties and ion flow across short–circuited sheep airways

Tissue	n	Flux direction	p.d. (mV)	I_{sc} μEq cm^{-2} h^{-1}	G (ms/cm²)	Na$^+$	Cl$^-$	K^{+*}
							Ion Fluxes μEq cm^{-2} h^{-1}	
Maternal bronchi	11	m → s	15.7 ±1.5	2.26 ±0.15	4.03 ±0.27	3.78 ±0.31	2.61 ±0.27	0.038 ±0.005
	10	s → m	17.9 ±1.4	2.32 ±0.14	3.62 ±0.28	1.69 ±0.21	3.05 ±0.26	0.138 ±0.040
		Net†				2.09‡ ±0.38	−0.44 ±0.38	−0.100‡ ±0.040
Maternal trachea	14	m → s	23.7 ±2.0	3.43 ±0.29	4.02 ±0.25	3.34 ±0.31	2.59 ±0.24	0.030 ±0.007
	14	s → m	25.6 ±2.7	3.45 ±0.31	3.85 ±0.36	1.19 ±0.19	2.84 ±0.31	0.060 ±0.024
		Net				2.15‡ ±0.37	−0.25 ±0.39	−0.30 ±0.025
Fetal trachea	20	m → s	12.1 ±0.9	1.65 ±0.10	3.88 ±0.24	1.82 ±0.17	1.64 ±0.12	0.052 ±0.016
	20	s → m	12.6 ±0.8	1.71 ±0.10	3.73 ±0.22	1.73 ±0.16	2.99 ±0.21	0.064 ±0.011
		Net				0.09 ±0.23	−1.35‡ ±0.24	−0.012 ±0.019

Values are means ± SE; n, no. of tissues; p.d., potential difference (lumen negative); I_{sc}, short-circuit current; G, conductance; m, mucosa; s, submucosa.
*$n = 6$.   † Indicates secretion.   ‡ Different from zero ($p < 0.05$).
Adapted, with permission, from the *Journal of Applied Physiology*[7]

EXCISED SHEEP AIRWAYS

Our first experiments dealt with the behaviour of tissue from sheep[7]. Table 6.1 compares the properties of excised maternal large airways with tracheas removed from 140–145-day fetuses. The direction of isotope movement was from the lumenal to interstitial-facing bath (mucosal to submucosal, M→S) or the opposite direction (S→M). Transepithelial p.d. was clamped at zero (i.e. short-circuited) by direct current from an external source, except for brief intervals when the circuit was opened to evaluate the magnitude of the transepithelial p.d.

Voltage across the adult airways, as we had previously noted for other species[8], was smaller in the more distal structures, and this resulted in a smaller short-circuit current because the conductances of epithelia from both regions were comparable. The p.d. and short-circuit current across fetal trachea were lower than those of the maternal tracheal barrier but the conductance was similar.

Na$^+$ moved more rapidly towards the interstitium (submucosa) than towards the lumen of both maternal airways. Since there was no elec-

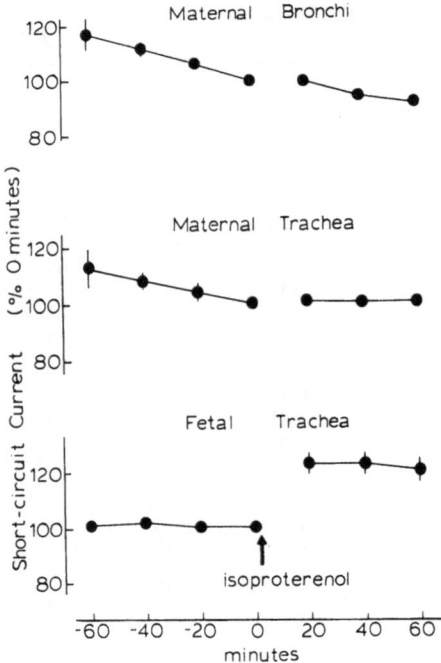

Figure 6.1 Effect of iosproterenol on short-circuit current. Tissues were maintained under short-circuit conditions except for 1 min every 20 min, when the circuit was opened and p.d. was measured. At the time indicated isoproterenol was added to interstitial-facing (submucosal) bath to achieve a final concentration of 10^{-6} mol/l. Short-circuit currents before exposure to drug were 2.3, 3.5 and 1.6 μEq/cm^2 per hour for maternal bronchi and trachea and fetal trachea, respectively. Mean $\pm$ SE; n = 10–20 tissues. Reprinted, with permission, from the *Journal of Applied Physiology*[7]

trochemical driving force, the flux asymmetry implies the existence of an active Na^+ absorptive process. In contrast, fluxes of Cl^- across both maternal airways were symmetric and compatible with passive diffusion.

On the other hand, Cl^- flow toward the lumen of fetal trachea clearly exceeded tracer flux in the opposite direction, a finding compatible with active secretion. There was no evidence for the flux asymmetry that would signal Na^+ absorption by the fetal trachea.

Some of the animal studies we will describe later were limited by the size and number of preparations. Moreover, conventional flux studies and voltage clamping of the epithelium of man *in vivo* is fraught with problems. Current passage across the epithelium has not been defined, and isotope flows across circumscribed areas of epithelium are difficult to control and not without risk. Accordingly, we must rely on the information that can be gleaned from bioelectric properties, or, sometimes, only the transepithelial p.d. Fortunately, a number of chemical agents or changes in bathing solution ion composition affect bioelectric properties and signal alterations in

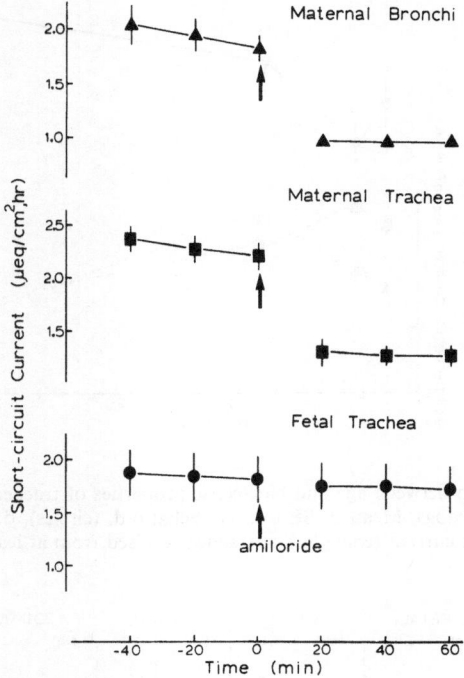

Figure 6.2 Effect of amiloride on short-circuit current of airway epithelia excised from maternal and fetal sheep. Tissues were short-circuited except for 1 min every 20 min, when the circuit was opened and p.d. was measured. Amiloride was added to the lumenal (mucosal) bath (final concentration = 10^{-4} mol/l) at the arrow. Mean ± SE; n = 6–8 tissues

ion permeation. An example of a drug-induced change in the short-circuit current of sheep airways is shown in Fig. 6.1. Exposure of the submucosal surface of the fetal trachea to 10^{-6} mol/l isoproterenol increased the current, whereas maternal airways were not affected by the drug. Analysis of ion fluxes revealed that Cl^- secretion by fetal trachea was stimulated selectively, but ion flows across maternal trachea and bronchi were not changed. In contrast, the Na^+ channel blocker, amiloride, inhibited p.d. and short-circuit current (Fig. 6.2) of maternal airways but did not affect either bioelectric property of fetal trachea appreciably. Again, flux analysis showed that Na^+ absorption by maternal airways was blocked by amiloride, but neither active Cl^- secretion nor the passive flow of Na^+ across fetal trachea was affected.

In summary, we found that active ion flow across large airways of the maternal sheep was dominated, in the basal state, by Na^+ absorption that could be blocked by amiloride but was not affected by isoproterenol. In contrast, only active Cl^- secretion was detected in studies of fetal trachea, and this transport was stimulated by isoproterenol but not affected by amioride.

81

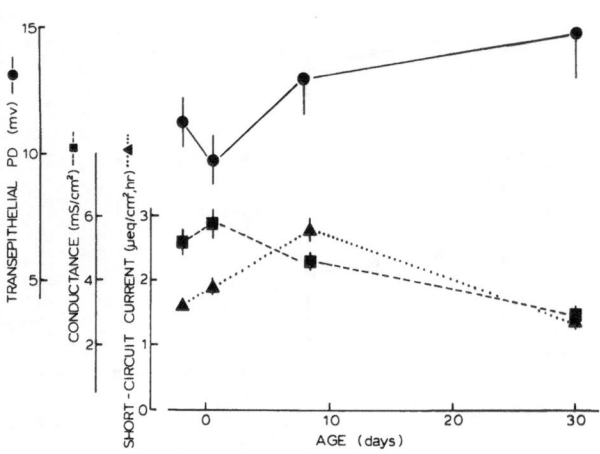

Figure 6.3 Relationship between age and bioelectric properties of tracheal epithelia excised from fetal and neonatal dogs. Mean ± SE transepithelial p.d. (circles), d.c. conductance (squares) and short-circuit current (triangles) of tracheas excised from at least 18 animals

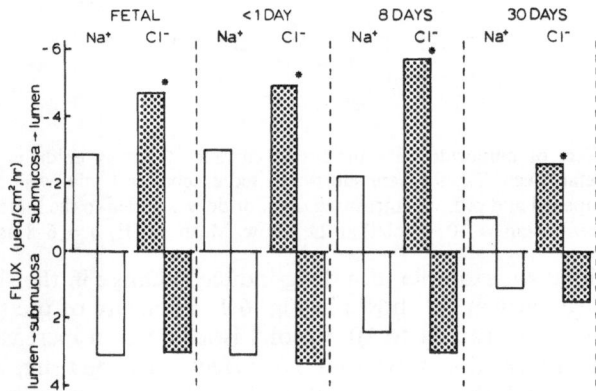

Figure 6.4 Relationship between age and unidirectional ion fluxes across tracheal epithelia excised from fetal and neonatal dogs. Histograms denote mean unidirectional Na^+ (open) or Cl^- (stippled) fluxes across tissues excised from at least nine animals

EXCISED CANINE AIRWAYS

We extended our study of the developing lung to the dog. Liquid sampled from lungs of fetal dogs was characterized by Na^+ and HCO_3^- concentrations that were similar to those of maternal and fetal plasma, whereas K^+ (9 mEq/l) and Cl^- (129 mEq/l) concentrations were significantly greater than those of plasma. Consequently, pulmonary liquid of fetal dogs, like that of fetal sheep, is rich in Cl^-.

When the airways of dogs were excised and mounted in flux chambers, we found the functional pattern of the fetal sheep, not only for the fetal trachea, but also for tracheas from pups that ranged in age from newborn to about 1 month[9]. Figure 6.3 summarizes the bioelectric properties of these tissues. In general, p.d. tended to rise with age and conductance tended to fall. Short-circuit current was somewhat higher in tracheas from 8-day neonates than in tissues from younger or older animals.

The ion flows reflected by these bioelectric properties are shown in Fig. 6.4. It is clear that Cl^- secretion (the difference between the unidirectional flows) by the trachea persisted for up to 1 month and paralleled the short-circuit current. The trend towards smaller conductances of tissues from older neonates (Fig. 6.3) was reflected in both smaller Na^+ fluxes and the passive flux of Cl^-.

Active Na^+ transport, which has been well documented by many studies of adult trachea, was missing from the fetal trachea and all neonatal tracheal epithelia. The lack of Na^+ transport does not appear to be a consequence of the 'noise' in the measurements. When we evaluated the relationship between electrical conductance (the aggregate of partial ionic conductances) and flux it was apparent that Na^+ flow in either direction described the same relationship. That is, lumen to interstitial (mucosal-submucosal) flow and interstitial to lumen (submucosal–mucosal) flows appeared to be part of the same population.

A comparable analysis of Cl^- flow across the fetal trachea demonstrated that points for interstitial to lumen flow routinely fell to the right, i.e. were greater than the best linear relationship that described the population of points for flow in the absorptive direction. Consequently, the Cl^- flux asymmetry and evidence for Cl^- secretion that was noted in Fig. 6.4 was accentuated by 'normalization' for overall ion conductance.

Flux studies showed that isoproterenol could stimulate Cl^- active transport by all fetal and neonatal tracheal preparations but amiloride had no effect. Again, bioelectric properties mirrored drug action on ion transport. When isoproterenol was added, short-circuit current nearly doubled. Similar changes were induced by β-adrenergic stimulation of neonatal trachea. These results suggest that the Na^+ transport process in the trachea which, along with Cl^- secretion, characterizes the adult epithelium, must mature very much later than the processes which transport Na^+ and help clear liquid from the lung around the time of birth.

We know that the epithelial cells of the immature trachea are not deficient in Na^+ pumps because exposure of the luminal surface to the cation pore-former, amphotericin B, induced a net Na^+ absorption of several $\mu Eq\ cm^{-2}h^{-1}$. It seems more likely that the appearance of amiloride-sensitive Na^+ channels is delayed in the trachea.

We have additional evidence for this thesis from studies with canine lobar bronchi. Because these bronchi are smaller in the fetus our flux chamber information is quite limited, and we were forced to draw conclusions that are based mostly on bioelectric properties. Exposure of bronchi from three fetuses to isoproterenol induced greater than 100% increases in short-circuit current that persisted for at least an hour, whereas exposure

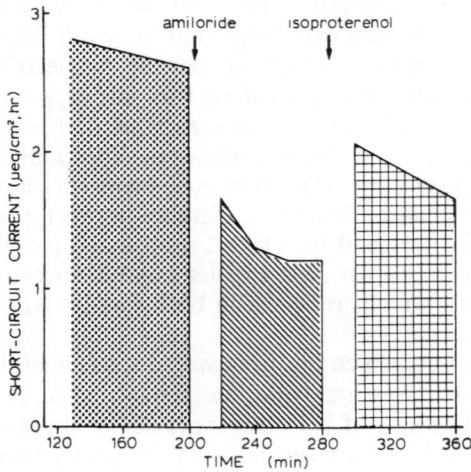

Figure 6.5 Effect of exposure of lobar bronchi excised from 30-day puppies to amiloride (10^{-4} mol/l, lumenal bath) and isoproterenol (10^{-5} mol/l, submucosal bath). Histograms represent mean short-circuit currents of tissues excised from 10 animals

of the luminal surface to amiloride did not induce a consistent change. In addition, the order of exposure of the two drugs did not affect the pattern of response. However, bronchi from 30-day pups behaved differently. The addition of amiloride caused a clear-cut inhibition of the mean short-circuit current of lobar bronchi, whereas subsequent exposure to isoproterenol stimulated the clamping current (Fig. 6.5). Once again, flux analysis confirmed that the inhibition of short-circuit current by amiloride was the consequence of a block of Na^+ absorption, whereas stimulation of current by isoproterenol resulted from a rise in Cl^- secretion. Moreover, the resting short-circuit current was carried largely by Na^+ absorption rather than by Cl^- secretion.

Since evidence for Na^+ absorption could not be found in studies of bronchi excised from fetal pups shortly before the end of gestation, it appears that the basal Na^+ absorption, which is the dominant active ion transport across large bronchi excised from 1-month neonates and adults, develops after birth.

HUMAN NASAL EPITHELIUM *IN VIVO*

From our studies of developing canine airways one might conclude that (1) maturation of ion transport in this region lags behind the processes which assist in clearing the lung of liquid at birth, and (2) distal airways mature more rapidly than proximal structures like the trachea. However, these animal studies do not necessarily allow us to predict the behaviour of airway epithelia in man.

Although the transepithelial p.d. across trachea and bronchi of conscious human subjects can be measured by a bridge that is positioned by a bronchoscope, it is much more convenient to restrict the evaluation to more proximal regions such as the nasal passages. The p.d. between the nasal surface and an indifferent bridge placed in the subcutaneous space can be measured with a small bridge of plastic tubing that is perfused slowly with Ringer solution[10]. The greatest p.d. is found across regions of the nasal epithelium, such as the inferior surface of the turbinate, that are populated mostly by ciliated cells. The morphology of the surface epithelium in these regions closely resembles that of the trachea and bronchi. Further, the electrical p.d. is about 30 mV, lumen negative, and the response of p.d. to drugs and changes in the composition of the perfusion solution follows the pattern for trachea and bronchi. Flux studies on pieces of resected turbinate revealed that ion transport across the nasal epithelium, like that across the bronchial epithelium of man and other mammals, is dominated by active Na^+ absorption[11].

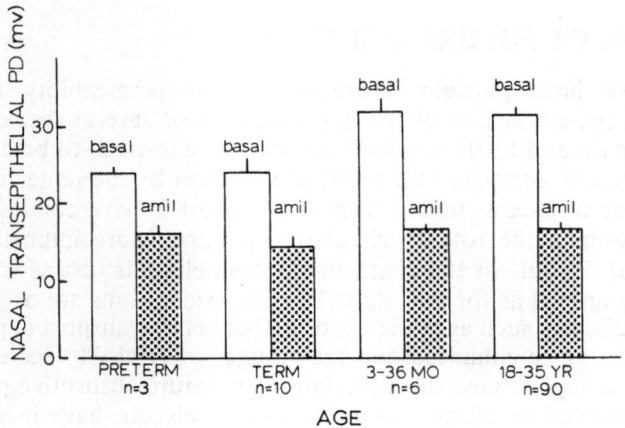

Figure 6.6 The effect of amiloride on the *in vivo* transepithelial p.d. of the nasal turbinate of neonates, children and adults. Open histograms represent mean maximum basal p.d. values from the inferior surface. Stippled bars denote the mean maximum steady-state p.d. that was measured after 2 min of perfusion of an amiloride (10^{-5} mol/l) solution over the turbinate surface. Vertical lines = SE

The magnitude of the maximal turbinate p.d. in neonates, children and adults is shown in Fig. 6.6. The open histogram on the right reiterates that the inferior surface of the adult turbinate is characterized by a transepithelial p.d. of about 30 mV. The p.d. values for term neonates and premature infants (26–36 weeks, mean gestation = 28.5 weeks) were about 22 mV when measured less than 24 h after delivery. These values remained stable for at least 72 h.

Regardless of the subject population, the transepithelial p.d. was inhibited by superfusion of a Ringer solution with amiloride over the surface in contact with the bridge[12]. The onset of a typical response was rapid and a

85

new steady p.d. was reached within seconds. Exposure of the luminal surface to amiloride induced about 40% inhibition of p.d. in adults and children. Although the response of term and preterm neonates may be marginally smaller, the effect of the drug is clearly evident. Consequently, we conclude that amiloride-inhibitable channels for Na^+ entry into the nasal epithelial cells and Na^+ transport are well developed not only in full-term neonates but in the premature infant population.

This conclusion clearly differs from the slow development of Na^+ transport we described for canine large airways. We do not know the importance of this apparent conflict but it must be emphasized that the studies in man and dog dealt with

1. different airway regions, and
2. a comparison of *in vivo* with *in vitro* results.

Either or both of these differences, along with species difference, could complicate our attempt to generalize.

DIRECTION OF FUTURE RESEARCH

Although we have partially characterized the permeability and ion transport of the epithelium of the upper airways of several species before and after the time of birth, it is obvious that there is much to be done. We have not carefully compared the mode of transport by the same airway region of different species under both *in vitro* and *in vivo* conditions and tried to determine the role of circulating factors. More important, our knowledge of the role of the distal airway epithelium is just as scanty for the maturing animal as for the adult. These considerations are of great importance in diseases such as cystic fibrosis where Na^+ transport in proximal airways seems to be enhanced and the vestiges of fetal Cl^- secretion appear to be missing[11,13]. One can postulate that mature absorptive processes normally restricted to distal structures, such as alveoli, have invaded the airways. However, until more direct methods are developed to assess the function of distal airways and alveolar epithelia, our attempts to understand the maturation of the pulmonary epithelial tract, the control of airways liquid, and derangement of this liquid in disease will continue to be based largely on speculation.

Acknowledgements

R. C. Boucher is an Established Investigator of the American Heart Association. M. R. Knowles is the recipient of a Clinical Investigator Award from the National Institutes of Health. Portions of this project were supported by research grants HL 16674, HL 22624 and HL 00787 from the National Institutes of Health. Some of the studies in this report were taken from a Ph.D. dissertation entitled 'Maturation of airway ion transport: studies of tracheal and bronchial epithelia excised from fetal, neonatal and adult dogs and sheep', that was submitted in 1984 to the University of North Carolina at Chapel Hill by C. U. Cotton.

References

1. Olver, R. E. and Strang, L. B. (1974). Ion fluxes across the pulmonary epithelium and the secretion of lung liquid in the fetal lamb. *J. Physiol. (Lond.)*, **241**, 327–57
2. Walters, D. V. and Olver, R. E. (1978). The role of catecholamines in lung liquid absorption at birth. *Pediatr. Res.*, **12**, 239–42
3. Olver, R. E. (1983). Fluid balance across the fetal alveolar epithelium. *Am. Rev. Respir. Dis.*, **127**, 533–6
4. Bland, R. D., Braun, D. and Boyd, C. A. R. (1985). Labor stimulates Na–K–ATPase activity in lung epithelial cells of fetal rabbits. *Fed. Proc.*, **44**, 640
5. McAteer, J. A., Cavanaugh, T. J. and Evan, A. P. (1983). Submersion culture of the intact fetal lung. *In Vitro*, **19**, 210–18
6. Kilburn, K. H. (1968). A hypothesis for pulmonary clearance and its implications. *Am. Rev. Respir. Dis.*, **98**, 449–63
7. Cotton, C. U., Lawson, E. E., Boucher, R. C. and Gatzy, J. T. (1983). Bioelectric properties and ion transport of airways excised from adult and fetal sheep. *J. Appl. Physiol.: Respirat. Environ. Exercise Physiol.*, **55**, 1542–9
8. Boucher, R. C., Stutts, M. J. and Gatzy, J. T. (1981). Regional differences in bioelectric properties and ion flow in excised canine airways. *J. Appl. Physiol.: Respirat. Environ. Exercise Physiol.*, **51**, 706–19
9. Cotton, C. U., Boucher, R. C. and Gatzy, J. T. (1984). Bioelectric properties and ion flows across excised fetal and neonatal dog trachea. *Fed. Proc.*, **43**, 830
10. Knowles, M. R., Carson, J. L., Collier, A. M., Gatzy, J. T. and Boucher, R. C. (1981). Measurements of transepithelial electric potential differences in the trachea and bronchi of human subjects in vivo. *Am. Rev. Respir. Dis.*, **124**, 484–90
11. Knowles, M. R., Stutts, M. J., Spock, A., Fischer, N., Gatzy, J. T. and Boucher, R. C. (1983). Abnormal ion permeation through cystic fibrosis respiratory epithelium. *Science*, **221**, 1067–70
12. Knowles, M. R., Gowen, C. W. Jr., Lawson, E. E., Gatzy, J. T. and Boucher, R. C. (1985). Nasal potential difference and amiloride sensitivity in neonates with cystic fibrosis. *C. F. Club Abstracts*, **26**, 7
13. Boucher, R. C., Stutts, M. J., Knowles, M. R., Cantley, L. and Gatzy, J. T. (1985). Na$^+$ transport in cystic fibrosis nasal epithelia: abnormal basal rate and response to adenylate cyclase activation. *Clin. Res.*, **33**, 467A

Discussion

Dr L. B. Strang   We have tended to assume that the ion transport observed in the fetal lung takes place across the epithelium of the thin-walled distal airways, but we have no direct evidence on which part of the epithelium is involved. However, you now tell us that adrenaline acts on the upper airways epithelium of both the adult and fetus to initiate or increase chloride secretion, and that it has no effect on sodium transport. Hence in the fetal lung the main effects observed - and particularly the absorptive effect of adrenaline - must be mediated by ion transport across a different part of the pulmonary epithelium, the peripheral airspaces.

Dr J. T. Gatzy   That is a point I was trying to make. The lung periphery would also appear to be involved from the experiments on cultured type 2 epithelial cells which show sodium absorption. This leads to the conjecture that, in the postnatal lung, liquid may be produced and absorbed by distal thin-walled airways. There is, presumably, a need for the cilia in small airways to be covered by liquid.

Strang   Surely chloride secretion by airway epithelium would see to that?

Gatzy   In most of the tracheal preparations from mammals other than dogs, and certainly in all the large bronchial preparations that we studied in the Ussing chamber, the dominant ion transport in basal conditions is sodium absorption. Now if you shut down sodium absorption by amiloride a curious phenomenon occurs. The apical membrane hyperpolarizes and chloride secretion begins - which is why, even though we can completely inhibit sodium transport by amiloride, there is always a residual short-circuit current. With amiloride the p.d. falls only by about 40–50% and the conductance does not change appreciably, so we are left with 50% of the original short-circuit current. Chloride secretion is now carrying that current. In most of these airway epithelia, except the trachea of the dog, the mechanism for chloride secretion is dormant because the electrochemical driving force across the apical membrane is not large enough to drive Cl^- out of the cell. As soon as we hyperpolarize the apical membrane with amiloride, which shuts down the sodium diffusion potential into the cell, chloride is ejected into the lumen and chloride secretion is observed. In the case of dog trachea this process is already present at rest - in tandem with sodium absorption - and the effect of amiloride accentuates the process.

Dr C. A. R. Boyd   Is there evidence that the apical membrane potential of the epithelium of the trachea is different between fetal and adult tissues?

Gatzy   Microelectrode studies have been done, and the results are consistent with the requirements for chloride secretion. Those epithelia, or stages of epithelial development, which show sodium absorption and no chloride secretion have a lower apical membrane potential than those that secrete chloride.

Dr J. A. Clements   Your short-circuit currents were over 40 to 80 $\mu A/cm^2$. Can you turn that into physiological dimensions?

Gatzy
The short-circuit current was very closely equal to the net transport of ions. If you take the microequivalents per cm^2 transported, add counterions, and multiply by surface area and an isosmotic water concentration (i.e. volume per unit osmoles) you can estimate net volume flow.

Clements
I calculate 2.4 ml kg^{-1} h^{-1} for the whole surface of the lung. Is that anywhere near right? It's not too far from the values given for fetal lung liquid secretion. Do you think that the volume rate of secretion matches up well enough in the upper airway with what is required for ciliary transport?

Gatzy
That's very difficult to answer because liquid swept by ciliomotion from lower structures adds to the contributions of absorption and secretion by the epithelium of the upper airways.

Strang
Does it follow that the cilia in the trachea have to work very much harder than the cilia further down? The total cross-sectional area of the lung lumen is getting rapidly narrower as we move towards the trachea, yet the cilia extend right down to very small bronchi.

Gatzy
This is a consideration that we took as one of the compelling arguments for expecting the existence of an absorptive process in upper airways, particularly at the point of smallest aggregate cross-sectional area. The rate of ciliary motion probably doesn't increase more than 3- to 10-fold on moving up the tracheobronchial tree, whereas a 100-fold increase in the velocity of liquid movement would be needed to keep the system from plugging up.

7
Analysis of Ion and Fluid Transport Across a Vertebrate Pulmonary Epithelium Studied *In Vitro*

M. R. WARD AND C. A. R. BOYD

INTRODUCTION

Over recent years the pioneering work of Strang and colleagues[1] on the driving forces of fetal lung liquid secretion and the subsequent perinatal regulation of the process has found an unexpected functional analogy in work on adult lung. Classically it is claimed that in the adult the airspaces are kept dry solely by Starling (bulk osmotic and hydraulic) forces. That this cannot be the whole story is shown by experiments, for example those of Matthay, Landolt and Staub[2], in which homologous serum added to the lung lumen may be shown to be absorbed. Clearly active transport in the sense implied by Weymouth Reid (1902) (who had performed the analogous experiment on small intestine[3]) is at work. This paper describes recent experiments which seek to address the mechanism(s) involved in this process. We start by justifying the experimental approach and the tissue preparation which we have chosen to use.

IS THERE A NEED FOR *IN VITRO* STUDIES ON ION TRANSPORT IN THE INTACT LUNG?

In order to open the black box of epithelial transport as far as the lung epithelium is concerned two developments are necessary. One is to further develop and characterize the properties of isolated lung epithelial cells, in particular with respect to changes of ion pumping and of ion 'leak' pathways that may occur during development[4]. Obviously the hetero-geneous nature of the epithelium of the mammalian lung (with type I and type II cells showing quite different morphological characteristics) means that it is going to be difficult to resolve the question as to the quantitative importance of these two cell types to transepithelial ion transport in the in-tact lung. The possibility of culturing isolated cell types following their separation, although attractive[5,6], suffers from the inherent problems of de-

91

or re-differentiation associated with culture of a particular cell. Second, and in addition to the problem of cell type, it will be important to characterize quantitatively the contribution of the paracellular pathway through this epithelium[7]. Electrophysiological evidence will be needed to describe the properties of the whole epithelium and of the apical and basal membranes of the epithelial cells when their normal anatomical relationship is preserved.

Necturus lung: structural studies

To this end we have sought to use a new pulmonary epithelial preparation composed of a homogeneous cell type which appears to be closely related to the mammalian type II cell. In this preparation the electrical properties of the epithelium studied both by short-circuit current measurements in Ussing chambers and by intracellular microelectrode recordings can be combined with flux studies in which transepithelial movement of ions may be related to changes in fluid absorption. The lung which shows this mixture of technically attractive possibilities is an unusual one, namely that of the urodele amphibian *Necturus maculosus* (the mudpuppy)[8].

The lungs of this amphibian form a paired structure, each of which is in the shape of a narrow, blind-ended sac some 5 cm long (see Fig. 7.1A). The surface of this lung is not subdivided into lobes. Rather when the lung is cut open it shows a smooth inner surface. Scanning electron microscopy (Fig. 7.1C) shows this to be composed of a continuous sheet of epithelial cells, all of which show the same surface characteristic of abundant short microvilli (Fig. 7.1D). The diameters of these cells lie between 8 and 16 μm. Figure 7.1B shows a cryostat section of the lung used for histochemical examination. The lung may be seen to be lined with a uniform columnar epithelium the cells of which are some 20 μm deep. No squamous cells have been found within this epithelium . On the outer (abluminal) surface of the epithelium there is a relatively thick layer of connective tissue in which scattered myoid elements may be identified. In contrast to what has been stated in the literature[9] the lung epithelium of *Necturus* is indeed very well vascularized. A dense network of capillaries lies just deep to the epithelium and indeed forms a plexus completely separating the epithelial surface from the connective tissue beneath. This vascular structure was in fact described (see Fig. 7.2B) by Suchard (1904) in the newt lung more than 80 years ago[10]. Figure 7.2A shows very clearly that similarly in *Necturus* a mass of nucleated erythrocytes lies in the dense capillary bed just beneath the epithelium. Transmission electron microscopy confirms previous reports[11] that this epithelium contains as intracellular organelles numerous osmiophilic lamellar bodies (Fig. 7.3) typical of the type II cell of the mammalian lung.

Necturus lung: biochemical evidence

We have examined the crude tissue extract from *Necturus* lung and have shown, using thin-layer chromatography, that it contains substantial quan-

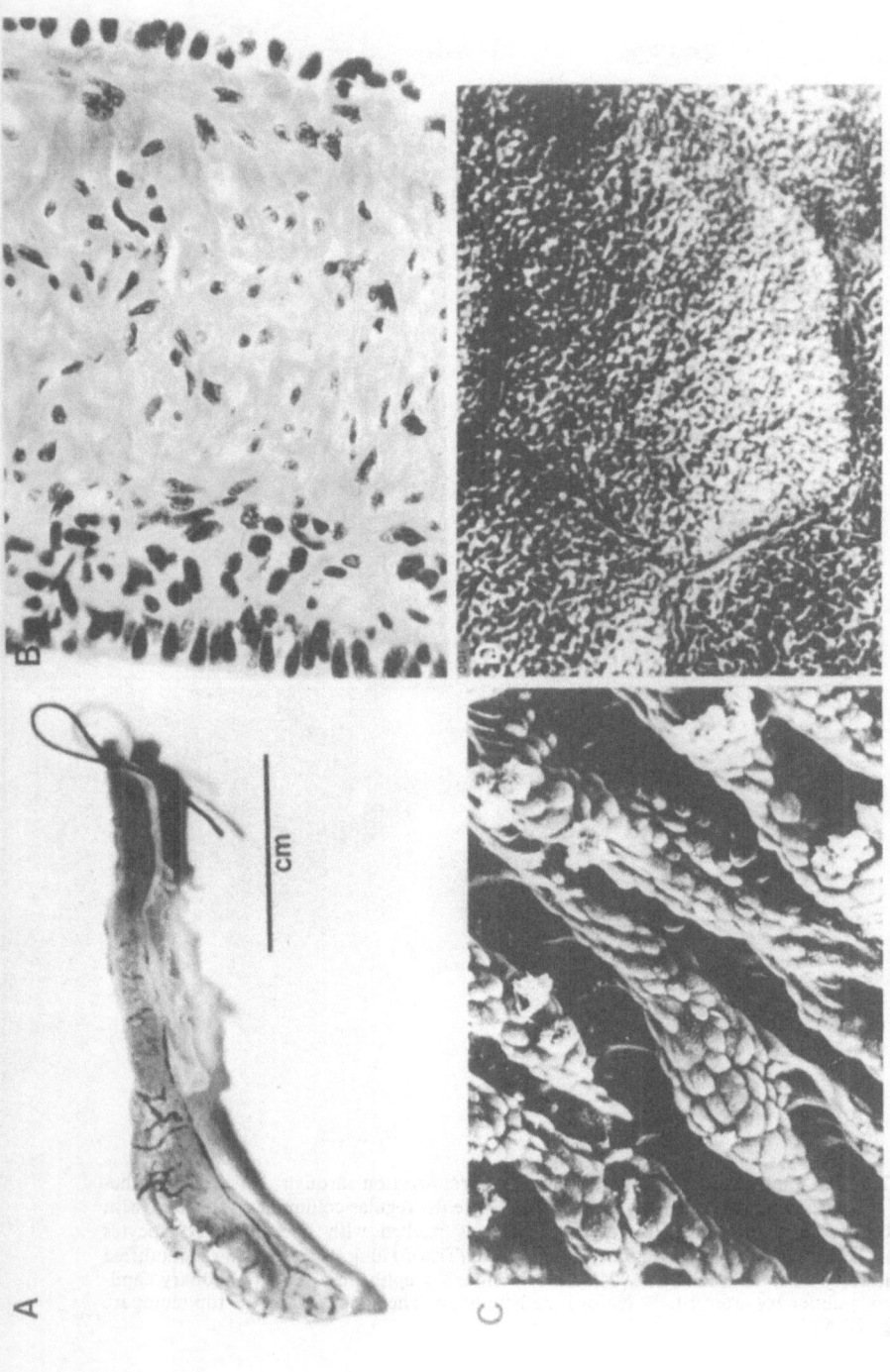

Figure 7.1 **(A)** External view of one lung of *Necturus maculosus*. **(B)** Full-thickness transverse section of *Necturus* lung (haematoxylin and Van Gieson, × 24). Note the pulmonary epithelium facing the lung airspace to the left of the figure. **(C)** Low-power scanning electron micrograph of the surface of the pulmonary epithelium of *Necturus* lung (× 60). Note pleating of cell surface and the occasional alveolar macrophage with ruffled cell surface. **(D)** High-power scanning electron micrograph of the surface of the pulmonary epithelium of *Necturus* lung. Note the hexagonal border of the epithelial cells and the surface lawn of stubby micovilli (× 3600)

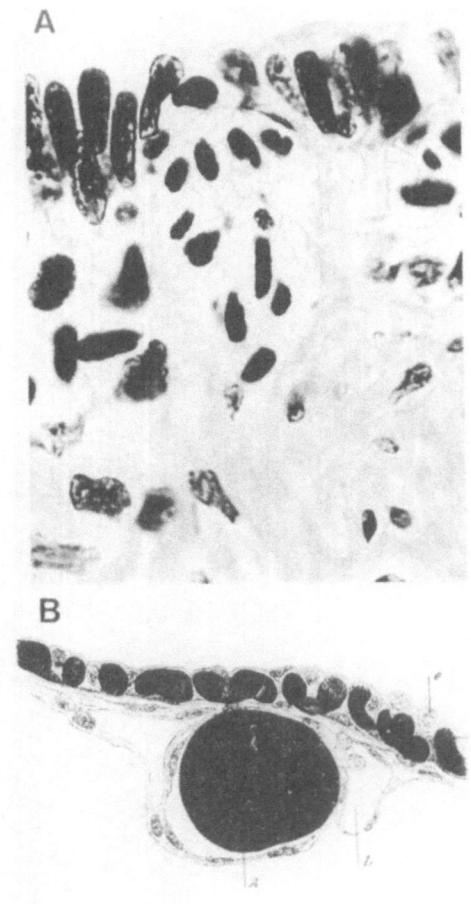

Figure 7.2 (A) Light micrograph (high-power) of cross-section through the surface epithelium of *Necturus* lung. The airspace is at the top. Note the regular columnar epithelium (with brush border) and the three underlying capillaries packed with nucleated erythrocytes (× 350). (B) Low-power cross-section through newt *(Triton)* lung. This drawing is modified from the early work of Suchard (1904)[10]: e = pulmonary epithelium; c = pulmonary capillary; A = pulmonary artery; L = major lung lymphatic. The airspace is at the top (compare with Fig. 7.2A).

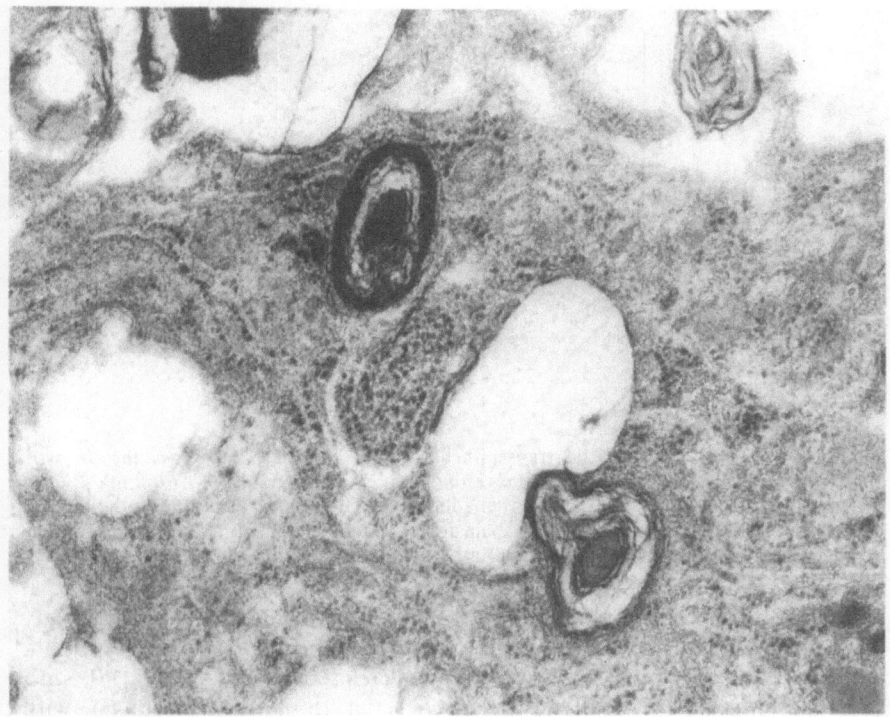

Figure 7.3 Electron micrograph at high power ($\times$ 50 000) showing two lamellar bodies (one in the process of exocytosis into a surface vacuole) in the pulmonary epithelium of *Necturus maculosus*

tities of both phosphatidylcholine and phosphatidylglycerol. Furthermore, preliminary experiments show that on a sucrose gradient this material resides predominantly in the pooled 0.40–0.55 mol/l sucrose fractions; further experiments should allow us to locate more precisely the lamellar body-containing fraction[12]. From these structural and biochemical studies we conclude that the epithelium lining the lumen of the lung of *Necturus maculosus* consists predominantly of a single cell type and that this cell is very similar to the mammalian type II alveolar cell both structurally and in its ability to synthesize and store surface-active material in lamellar bodies. Since this epithelium may readily be opened out as a flat sheet it is highly accessible to physiological studies.

Necturus lung: electrophysiology

Transepithelial properties

Figure 7.4 shows electrophysiological findings once this epithelium is

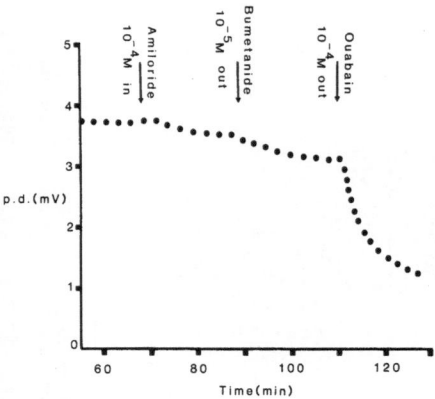

Figure 7.4 Figure showing the transepithelial potential difference across the *in vitro* preparation of *Necturus* lung. Note the resting transepithelial potential of 3.8 mV (lumen negative) and the small depolarization that follows the addition of amiloride to the luminal surface. Note also that addition of ouabain to the external (abluminal) surface causes the rapid collapse of the transepithelial potential

mounted in an Ussing chamber so that the inner and outer surfaces may separately be bathed with appropriate artificial *Necturus* Ringer solution[13]. The potential difference observed across such preparations is 3.8 ± 0.4 mV (mean $\pm$ standard area of mean in 33 preparations from 12 lungs), with the inside being negative with respect to the serosal surface. The mean transepithelial d.c. resistance after compensation for fluid resistance is 592 ± 84 ohm cm^2 ($n = 33$) which means that this lung epithelium is moderately tight. We cannot at present totally exclude the possibility that some of the smaller p.d. values and resistances were from edge-damaged preparations. Our preparations are 0.3 cm in diameter, and any edge damage would create a particularly dominant shunt pathway across such a small-diameter tissue. Every precaution was taken to minimize such damage, and transepithelial resistance was monitored as the two halves of the chamber were tightened. Visible edge damage resulted in very low (50 ohm cm^2) resistances and such preparations were excluded from the analysis. All other preparations are included. No obvious bimodal distribution of resistances was obtained, and although three preparations had resistances > 1400 ohm cm^2, their p.d. values were only 9–10 mV. Even if these three higher resistance epithelia turn out to be representative of the tissue, the p.d. is clearly not going to be as great as that generated by bullfrog alveolar epithelia[14]. Edge damage is thus a possible problem which may require that the distribution of results be shifted to the right.

Short-circuit current

If the p.d. across the epithelium is made zero by passing current from an external source, and if the solutions on either side of the preparation are identical, no electrical or chemical gradient exists across the tissue. Under these conditions remaining net ion transport must be by active transport[15]. The current applied to clamp the p.d. to zero, the short-circuit current, reflects the active transport processes occurring within the epithelial cell. Both resting p.d. and the short-circuit current across the *Necturus* lung epithelium are abolished by application of ouabain 10^{-4} mol/l to the outer (abluminal) aspect of the lung (Fig. 7.5). Application of ouabain to the apical (lumen) surface has little effect. Since ouabain blocks sodium pump activity this clearly indicates that the active p.d. and short-circuit current observed in this preparation are a consequence, whether directly or indirectly, of the activity of the sodium potassium ATPase located in the abluminal surface of the epithelium. Amiloride, a drug which blocks sodium transport across many tight epithelia, has a partial inhibitory effect at 10^{-4} mol/l on both transepithelial p.d. and short-circuit current, but this is found only when the drug is applied to the apical (luminal) aspect of the epithelium (Fig. 7.5).

Intracellular recordings

Intracellular recordings of membrane potential and of input resistance have been made from the epithelial cells using the same electrophysiological protocol as that used on small intestinal epithelium[13]. The cells are impaled under visual control from the apical surface with a KCl-filled microelectrode. The mean resting potential across the apical membrane is -32 ± 2.2 mV ($n = 17$). These potentials are recorded immediately after impalement of the cells, since, quite unlike our experience with intracellular recording from *Necturus* small intestinal epithelium[13], we find that the membrane potential of these lung cells spontaneously fluctuates and shows transient depolarizations of 2–3 mV occurring up to 10 times per minute. This we have attributed to the spontaneous contraction of sub-epithelial myoid elements giving rise to a movement artefact in the recordings from the small epithelial cells, but we have not ruled out the possibility that these fluctuations arise within the epithelial cells themselves (exocytosis of lamellar bodies is one rather intriguing possibility). As is shown in Fig. 7.6 the membrane is hyperpolarized by the application of 10^{-4} mol/l amiloride to the apical surface. This indicates that there is amiloride-sensitive electrogenic entry of sodium ions across the apical membrane of the cell. Moreover it appears that sodium absorption must contribute both to the transepithelial p.d. and to the short-circuit current across the tissue: however, and in contrast for example to frog skin, sodium absorption does not account totally for the generation of the short-circuit current.

Effects of transport inhibitors

Figure 7.5 shows that the loop diuretic bumetanide reduces the resting p.d. only when applied to the basolateral (abluminal) surface. This is consistent with the presence of diuretic-sensitive sodium chloride cotransport in the basolateral membrane as, for example, has been found in many secretory

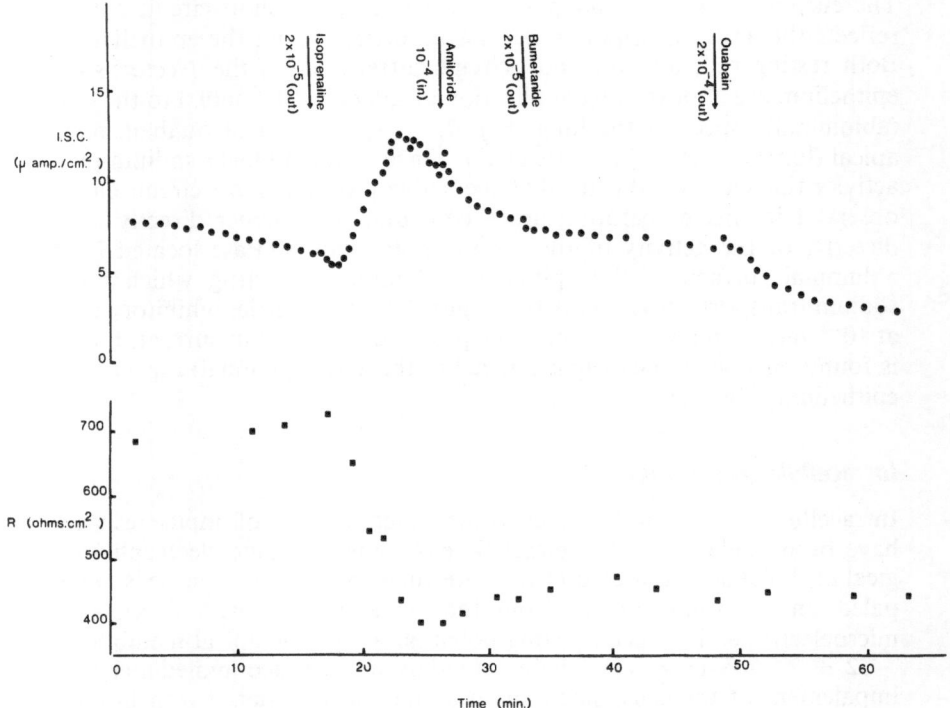

Figure 7.5 Figure showing the short-circuit current (I.S.C, upper trace) and transepithelial resistance (lower trace) of *Necturus* lung *in vitro.* Note that ouabain inhibits the short-circuit current

epithelia. It appears that such a diuretic-sensitive cotransport system contributes to the generation of both the p.d. and the short-circuit current in *Necturus* lung, and ion replacement studies will be needed to investigate the mechanism of such cotransport systems in more detail. Thus, although sodium absorption and chloride secretion are implicated in the generation of the transepithelial p.d., a quantitative description of the origin of the p.d. awaits the results from our isotope flux studies. Our experiments on fluid transport (see below) lead us to believe that a net absorption of ions occurs across the epithelium. The β-adrenergic agonist isoprenalin increases the transepithelial p.d. and the short-circuit current, and also produces complex changes in resistance (see Fig. 7.7) the basis of which is at present unclear. It may be associated both with changes in epithelial properties and also with changes in resistance of the underlying connective tissue layer (in which, as pointed out above, smooth muscle is present).

Necturus lung: fluid transport

Recent results (Fig. 7.8) show that this epithelium is capable of performing

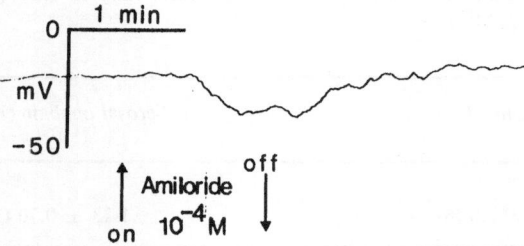

Figure 7.6 Intracellular record of membrane potential recorded from the pulmonary epithelium of *Necturus maculosus in vitro*. Note the initial membrane potential (with typical small fluctuations) of some -20 mV and the pronounced reversible hyperpolarisation that follows exposure of the luminal surface to amiloride (10^{-4}M). Note also the return of the recorded potential to zero mV following the withdrawal of the microelectrode from the epithelial cell at the end of the trace

net transepithelial water transport. Using a simple gravimetric assay similar to that used by Diamond[16] it has been possible to show that there is a net absorptive water flux across the epithelium when the lung is studied *in vitro* with isotonic *Necturus* Ringer inside and outside. As shown in Fig. 7.8, addition of ouabain rapidly reduces the rate of water absorption from the lung lumen. Table 7.1 confirms that this finding is a consistent one. The magnitude of the observed s.c.c. (Figs 7.5 and 7.7) and water fluxes (Table 7.1) shows that the absorbate is approximately isotonic. Using the data shown in Fig. 7.7 (s.c.c.) and Table 7.1 (water flux) it is possible to calculate the tonicity of the absorbate. Thus a short-circuit current of 10 μA cm^{-2} (assuming Na$^+$ to be the only ion which is actively transported under control conditions) is equivalent to a flux of Na$^+$ of 0.36 μmol cm^{-2} h^{-1}; with *Necturus* Ringer containing 105 mmol Na$^+$ litre^{-1} this would require an isotonic volume flow of about 3 μl cm^{-2} h^{-1}, whereas the water flux observed (15 μl 100 mg^{-1} h^{-1}) is equivalent to a volume flow of approximately 2 μl cm^{-2} h^{-1}. Similarly ouabain (Fig. 7.9) is able to inhibit water transport from the gallbladder lumen when the same method is used. Although the rate of fluid transport is considerably higher in *Necturus* gallbladder than in lung, it should be noted that the gallbladder does not have the thick connective tissue layer which is present in *Necturus* lung, and which is important, since these fluxes are expressed in units of volume per unit weight of tissue. Additional experiments using ^{14}C sucrose and ^{3}H$_2$O added to the lung lumen confirm that fluid is absorbed from *Necturus* lung *in vitro*. Very preliminary studies have been carried out to investigate the influence of both amiloride and isoprenalin on fluid movement across Necturus lung. Amiloride (10^{-4} mol/l in the lumen) was found to inhibit fluid transport by some 30% as compared to control: isoprenaline (5 x 10^{-5}mol/l) added to the external (abluminal) surface appeared to roughly halve the rate of fluid absorption from the lumen. These findings warrant further investigation, as does the finding that indomethacin (10^{-5}mol/l) appears to act as a secretogogue.

Table 7.1 Measurement of fluid absorption by *Necturus* lung *in vitro* (μl (100 mg wet weight)$^{-1}$ h^{-1}) mean $\pm$ SEM

Control	+ Serosal ouabain (10^{-4} mol)
15.2 $\pm$ 1.0 (6)	1.13 $\pm$ 0.70 (3)

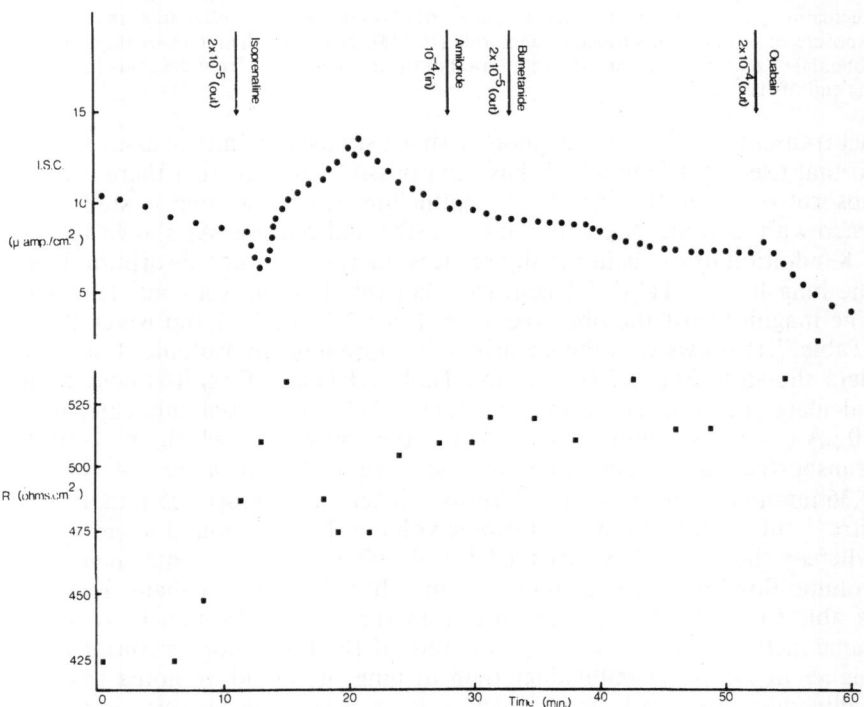

Figure 7.7 Record showing short-circuit current (I.S.C., upper trace) and transepithelial resistance (R) (lower trace) of *Necturus* lung studied *in vitro*. Note the biphasic change in short-circuit current which is associated with complex changes in resistance which follows exposure of the tissue to the β-adrenergic stimulant isoprenalin

CONCLUSION

Necturus lung should provide useful information about the mechanisms and their regulation that are involved in the transport of fluid and electrolytes between the airspaces and the circulation. Because of its unique and

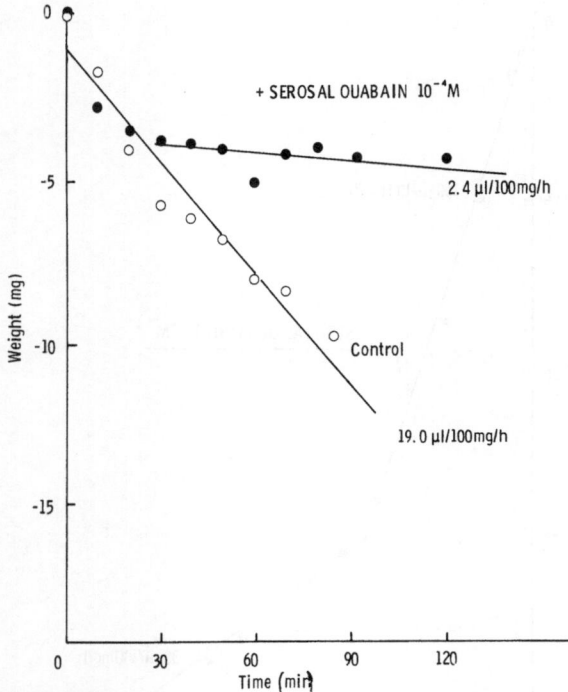

Figure 7.8 Fluid absorption from *Necturus* lung studied *in vitro*. Ouabain (10^{-4} mol) was added to the external (abluminal) surface to one of the two paired lungs. Note the profound inhibition of fluid transport seen in the presence of ouabain as compared to the control

simple structural basis this epithelium, composed of cells similar to the mammalian type II cell, will be useful as a model in the study of agents that modify or regulate fluid transport between the lung and the interstitium. In particular the prospect of intracellular epithelial analysis of membrane resistance of the apical and basal surfaces during conditions of fluid absorption, and the modification of this process by hormonal agonists and by pharmacological intervention, offers very attractive possibilities for studying the interactions between the fundamental membrane transport processes which must underlie the whole process of transepithelial ion transport in this tissue.

References

1. Olver, R. E. and Strang, L. B. (1974). Ion fluxes across the pulmonary epithelium and the secretion of lung liquid in the foetal lamb. *J. Physiol.*, **241**, 327–57
2. Matthay, M. A., Landolt, C. C. and Staub, N. C. (1982). Differential liquid and protein clearance from the alveoli of anaesthetised sheep. *J. Appl. Physiol.*, **53**, 96–104
3. Reid, E. W. (1902). Intestinal absorption of solutions. *J. Physiol.*, **28**, 242–56
4. Bland, R. D. and Boyd, C. A. R. (1986). Cation transport in lung epithelial cells derived from fetal, newborn and adult rabbits. *J. Appl. Physiol.* (In press)

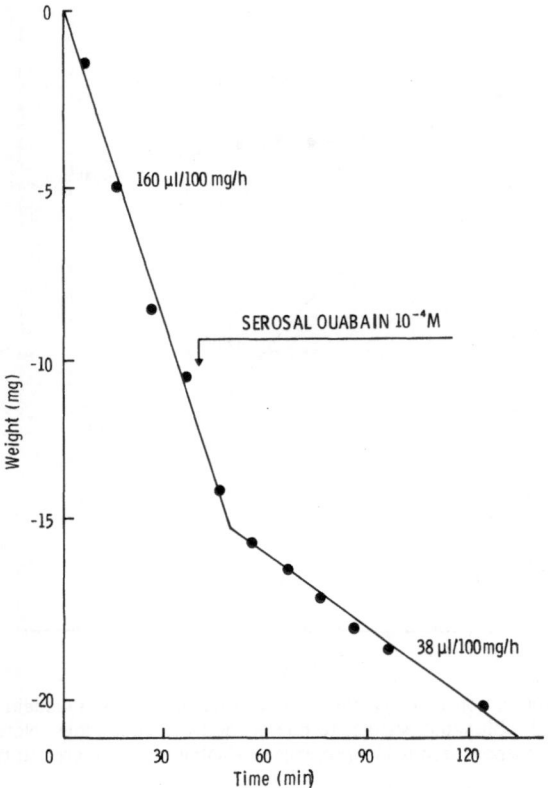

Figure 7.9 Fluid absorption by *Necturus* intact gallbladder studied *in vitro*. Note that the effect of ouabain on fluid transport is similar to that shown in Fig. 7.8

5. Mason, R. J., Williams, M. C., Widdicombe, J. H., Sanders, U. J., Misfeldt, D. S. and Berry, L. C. (1982). Transepithelial transport by pulmonary alveolar type II cells in primary culture. *Proc. Natl. Acad. Sci. USA.*, **79**, 6033-7
6. Schneider, G. T., Cook, D. I., Gage, P. W. and Young, J. (1985). Voltage sensitive high conductance chloride channels in the luminal membrane of cultured pulmonary alveolar (type II) cells. *Pflugers Archiv.*, **404**, 354-7
7. Basset, G., Crone, C. and Saumon, G. (1986). The rat alveolar membrane – an epithelium performing sodium-coupled water transport. *J. Physiol.* **371**, 168P
8. Boyd, C. A. R., Steele, L. W. and Ward, M. R. (1984). The mudpuppy lung epithelium: a preparation for the study of lung electrolyte and fluid transport. *J. Physiol.*, **358**, 113P
9. Guimond, R. W. and Hutchinson, V. K. (1976). Gas exchange of the giant salamanders of North America. In Hughes, G. M. (ed.) *Respiration of Amphibian Vertebrates*. pp. 313-338. (New York: Academic Press)
10. Suchard, E. (1904). Structure du poumon du triton et de la salamandre maculee. *Arch. d'Anat. Microscop.*, **6**, 170-9
11. Brooks, R. E. (1970). Lung alveolar cell cytosomes: a consideration of their significance. *Z. Zellforsch.* **106**, 484-97
12. Gil, J. and Reiss, O. K. (1973). Isolation and characterization of lamellar bodies and tubular myelin from rat lung homogenates. *J. Cell Biol.*, **58**, 152-71

13. Boyd, C. A. R. and Ward, M. R. (1982). A microelectrode study of oligopeptide absorption by the small intestinal epithelium of *Necturus maculosus*. *J. Physiol.*, **324**, 411–28

14. Crandall, E. D. and Kim, K. J. (1981). Transport of water and solutes across bullfrog alveolar epithelium. *J. Appl. Physiol.*, **50**, 1263–71

15. Ussing, H. M. and Zerahn, K. (1951). Active transport of sodium as the source of electric current in the short circuited frog skin. *Acta Physiol. Scand.*, **23**, 110–27

16. Diamond, J. M. (1962). The reabsorptive function of the gallbladder. *J. Physiol.*, **161**, 442–73

Discussion

Dr J. T. Gatzy	What do you think the ouabain-insensitive flow indicates?
Dr C. A. R. Boyd	In part it shows that there is a potassium permeability in the cells.
Gatzy	How did you deal with the possibility of a potassium isotope self-exchange?
Boyd	We have the same problem as everyone else who looks for isotopic flux in isolated cells. The useful things to do are to change the external or the internal potassium concentrations or the external or internal sodium concentrations, and we have done experiments of that sort. As the constant for half-maximal activation of the ouabain-sensitive potassium in flux is about 1.5 mmol/l, the major portion of the ouabain-sensitive flux appears to be going through a quite orthodox sodium pump. The ouabain-insensitive flux also shows saturation, interestingly enough, but with a much higher external concentration of 20–25 mmol/l potassium. The fact that you can inhibit much of that ouabain-insensitive flux with loop diuretics suggests again that it is not an exchange flux.
Gatzy	What do you think is happening when this ouabain-inhibitable portion increases as a funcion of gestation or labour?
Boyd	Either there is an increased delivery of sodium into the cells, with increased pumping as a secondary consequence following the rise of internal sodium, or there must be an increase in the number of sodium pumps. To distinguish between these possibilities we have tried to look at ouabain binding by isolated type II cells at different stages of gestation. Preliminary experiments suggest that both processes (increased Na entry and increased Na pump number) are taking place as gestation advances. The primary change appears likely to be in the number of sodium entry sites at the apical surface of the cell: increasing sodium delivery to the cell may induce secondary effects on the number of pumps.
Dr J. A. Clements	Mason and others[1,2] have shown that if type II cells isolated from the adult lung are kept in culture for 4 or 5 days, they form a continuous sheet with tight junctions and then show dome formation, this being inhibitable by amiloride. The domes are taken as direct evidence of fluid transport. At the same time the cells seem to be taking on characteristics, shown by lectin binding and electron microscopy, which relate them perhaps more closely to type I than to type II cells. Do you have any data with the fetal cells which would indicate similar changes?
Boyd	I can't really give you any hard information. An interesting possibility in the intact lung would be that there are gap-junctional channels, permeable to ions, which connect type I and type II cells. It's at least possible that the type II cells are the powerhouse but that the type I cells provide the surface area across which ion exchange can occur. Under the electron microscope type I cells do not look like epithelial cells specialized for active transport, yet make up 90% or so of the lung surface. Is it possible that ions may leak into these cells, enter type II cells by means of gap junctions, and then be powered out of the epithelium by pumps in the type II cells?

References

1. Mason, R. J., Williams, M. C., Widdicombe, J. H., Sanders, M. J., Misfeldt, D. S. and Berry, L. C. (1982). Transepithelial transport by pulmonary alveolar type II cells in primary culture. *Proc. Natl. Acad. Sci. USA*, **79**, 6033–7
2. Goodman, B. E., Brown, S. E. S. and Crandall, E. D. (1984). Regulation of transport across pulmonary alveolar epithelial cell monolayers. *J. Appl. Physiol.*, **57**, 703–10

8
The Maturation of the Control of Respiration in Infancy

P. J. FLEMING, M. R. LEVINE, A. M. LONG AND J. CLEAVE

ABBREVIATIONS USED

$\dot{V}_E$ = Minute ventilation.
QS = Quiet sleep.
REM = Rapid eye movement sleep.
$\dot{Q}$ = Cardiac output.
T = Transit time from lung to carotid body.
VA = Volume of the lung compartment.

During fetal life the control of gas exchange by the placenta is largely under maternal control[1]. The fetus responds to fluctuations in supply or demand of oxygen by chemoreflex modulation of regional blood flow[1]. The fetus thus makes active responses to fluctuations in blood gas tensions, but they are mediated almost entirely by cardiovascular adaptations. In contrast the adult responds to alterations of blood gas tensions by mechanisms which are almost entirely respiratory.

Thus not only is there a change of the organ responsible for gas exchange at birth, but there is also at some stage in postnatal life a complete change in the pattern of response to disturbances of gas exchange.

For over 50 years there has been an appreciation that the breathing pattern of newborn infants is different from that of adults, but the importance of many of the factors influencing breathing pattern – such as gestation, temperature, sleep state and postnatal age – has only slowly become apparent. The huge literature on this subject has been well summarized elsewhere[2-5]. In this paper we will attempt to discuss briefly some of the more important observations, some of the results of stimulation or perturbation of presumed control mechanisms, and the ways this information may fit into some of the more complex mathematical models which have recently been described.

Before discussing the results of recording infant respiration it is important to briefly consider the methods used. Since the description by

Cross in the 1940s of a plethysmograph for recording the rate and depth of breathing in infants[6] a variety of methods have been used. No one method can be said to have overwhelming advantages. All methods currently available have potential limitations. For example, the face of an infant is highly sensitive to being touched, even during sleep, and methods of recording respiration which rely on the use of a face mask or face seal may significantly alter breathing pattern[7]. There is a variable slowing of respiration, accompanied by a rise in tidal volume. The overall effect is to produce little change in minute ventilation, but probably a slight rise in alveolar ventilation. Such effects are most marked (but most variable) in REM sleep, and are affected by other factors, such as maternal epidural anaesthesia, which significantly decreases the effects of facial stimulation.

The barometric plethysmograph[8] is a direct method of recording respiration which relies upon the measurement of the very small pressure change which results from the warming and humidification of inspired air within the airways and lungs. The infant is unrestrained and can adopt a position of comfort, but access to the baby is limited. The method is complex and expensive to install, but is accurate, reliable and relatively simple to use. Calculation of absolute values of tidal volume requires the use of complex formulae involving inspired gas humidity, nasal temperature, and inspiratory and expiratory times.

Indirect methods of recording respiration, such as impedance or inductance plethysmography[7,9] have the advantage that they allow semiquantitative measurements of rate and depth of breathing in unrestrained infants in the nursery or at home. Impedance signals are greatly affected by movements and posture, and are thus only suitable for comparing changes in respiration over short periods of time[7]. The difficulties involved in the calibration of inductance plethysmography limit its usefulness at present[9].

Thus interpretation of the results of any study of infant respiration requires some understanding of the potential limitations of the method employed.

The importance of sleep or waking state on the pattern of respiration has been recognized for several years, largely as a result of the work of Phillipson[10], who showed in adult dogs that respiration in QS was largely dependent on chemical and vagal reflex inputs, whilst in REM sleep or the awake state such inputs were of much less importance. The effect of sleep state on the control of respiration in newborn infants or animals seems to be rather more complex, but some of the apparently conflicting results may be related either to problems with the definition of state, or to methodological differences.

Several sets of standardized criteria for the definition of sleep state in term or preterm infants have been described[5,11-13], but commonly slightly different criteria are used by different investigators. The precise choice of criteria may make sustantial differences to the labelling of particular periods of recording as REM, QS or indeterminate sleep. For example, one widely used criterion of QS is that respiration is regular, with only occasional deep breaths or gross movements[13]. Such a classification may result in episodes of periodic breathing, which commonly occur in QS, being labelled as always occurring in REM or indeterminate sleep. We suggest that for the definition of sleep state in studies of the control of respiration, respiratory pattern should not be a criterion of state.

A further problem in the definition of state is illustrated by the work of Heinz Prechtl and John O'Brien, who showed that the proportion of time during sleep identified as being in any particular state depended on the length of the time window used – e.g. with a 1 min window many short periods of REM or quiet waking were identified which would have been missed using a 3 min window[14].

State definition is further complicated when the preterm infant is considered. Stefanski has recently described a scoring system for the definition of state in preterm infants which combines behavioural and EEG criteria, but does not include respiratory pattern[15]. If widely adopted, such a system might avoid many of the difficulties described.

The effect of sleep state on the response to hypoxia in the newborn period has been studied by several groups, on different species, with apparently conflicting results[4,16-18]. The human infant in thermoneutral conditions shows a biphasic or triphasic response to sustained hypoxia. After a variable immediate small fall in ventilation, there is a rise which is sustained for a minute or two, followed by a further fall, commonly to values below baseline[2,4].

The effect of sleep state on this pattern seems to be species-dependent, as shown in Table 8.1. Haddad, studying puppies, found that the late reduction in ventilation was only present in QS in the first 2 weeks of life. Beyond this age in QS, and at all ages in REM, there was a sustained increase in ventilation[16]. Similarly, McGinty, studying kittens, found that hypoxia led to marked respiratory depression in QS but the onset of REM sleep always led to increased ventilation[17]. These results suggest that for these species, which are relatively immature at birth, REM sleep, an ontogenetically older state than QS, may provide some protection from the potential effects of hypoxia, and McGinty has speculated on the importance to such species of spending a large proportion of time in the newborn period in REM sleep[17].

Results from the calf and the human infant are different[4,18]. The initial increase in ventilation with hypoxia, which occurs in all states, is best sustained in QS. Rigatto showed that the initial increase in tidal volume in the human infant is well sustained in all states, but in all states there is a subsequent fall in respiratory frequency to below baseline values. In QS the overall effect is for minute ventilation to be maintained close to or slightly above resting values, whilst in REM or when awake there is a net fall in minute ventilation[4].

Tenney and Ou described separate neural pathways from the cerebral cortex and the hypothalamus to the medulla[19]. Hypoxia leads to respiratory inhibition via the former, and facilitation via the latter pathways. Thus in the mature animal there is a balanced effect. The very low levels of CNS noradrenaline (a facilitatory neurotransmitter) in the newborn period may reduce the facilitatory effect of the hypothalamic pathway.

Table 8.1 The effects of hypoxia on ventilation during sleep in the newborn

Investigator	Species	Effects of sustained hypoxia
Haddad et al.[16]	Puppies	$\downarrow \dot{V}_E$ in QS up to 14 days $\uparrow \dot{V}_E$ in REM at all ages
Baker and McGinty[17]	Kittens	$\downarrow \dot{V}_E$ in QS, transitional and awake states $\uparrow \dot{V}_E$ in REM at all ages $\downarrow$ Time in REM
Jeffrey and Read[18]	Calves	$\uparrow \dot{V}_E$ more sustained in QS than in REM
Rigatto[4]	Human infants	$\uparrow \dot{V}_E$ in all states initially: subsequent $\dot{V}_E$ in REM or awake; sustained $\dot{V}_E$ in QS

Other possible mechanisms for the late respiratory depression with hypoxia include the release of inhibitory neuromodulators such as adenosine or endorphins. Preliminary results from Darnall suggest that adenosine may be important[20]. He showed in piglets that theophylline, a specific competitive inhibitor of adenosine, led to a marked reduction in the late hypoxic ventilatory depression. Rigatto's group have shown a similar effect in infants given intravenous naloxone, suggesting that endorphin release may also contribute to the late ventilatory depression[21].

Recently the work of Hanson and his group has shown evidence of another important mechanism in the differences between newborn and adult animals' responses to hypoxia[22]. They showed that in the sheep fetus close to term carotid chemoreceptor activity can be recorded, and is increased by hypoxia. At birth the marked increase in PaO_2 leads to a fall in chemoreceptor activity, which is then 'reset' to adult values by a shift to the right over the next few days. In sheep fetuses ventilated *in utero* for 24 h to produce hyperoxia there was no consistent difference from controls in chemoreceptor sensitivity after birth, suggesting that the process of 'resetting' is determined by factors other than PaO_2 alone. However, one fetus did show a response far to the right of the normal fetal range, which may represent the beginning of the resetting process[23]. The same investigators have shown in newborn rats that the response to hypoxia can be modified by prevention of the normal rise in PaO_2 after birth[24]. Rats reared in an FiO_2 of 0.15 showed no increase in ventilation when the FiO_2 was further reduced to 0.12 at any age from birth to 10 weeks. Whether this effect is mediated via alteration of postnatal peripheral chemoreceptor resetting or via changes in the maturation of central nervous processes is unclear.

The clinical implications of these studies may be important. If chronic hypoxia in the immediate neonatal period affects the subsequent ventilatory response to acute hypoxia then infants with neonatal respiratory distress, particularly those who go on to develop chronic lung disease, may have chemoreceptor responses different from those of normal infants. The finding[25] that many apparently healthy growing preterm infants have chronic or recurrent mild hypoxia may thus be of particular relevance to the increased risk of death from SIDS in such infants.

Despite significant falls in ventilation during hypoxia in puppies the PCO_2 was lower than during normoxia, which implies either a reduction in metabolic rate or more efficient gas exchange[16]. During hypoxia oxygen consumption fell during both QS and REM in puppies, whereas in adult dogs there was no change.

The strategy adopted by the newborn to cope with hypoxia is thus quite different from that of the adult, and it may be quite inappropriate to regard the late hypoxia depression of ventilation in the newborn as a maladaptive, primitive or immature response. Teleologically it would be very surprising if nature had left newborn animals completely vulnerable to the effects of what must constitute one of the major risks of early life – i.e. hypoxia – at an age when most are quite unable to make the sort of behavioural response (e.g. moving to a safer environment) that would be characteristic of the adult.

This concept is supported by the presence in the newborn of the complex physiological phenomenon of active thermoregulation in all states, compared to the adult, in whom such mechanisms are greatly depressed in REM sleep[26].

Thus the interaction between mild cold stress and the ventilatory response to hypoxia[27] may reflect the operation of complex mechanisms which are attempting to respond to the combined stimuli in the most economical way in terms of the preservation of oxygen supply to vital organs.

Beyond the immediate newborn period, technical difficulties have limited the number of detailed studies of the development of the control of breathing in human infants. The wide inter-species differences mean that generalizations from studies of other animals are of limited value.

The difficulties in obtaining quantitative recordings of ventilation and sleep state in older infants have led most investigators to record only respiratory rate rather than tidal volume, and assessments of minute ventilation have been indirect – e.g. by recording $TCPO_2$ and $ETCO_2$.

Changes in respiratory frequency by sleep state at ages from 1 week to 6 months have been studied by several groups[28-30]. There is a slight fall in respiratory frequency with increasing age, in both REM and QS. The study by Hoppenbrouwers[30] showed more marked changes in both states than the other studies, and perhaps of relevance is the fact that in this study the infants were restrained, whereas in the other two studies the infants were put into their usual sleeping position and allowed to assume a position of comfort. The other important difference is that in this study respiratory pattern was used as a criterion of sleep state, which was not the case in the other two studies. Haddad et al.[31] showed that the fall in respiratory frequency was accompanied by a slight rise in tidal volume per kg body weight, so the overall effect was of very little change in minute ventilation.

Carse et al.[29] showed a rise in $TCPO_2$ between 1 week and 1 month, and steady values thereafter, with no significant difference between REM and QS. They also showed that $ETCO_2$ remained constant throughout this period.

The reduction in respiratory rate with age thus probably represents a strategy to minimize the work of breathing in the presence of decreasing specific airways conductance. There is certainly no evidence from these studies that metabolic rate changes significantly with age.

The incidence of periodic breathing was found[13,29] to be highest at 1 month of age. Carse *et al.*[29] found brief episodes of periodic breathing in all infants in QS at 1 month, and in many infants at 1 week and 3 months, more commonly in REM. Hoppenbrouwers *et al.*[13] found that periodic breathing was rare in QS, but, as noted above, the definition of sleep state in this study included regularity of breathing.

One interesting observation in all three studies was that heart rate rose between 1 week and 1 month, in both QS and REM, before progressively falling with further increase in age[31,32].

The techniques used in all these studies to extract information from respiratory recordings were crude, and recently several investigators have used more sophisticated signal processing techniques to identify patterns superimposed on the respiratory signals.

Hathorn[33] used the technique of autocorrelation to demonstrate the presence of oscillations in tidal volume and respiratory rate in newborn infants. These oscillations had a period of 8–12 seconds, and were more marked in REM than in QS. Cross-covariance analysis showed that the oscillations in tidal volume were usually out of phase with those in frequency, particularly in QS. In a subsequent elegant ultrasound study of human fetuses *in utero* close to term, Gennser and Hathorn[34] showed very similar patterns of breathing movements – i.e. regular oscillations, of period 6–12 seconds, and a negative cross-covariance at zero lag. These findings suggest that these oscillations – at least in REM sleep – may be not just the result of chemoreceptor feedback loops.

Waggener *et al.*[35] have shown in a series of studies using digital comb filtering of respiratory recordings that the pattern of respiration in REM sleep in term and preterm infants can be closely approximated by the effects of numerous superimposed oscillations of period 6–87 seconds. The occurrence of apnoea in REM sleep, an apparently random event, is shown to correlate closely with the trough of one or more of these oscillations. These oscillations may represent the activity of chemoreceptors, together with interactions with other physiological systems such as blood pressure control. No information is yet available on changes in the patterns of such oscillations with age.

One important limitation of these studies of respiratory oscillations is that they assume relatively constant operation of the control system, and are of limited value in the analysis of transient disturbances.

One of the commonest such disturbances is a spontaneous sigh. Sighs are common in human infants, are vagally mediated, and are important in maintaining lung compliance through recruitment of atelectatic alveoli[36]. Whatever the cause, however, one predictable effect of a sudden deep breath will be to produce a transient fall in $PaCO_2$ and probably a rise in PaO_2.

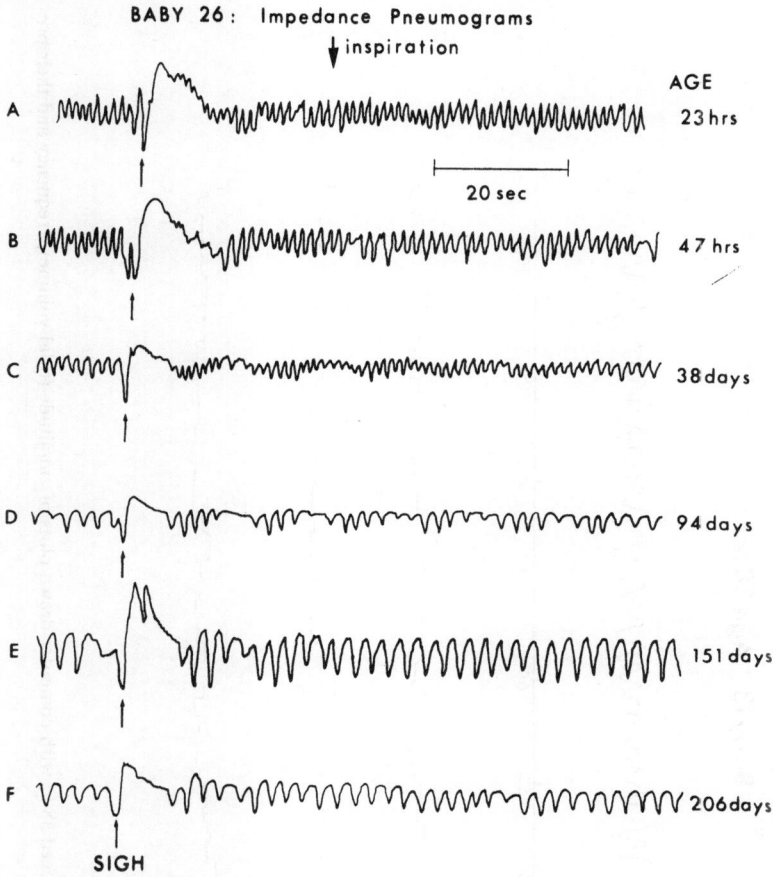

Figure 8.1 Sections of respiratory recordings from one infant in QS at ages 23 h–206 days, to show the changing patterns after a sigh. (Reproduced from *J. Physiol.* (1984), **347**, 1–16)

We have carried out a series of recordings of respiration and sleep state in normal infants and examined the responses to spontaneous sighs in QS[37]. Figure 8.1 shows a series of six recordings taken from one infant, at ages from 23 hours to 206 days. In the first recording the sigh is followed by a brief apnoea and a slow return to baseline ventilation. By 48 hours of age the return is more rapid, with an overshoot and slight oscillation. With increasing age to 94 days the pattern becomes increasingly oscillatory, and beyond that age the pattern becomes more damped, with a rapid return to regular respiration.

Figure 8.2 shows a section of respiratory recording from an infant aged 38 hours in QS, together with computer-generated breath-by-breath plots of tidal volume, frequency and their product minute ventilation. The oscillation which is apparent in the raw tracing clearly affects tidal volume, but there is also an oscillation, of longer period and different phase, in frequency. The overall effect is of an oscillation in minute ventilation,

113

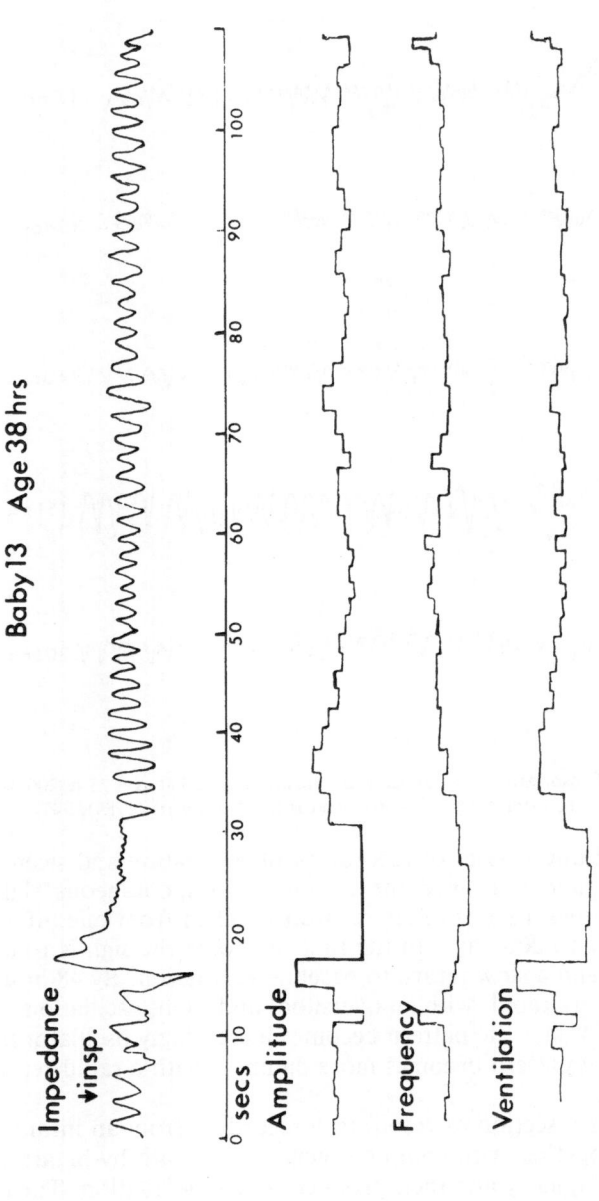

Figure 8.2 A section of respiratory recording from an infant aged 38 h, with computer-drawn plots of amplitude (tidal volume), frequency and their product breath-by-breath minute ventilation

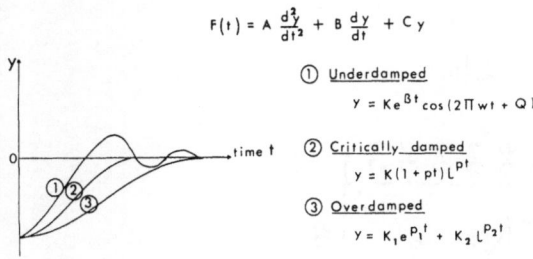

Figure 8.3 Equations describing the possible responses of a linear second-order system to a disturbance

which is similar but not identical to that in tidal volume. The simplest way to mathematically describe such an oscillation is by a linear second-order equation (see Fig. 8.3). There are three possible solutions, which give an underdamped, overdamped or critically damped pattern of response.

Figure 8.4 shows computer-drawn plots of breath-by-breath minute ventilation for the same six sections of respiratory recording shown in Fig. 8.1. Curves derived by a least-squares fitting programme are superimposed, and the values are given for the damping factor, β, and the period of oscillation, T. The pattern at 23 hours approximates critical damping, by 47 hours a period of oscillation, (T), of 22.5 seconds emerges, though the damping factor remains high. With increasing age there is a progressive shortening of the period of oscillation and a fall in the damping factor to a minimum at 94 days. Beyond this age the period of oscillation continues to shorten, but the damping factor increases, to a value close to that on the first day. One way of describing these changes is to plot the damping factor β against the angular frequency of oscillation, $2\pi/T$, equivalent to the polar coordinates ω_n and θ, as shown on the right of Fig. 8.4. The values from these sighs have been plotted. If the equations fitted represent the operation of a feedback control system, then the stability of that system depends on the damping factor ($\cos \theta$), and the undamped frequency of oscillation (ω_n). Thus point a represents a highly stable but slow response; point b a stable but faster response; points c and d relatively unstable responses, and points e and f represent a more stable response, with rapid recovery. Points e and f may be considered to represent optimal control, since disturbances are rapidly corrected with minimal oscillation. Points c and d indicate relatively unstable respiratory control, since a small increase in β such that it became zero or positive would be associated with persistent respiratory oscillation with maintained or increasing amplitude respectively.

Similar patterns of change with age have been seen in all normal-term infants studied, though there is some variation in the ages at which changes occur.

115

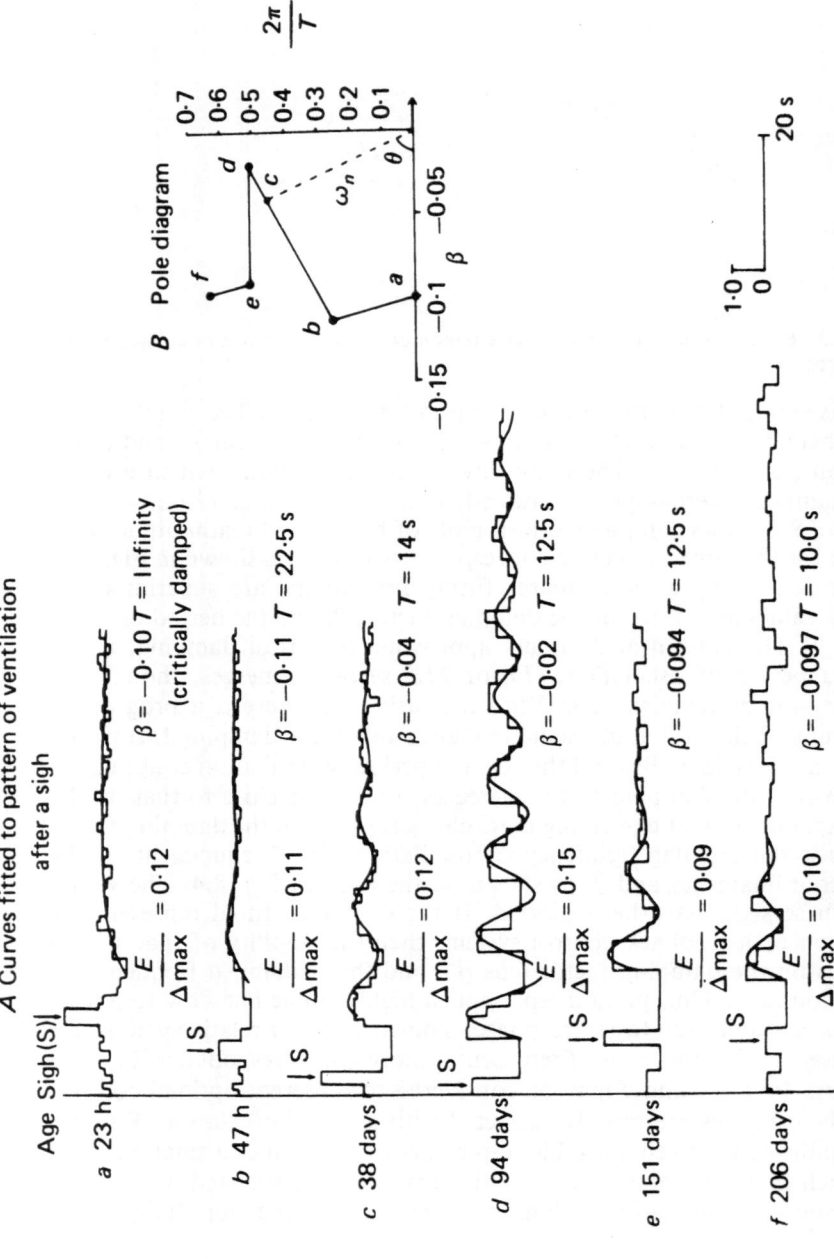

Figure 8.4 Plots of breath-by-breath minute ventilation for the same sections of recording shown in Fig. 8.1. Curves have been fitted and the constants B and T plotted on a pole diagram (see text). (Reproduced from *J. Physiol.* (1984), **347**, 1-16)

Table 8.2 Postnatal development of respiratory control

Stage 1 : birth–48 hours	Relatively insensitive
	Sluggish
	Stable
Stage 2 : 48 hours–3 months	Increasing sensitivity
	Increasing rapidity
	Decreasing stability
Stage 3 : > 4 months	Highly sensitive
	Rapidly responding
	Highly stable

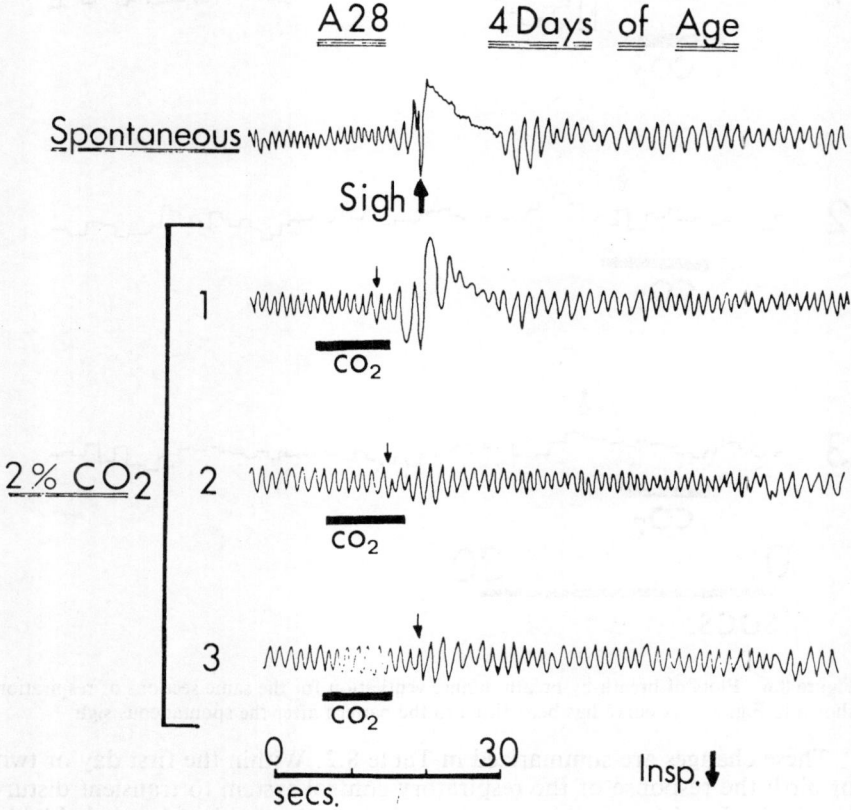

Figure 8.5 Four sections of respiratory recording, from an infant aged 4 days, to show the effect of a spontaneous sigh and of a few breaths of 2% CO_2 in air (see text)

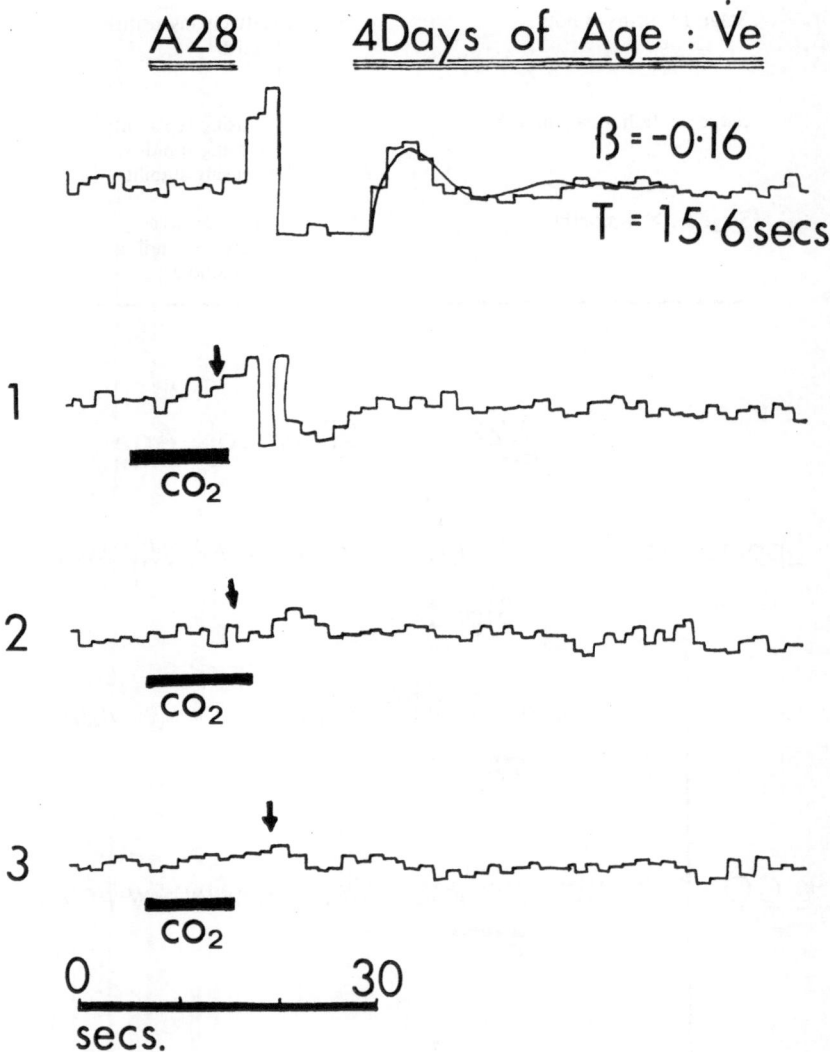

Figure 8.6 Plots of breath-by-breath minute ventilation for the same sections of respiration shown in Fig. 8.5. A curve has been fitted to the pattern after the spontaneous sigh

These changes are summarized in Table 8.2. Within the first day or two of birth the response of the respiratory control system to transient disturbances is sluggish and the system is relatively insensitive, but it is highly stable. From around 48 hours until around 3 months there is a progressive change in the control system, with increasing sensitivity to disturbances, increasing rapidity of response, and decreasing stability, which reached minimum values between 1 and 3 months in all term infants in this study. After about 4 months of age the system remains highly sensitive and rapidly responding, but the stability increases, to reach adult values by around 5 or 6 months of age.

The characteristics of these oscillations make it likely that they result from the carotid body mediated CO_2 response.

Oscillations of similar period can be produced by the administration of a few breaths of CO_2, as shown in Fig. 8.5. This shows four sections of recording from an infant aged 4 days. The top section shows a spontaneous sigh, followed by a pattern of damped oscillation. The other three sections show the effects of giving a few breaths of 2% CO_2. In each recording the first breath after the start of the CO_2 stimulation to show a significant rise in tidal volume is marked with an arrow. The lag varied from 8 to 12 seconds. Figure 8.6 shows the changes in breath-by-breath minute ventilation for the same sections of recording. The best-fit curve has been fitted to the pattern after the spontaneous sigh, and shows a period of oscillation of 15.6 seconds. This is consistent with the operation of a feedback loop with a response time of 8 seconds, which is exactly that observed with the most rapid response to CO_2. The longer delay in the response in the third section may be due to the small size of the stimulus, and to difficulty in synchronizing the beginning of the stimulus with inspiration. The results of similar CO_2 stimulation studies in 12 normal-term infants, in sequential studies at ages from 7 hours to 164 days, have shown wide variation. There are at least two different mechanisms involved in the response to transient CO_2 stimulation. If more than 3-4% CO_2 is given there is usually a response within 2 seconds, commonly accompanied by evidence of arousal. This is too rapid to be a carotid body response, and is probably mediated through airway receptors[38]. At lower levels of CO_2 the time to respond seems partly to depend on the magnitude of the stimulus (Fig. 8.6), suggesting a ramp effect. The response may take the form of a sigh or an increase in tidal volume of smaller magnitude. As shown in Fig. 8.5, these increases in tidal volume are commonly followed by damped oscillations of similar period, but different damping from those shown after spontaneous sighs.

These results suggest that the pattern of response to spontaneous sighs, whilst related to the carotid body CO_2 response, is far more complex than the operation of a single linear feedback system.

We have now carried out similar prospective sequential studies of the development of patterns of response to spontaneous sighs in 14 preterm infants, of gestation 30-36 weeks, at ages from 4 days to 222 days. Examination of the results reveals interesting differences from the term infants.

The most striking difference is in the variability of the responses within a single period of QS. The term infants showed quite consistent responses to sighs during any one recording after the first few days of life. The patterns in the preterm infants vary from one sigh to the next. As shown in Fig. 8.7, periodic breathing can be followed by a highly damped response, and viceversa.

In looking for a pattern of development with age in preterm infants it is usual to consider postconceptional age rather than postnatal age. However in this study a clearer pattern emerges if postnatal age is used, suggesting perhaps that postnatal environment has an important influence on the

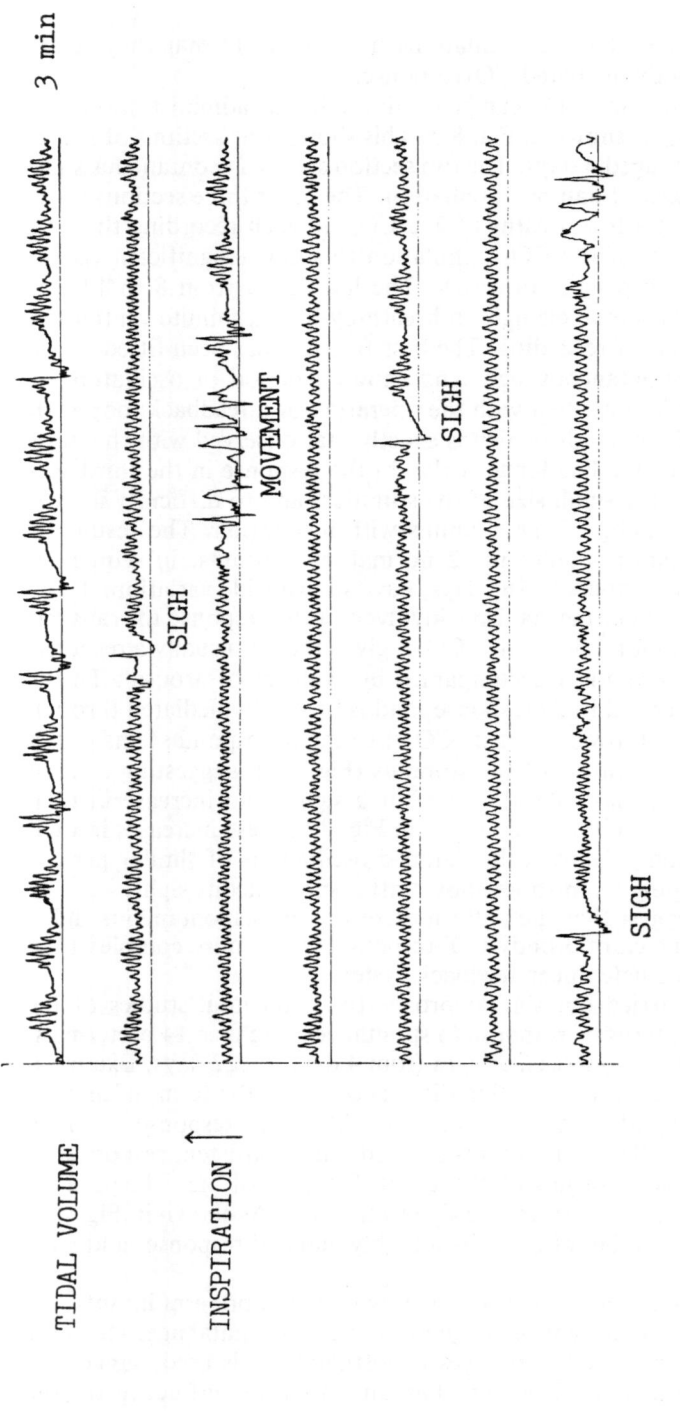

Figure 8.7 A 21-min recording of respiration from an infant of 34 weeks gestation, aged 17 days, in QS, to show the marked variation in the damping of the oscillations after sighs

maturation of the control of respiration. The 12 infants in this study who were of less than 35 weeks gestation at birth consistently showed the 'mature' response to sighs, with a rapid return to baseline and a highly damped oscillation in recordings after 90 days of age, which for all of them constituted a postconceptional age of less than 30 days past term. The two infants of 35 and 36 weeks gestation showed patterns more similar to the term infants. It thus appears that for the more immature preterm infants, the development of stability of the control of respiration is not only shifted to the left on the age scale, but it may also be compressed into a shorter age span. It is interesting to speculate on the possible adverse consequences of such a shifted and altered developmental pattern.

One way of trying to understand and predict the behaviour of such a complex physiological control system as the response to transient disturbances such as sighs is to design a mathematical model incorporating the known physiology, and simulate the known responses. We have described such a model, which incorporates the simplest possible expressions for the responses of the central and peripheral chemoreceptors to transient disturbances of $PaCO_2$. The model does not deal explicitly with the responses to changes in PaO_2, which are assumed to act through an effect on the gain of CO_2 responses[39]. This model was able to account qualitatively for the observed patterns of respiration.

A combination of mathematical investigation and computer simulation guided by the mathematical results has enabled us to go some way towards understanding the likely consequences of instability[40,41]. It turns out that on transition from stability to instability the model system responds to a disturbance by going into a limit cycle – i.e. a sustained undamped oscillation in ventilation (Fig. 8.8). The oscillation can be so great that the CO_2 level falls below the threshold for respiration during each cycle, giving rise to apnoea. This is periodic respiration, which, as described above, is commonly seen in both term and preterm infants. It is unstable in the technical sense that ventilation does not settle down to the equilibrium value, but it is a stable phenomenon in the sense that if the system is disturbed from the limit cycle it will return to it. The condition which we derived for the transition point depends on the gains of the central and peripheral chemoreceptors being different. This appears to be fulfilled when PaO_2 is low[42]. Thus intermittent or continuous mild hypoxia might lead to respiration which alternated between a pattern of damped oscillation and frank periodic breathing.

Thus we now have a single framework within which to discuss both stable damped oscillations and continuous periodic oscillations. Further investigation of a more complex model may predict other instabilities, and perhaps chaotic behaviour. Such studies may allow understanding of the complex ways in which the intact respiratory control system functions in the normal infant, and give some insight into the ways in which the system may malfunction with potentially disastrous effects.

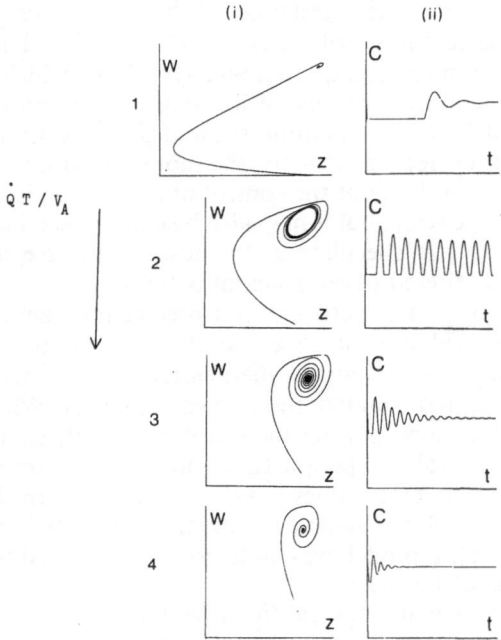

Figure 8.8 Computer-drawn simulations of the response of a mathematical model of the control of respiration to a sigh[39]. Column (i) shows the effects of a progressive increase (from (i)1 to (i)4) in $\dot{Q}T/VA$ on the relationship between W ($P\,CO_2$ in the lung) and Z ($P\,CO_2$ at the carotid body). Column (ii) shows the effects of the same changes on the output of the controller *(C)*, plotted against time *(t)*. An increase in cardiac output as a proportion of lung volume, or an increase in transit time, or a combination of these changes, could result in changes in the patterns of controller output in response to a sigh, similar to those observed in infants with increasing age[37]

Acknowledgements

These studies were supported by a grant (project no. 45) from the Foundation for the Study of Infant Deaths, and by a grant from the South West Regional Health Authority Research Committee.

References

1. Dawes, G. S., Duncan, S., Lewis, B. V., Merlet, C. L., Owen-Thomas, J. B. and Reeves, R. T. (1969). Hypoxaemia and aortic chemoreceptor functions in fetal lambs. *J. Physiol.*, **201**, 105-16
2. Haddad, G. G. and Mellins, R. B. (1984). Hypoxia and respiratory control in early life. *Ann. Rev. Physiol.*, **46**, 629-43
3. Walker, D. W. (1984). Peripheral and central chemoreceptors in the fetus and newborn. *Ann. Rev. Physiol.*, **46**, 687-703
4. Rigatto, H. (1984). Control of ventilation in the newborn. *Ann. Rev. Physiol.*, **46**, 661-74
5. Read, D. J. C. and Henderson-Smart, D. J. (1984). Regulation of breathing in the newborn during different behavioural states. *Ann. Rev. Physiol.*, **46**, 675-85

6. Cross, K. W. (1949). The respiratory rate and ventilation in the newborn baby. *J. Physiol.*, **109**, 459–74
7. Fleming, P. J., Levine, M. R. and Goncalves, A. (1982). Changes in respiratory pattern resulting from the use of a facemask to record respiration in newborn infants. *Pediatr. Res.*, **16**, 1031–4
8. Fleming, P. J., Levine, M. R., Goncalves, A. and Woollard, S. (1983). Barometric plethysmograph: advantages and limitations in recording infant respiration. *J. Appl. Physiol.*, **55**, 1924–31
9. Dufty, P., Spriet, L., Bryan, M. H. and Bryan, A. C. (1981). Respiratory inductance plethysmography (Respitrace): An evaluation of its use in the infant. *Am. Rev. Respir. Dis.*, **123**, 542–6
10. Phillipson, E. A. (1978). Respiratory adaptations during sleep. *Ann. Rev. Physiol.*, **40**, 133–56
11. Anders, T., Emde, R. and Parmelee, A. (1971). *A Manual of Terminology, Techniques and Criteria for Scoring of States of Sleep and Wakefulness in Newborn Infants.* UCLA Brain Information Service, BRI Publications Office, California
12. Prechtl, H. F. R. (1974). The behavioural states of the newborn infant (a review). *Brain Res.*, **76**, 1304–11
13. Hoppenbrouwers, T., Hodgman, J. E., Harper, R. M., Hofman, E., Sterman, M. B. and McGinty, D. J. (1977). Polygraphic studies of normal infants during the first 6 months of life. III: Incidence of apnea and periodic breathing. *Pediatrics*, **60**, 418–25
14. Prechtl, H. F. R. and O'Brien, M. J. (1982). Behavioural states of the full-term newborn. The emergence of a concept. In Stratton, P. (ed.) *Psychobiology of the Human Newborn.* pp. 53–73 (New York: Wiley)
15. Stefanski, M., Schulzek, K., Bateman, D., Kairam, R., Pedley, T. A., Masterson, J. and James, L. S. (1984). A scoring system for states of sleep and wakefulness in term and preterm infants. *Pediatr Res.*, **18**, 58–62
16. Haddad, G. G., Gandhi, M. R. and Mellins, R. B. (1982). Maturation of ventilatory response to hypoxia in puppies during sleep. *J. Appl. Physiol.*, **52**, 309–14
17. Baker, T. L. and McGinty, D. J. (1977). Reversal of cardiopulmonary failure during active sleep in hypoxic kittens: implications for sudden infant death. *Science*, **198**, 419–21
18. Jeffrey, H. E. and Read, D. J. C. (1980). Ventilatory responses of newborn calves to progressive hypoxia in quiet and active sleep. *J. Appl. Physiol.*, **48**, 892–5
19. Tenney, S. M. and Ou, L. C. (1977). Ventilatory response of decorticate and decerebrate cats to hypoxia and CO_2. *Resp. Physiol.* **29**, 81–92
20. Darnall, R. A. (1983). The effect of opioid and adenosine antagonists on hypoxic ventilatory depression in the newborn piglet. *Pediatr. Res.*, **17**, 374A
21. DeBoeck, C., Reempts, P. V., Rigatto, H. and Chernick, V. (1983). Endorphins and the ventilatory depression during hypoxia in newborn infants. *Pediatr. Res.*, **17**, 374A
22. Blanco, C. E., Dawes, G. S., Hanson, M. A. and McCooke, H. B. (1984). The response to hypoxia of arterial chemoreceptors in fetal sheep and newborn lambs. *J. Physiol.*, **351**, 25–37
23. Blanco, C. E., Hanson, M. A. and McCooke, H. B. (1985). Studies in utero of the mechanism of chemoreceptor resetting. In Jones, C. J. (ed.) *Physiological Development of the Fetus and Newborn.* pp. 639–41. (London: Academic Press)
24. Eden, G. J. and Hanson, M. A. (1985). The effect of hypoxia from birth on the biphasic response of the newborn rat to acute hypoxia. *J. Physiol.* (In press)
25. Carse, E. J., Wilkinson, A., Whyte, P., Henderson-Smart, D. J. and Johnson, P. (1981). Oxygen tension, heart rate, breathing and sleep state following preterm birth. *Pediatr. Res.*, **15**, 1187A
26. Darnall, R. A. and Ariagno, R. L. (1982). The effect of sleep state on active thermoregulation in the premature infant. *Pediatr. Res.*, **16**, 512–14
27. Brady, J. P. and Ceruti, E. (1966). Chemoreceptor reflexes in the newborn infant. *J. Physiol.*, **184**, 631–45
28. Haddad, G. G., Epstein, R. A., Epstein, M. A. F., Leistner, H. L., Mario, P. A. and Mellins, R. B. (1979). Maturation of ventilation and ventilatory pattern in normal sleeping infants. *J. Appl. Physiol.*, **46**, 998–1002

29. Carse, E. A., Wilkinson, A. R., Whyte, P., Henderson-Smart, D. J. and Johnson, P. (1981). Oxygen and carbon dioxide tensions, breathing and heart rate in normal infants during the first six months of life. *J. Dev. Physiol.*, **3**, 85-100

30. Hoppenbrouwers, T., Harper, R. M., Hodgman, J. E., Sterman, M. B. and McGinty, D. J. (1978). Polygraphic studies of normal infants during the first six months of life. II: Respiratory rate and variability as a function of state. *Pediatr. Res.*, **12**, 120-5

31. Haddad, G. G., Epstein, R. A., Epstein, M. A. F., Leistner, H. L. and Mellins, R. B. (1980). The R-R interval and R-R variability in normal infants during sleep. *Pediatr. Res.*, **14**, 809-11

32. Harper, R. M., Hoppenbrouwers, T., Sterman, M. B., McGinty, D. J. and Hodgman, J. (1976). Polygraphic studies of normal infants during the first 6 months of life. I: Heart rate and variability as a function of state. *Pediatr. Res.*, **10**, 945-51

33. Hathorn, M. K. S. (1978). Analysis of periodic changes in ventilation in newborn infants. *J. Physiol.*, **285**, 85-99

34. Gennser, G. and Hathorn, M. K. S. (1979). Analysis of breathing movements in the human fetus. *Lancet*, **1**, 1298

35. Waggener, T. B., Stark, A. R., Cohlan, B. A. and Frantz, I. D. (1984). Apnea duration is related to ventilatory oscillation characteristics in newborn infants. *J. Appl. Physiol.*, **57**, 536-44

36. Thach, B. T. and Taeusch, H. W. (1976). Sighing in newborn human infants: role of inflation-augmenting reflex. *J. Appl. Physiol.*, **41**, 502-7

37. Fleming, P. J., Goncalves, A. L., Levine, M. R. and Woollard, S. (1984). The development of stability of respiration in human infants: changes in ventilatory responses to spontaneous sighs. *J. Physiol.*, **347**, 1-16

38. Johnson, P. (1976). Evidence for lower airway chemoreceptors in newborn lambs. *Pediatr. Res.*, **10**, 462

39. Cleave, J. P., Levine, M. R. and Fleming, P. J. (1984). The control of ventilation: a theoretical analysis of the response to transient disturbances. *J. Theor. Biol.*, **108**, 261-83

40. Cleave, J. P., Fleming, P. J., Levine, M. R. and Long, A. M. (1985). Stability of the control of breathing in newborn infants: a non-linear mathematical analysis. In Jones, C. J. (ed.) *Physiological Development of the Fetus and Newborn.* pp. 267-72. (London: Academic Press)

41. Cleave, J. P., Fleming, P. J., Levine, M. R. and Long, A. M. (1985). A mathematical study of the ventilatory response to a deep sigh. *J. Physiol.*, **364**, 68P

42. Cherniack, N. S., von Euler, C., Homma, I. and Kao, F. F. (1979). Experimentally induced Cheyne Stokes breathing. *Resp. Physiol.*, **37**, 185-200

Discussion

Dr C. J. Morley	Can you comment on the influence of environmental temperature?
Dr P. J. Fleming	The effect is crucial. One of the ways the baby responds to hypoxia seems to be to go into a state of near-hibernation. If you add a cold stress, the pattern of response changes. However, the newborn has active thermoregulation in all states, which the adult does not. Thus the baby seems better adapted to cope with thermoregulatory stress than it does to alterations of blood gas tensions. Paul Johnson[1] has shown that in lambs a very stable pattern of respiration can be destabilized by changing the thermal environment when a highly damped response to disturbances can become an oscillatory one. The temperature at which this change occurs is age-dependent, hence what is thermoneutrality at one age might be heat stress at another.
Dr A. C. Bryan	I don't like the way you swing from the word 'damped' to the more pejorative 'unstable'. You imply that if there is underdamping the system is in bad shape. The carotid body responds perfectly to hypoxic stimuli in the infant. It is the rest of the system which determines damping – the lung volume in relation to metabolic rate. The relationship in the newborn is such that oscillations are not damped out, but I don't see that as unstable. An underdamped system can be very stable.
Fleming	I agree. The computer oscillation, the limit cycle, is technically unstable because it doesn't return to the point from which it originated. But it is stable in a way that really matters; it doesn't go anywhere else, and if you disturb it, it comes back to the same oscillation again.
Dr L. B. Strang	I don't know what's meant by overdamped, underdamped, critically damped, stable or unstable.
Fleming	If there is a control system which on disturbance returns back to its pre-set values in a smooth 'monotonic' way in the shortest possible time, that's critical damping.
Strang	What is the shortest possible time?
Fleming	It depends on the system. If you have the equation that defines the system, you can say what is the shortest possible time. A system that is overdamped has a similar but slower pattern of return. Underdamping means a quick return to baseline followed by an overshoot and oscillation. Optimal control is when the area under the curve between the baseline and the curve is as small as possible. Optimal control is always slightly underdamped.
Bryan	I don't think that is necessarily optimal. You keep slipping between 'critical damping' and 'optimal damping' but the latter certainly depends on what you want the system to do.

Fleming If the system exists to minimize error signal that must be what the controller in the system is trying to do. We are trying to apply fairly complex control systems analysis to a system we don't really understand. Even though we don't know what's being controlled, it is still a reasonable supposition that the error signal should be kept to a minimum.

Dr J. P. Mortola I do not see why the breathing pattern has to be stable. For example, during acute hypoxia in the newborn oxygen consumption decreases. Let us assume, for the sake of argument, that it dropped to zero. Ventilation also would decrease significantly, which may look like an extreme situation of 'instability'; however the drop in ventilation, in such a case, would simply represent the appropriate response to the drop in oxygen consumption. From your presentation you seem convinced that respiration has to be as regular as possible while I find no requirement for the breathing pattern to be regular.

Fleming If I gave that impression, I apologize. If you are looking at regular respiration and quiet sleep when we must assume that the metabolic rates do not change in the short term, variations in breathing pattern should be unrelated to changes in metabolic rate.

Mortola I do not think that it would be difficult to list other situations which influence the breathing pattern in the short term. Many inputs come from the periphery to the 'respiratory controller' within a breath to determine appropriate changes in ventilation.

Fleming If you apply a short unit impulse, the control system should respond, and the way it responds tells you something about the system. We are trying to analyse the nature of that feedback. If there are multiple inputs, a control system whose response is not stable in terms of returning to the preset value quickly might well result in positive feedback – tipping over into instability which would set off an indefinite oscillation.

Dr C. L. Gaultier Dr Fleming, you describe the response to a sigh in a normal population of infants. Did you have the opportunity to look at the same thing in sudden infant death syndrome (SIDS) babies?

Fleming We have recordings of 30 infants who subsequently died of SIDS and we are in the process of going through these as well as recordings from age- and sex-matched controls. We have already looked at prospective longitudinal studies of 10 subsequent siblings of SIDS victims, and at four identical twins of children who died of SIDS who were studied within 48 hours of their sibling's death. For what it is worth, two of these four infants showed very highly oscillatory patterns even though one of them was well beyond the age when we would expect to see such a pattern. The subsequent siblings of SIDS victims all shared developmental patterns very similar to the normal infants.

Dr J. A. Clements I wonder if it would be useful to consider whether a system that behaves chaotically is more energy-dispersive than one which behaves with a regular oscillation? I would like you to discuss whether a respiratory system which leads to the most regular kind of breathing pattern while dealing with the various metabolic and other stresses that fall on the respiratory system may not be the most energy-conserving system. Would that not be a reasonable riposte to Dr Mortola?

Fleming I agree, if the response to a disturbance is regular and highly damped, that would be energy-efficient and a desirable response by the control system.

126

Mortola	Energetic aspects should not play an important role in the choice between stability and instability, since the energy cost of breathing, at least from what we know in the adult, seems a very small component of the total body energy requirements whatever the breathing pattern.
Strang	The real significance of Dr Fleming's approach is perhaps quite different. Our knowledge of the control of breathing tells us that it is hopelessly complex. What we are at present seeking is not yet another entry into that labyrinth but rather a practical insight into a clinical phenomenon – periodic breathing (call it instability). The approach in these studies seems to be a pragmatic attempt to describe what happens in periodic breathing.
Bryan	Periodic breathing is a very common phenomenon in adults at the entry into sleep. I don't regard it as unstable.
Strang	But if it goes too far and you stop breathing too long, you can do your central nervous system some damage.
Bryan	I've been doing it for over 50 years. The essential control element is the response of the peripheral chemoreceptors. Thus if I have a high gain on my carotid body, I don't need to worry about apnoea because breathing will be initiated at the first hint of hypoxia. The other side of the control loop contains the damping factor – the store of O_2 in the lungs. The reason the baby has a more oscillatory breathing pattern than the adult is simply that the amount of oxygen in the lungs (which determines damping) is relatively small. Lung volume in the newborn infant is small relative to metabolic rate but the relationship changes around 3 months of age – when the lungs become relatively larger. The oscillatory breathing pattern of the young infant reflects a high gain in the carotid chemoreceptors and a small damping effect due to the small volume of the lungs. This poor damping is not, I think, critical to the system.

Reference

1. Johnson, P. (1985). The development of breathing. In Jones, C. J. (ed.) *The Physiological Development of the Fetus and Newborn.* pp. 201–10. (London: Academic Press)

9
Establishment of the End-Expiratory Level (FRC) in Newborn Mammals

J. P. MORTOLA

ABSTRACT

The establishment of FRC at birth represents one of the important aspects of the respiratory adaptation. In the immediate perinatal period the tensioactive properties of the pulmonary surfactants and other purely mechanical factors (related to the progressive aeration of the lung and the decrease in chest wall compliance) are the main contributors to the formation of FRC. In addition, in the first hours after birth total closure of the larynx during the expiratory phase represents an effective mechanism to keep the lungs inflated. After the first hours FRC is maintained elevated above the resting·volume of the respiratory system V_r through a combination of dynamic factors which include the high breathing frequency, the narrowing of the larynx and the braking action of the inspiratory muscles during expiration. Despite the obvious advantages of an elevated FRC, such a pattern implies a prolongation of the expiratory time, hence a decrease in breathing rate which may not be desirable in small newborn species with large metabolic demands and needs of high ventilatory rates. Indeed, in newborn rats expiratory laryngeal closure is retained only in the first hours, when it is probably important for lung expansion and fluid reabsorption. Afterwards it is abandoned and the FRC–V_r difference is almost nil. The control of FRC therefore appears to be an important aspect of the neonatal adaptation at birth, finely controlled and matched to the ventilatory requirements of the animal.

INTRODUCTION

A comparative view of the functional and structural properties of the respiratory system among animals often reveals striking similarities. One example is the functional residual capacity (FRC), i.e. the amount of air left in the lung at end-expiration, which not only is a characteristic of all mammals but is also a fixed proportion of the animal's size[1]. The presence of an FRC substantially increases the efficiency of the breathing act by reducing the elastic and resistive components of the external work of breathing and improving the distribution of ventilation. In addition, the oscillations in alveolar gases, and therefore in blood gases, are not as large as one would expect in the absence of FRC.

Newborn mammals initiate their extrauterine ventilatory activity with fluid-filled lungs, and it therefore seems reasonable to consider the establishment of FRC an important priority at birth, along with the onset of an adequate external ventilation and the clearance of the pulmonary fluid. The aim of this paper is a brief review of the factors involved in the establishment and control of FRC in the newborn period.

If one attempts to measure the changes in lung volume during the first breaths immediately after birth, as Karlberg and co-workers[2] did about 25 years ago, records such as those presented in Fig. 9.1 are obtained. It is apparent, despite the large individual variability, that the amount of air exhaled after the first breath is less than that inhaled, the difference representing the first establishment of FRC. This is mainly the result of the tensioactive properties of surfactants, which, by reducing surface tension in expiration, also decrease lung recoil. The physiological role of lung surfactants is addressed in much detail in other chapters of this book. In part, the stress relaxation (determined by the viscoelastic nature of the lung tissue) could also favour air trapping, by reducing the recoil pressure during expiration. The progressive aeration of the lung, and the probable increase in chest wall stiffness which accompanies the increase in muscle tone and geometrical changes of the respiratory structures, are additional factors contributing to the rise in FRC. In summary, several combined mechanical factors (tensioactive properties of surfactant, lung tissue stress relaxation, increase in lung compliance and drop in chest wall compliance) represent the most relevant determinants of the immediate establishment of FRC with the onset of breathing.

In several adult mammals, including man, FRC is very close to the resting passive volume of the respiratory system (V_r), which is set by the balance between the expanding pressure of the chest and the collapsing tendency of the lung. In newborns, the large chest wall compliance and the relatively stiff lungs do not favour a large V_r. About 10 years ago Olinsky and co-workers[4] pointed out that in a few-days-old infant, during short periods of apnoea, the end-expiratory level decreased, suggesting that during resting breathing (a) FRC was maintained above V_r, and (b) the high breathing frequency, characteristic of the neonatal period, determined the FRC–V_r difference. In subsequent studies it has been possible to compute the FRC–V_r difference from analysis of the pressure–volume curve of the whole respiratory system[5-7] or the expiratory volume-flow relation during resting breathing[6-8]. Despite the rather high individual variability, which is in part expected considering that some factors (namely sleep state and muscle relaxation) are known to influence the measurements, both approaches gave similar results, the FRC–V_r difference in a few-days-old infant averaging approximately 10–15 ml, or 3 ml/kg. Such a value cannot be explained only as the result of the newborn's high respiratory rate. In fact, if the whole expiration were a purely passive process, and assuming that the compliance and resistance of the respiratory system are linear in the tidal volume (V_T) range[9], the amount of air left in the lung at end-expiration (i.e. the FRC- V_r difference) could be computed as

$$\text{FRC} - V_r = V_T \exp(-T_E/T_{rs}),$$

T_E being the expiratory time and T_{rs} the passive time constant of the respiratory system. Once the appropriate values are entered, the resulting FRC- V_r difference would be only 2-3 ml[10]. In other words, if the dynamic elevation of FRC were only determined by the interaction between breathing pattern (V_T, T_E) and the *passive* properties of the respiratory system, the FRC- V_r difference should be much less than actually measured. Therefore it must be concluded that during breathing in infants some mechanisms are effective in retarding the emptying of the lung during expiration, determining an expiratory time constant (T_{exp}) longer than T_{rs}. Two mechanisms appear particularly relevant during expiration in infants in prolonging T_{exp}; the increase in upper airway resistance and the braking action of the inspiratory muscles.

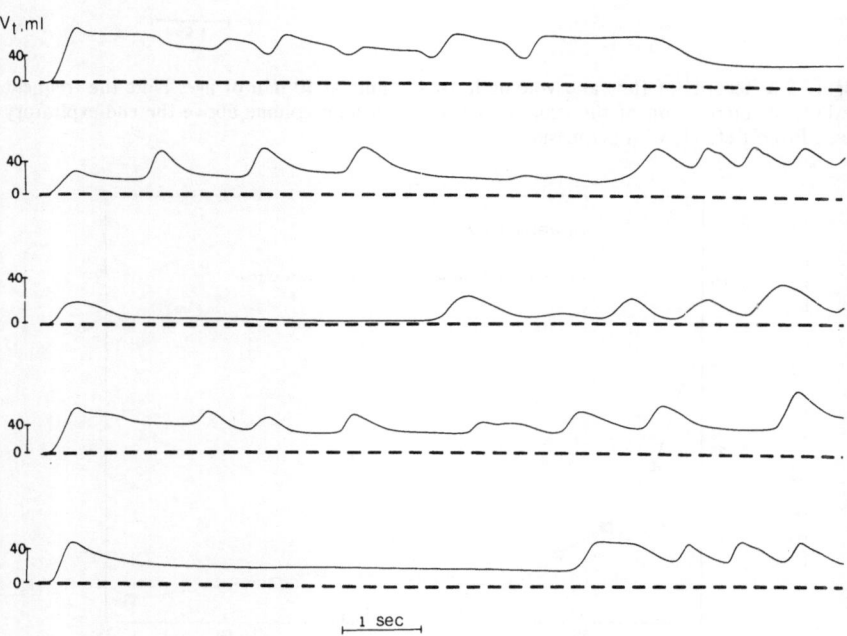

Figure 9.1 Spirometric records obtained in five infants immediately after delivery. Each record begins with the first breath after birth. Note the progressive formation of the functional residual capacity. From Ref. 3, with permission

131

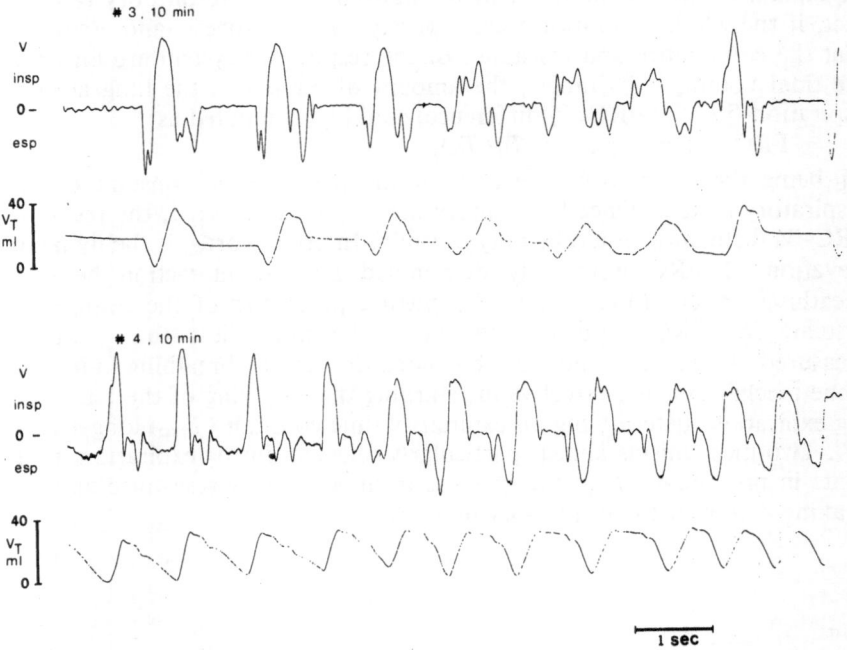

Figure 9.2 Records of flow and volume in two infants at 10 min of age. Note the frequent periods of interruption of the expiratory flow, with lung volume above the end-expiratory level. From Ref. 11, with permission

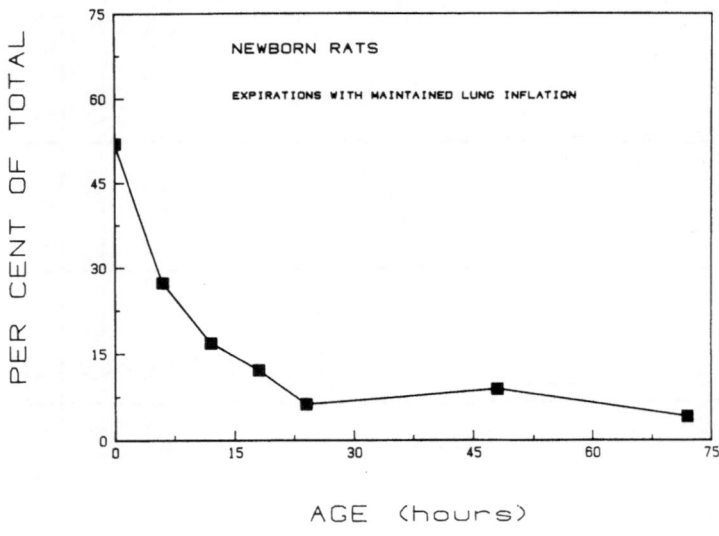

Figure 9.3 Percentage occurrence of breaths with interruptions of the expiratory flow as a function of postnatal age. Each data point is the mean of 9 to 14 rats (from de Saint-Rome and Mortola, unpublished)

UPPER AIRWAY CONTROL OF EXPIRATORY FLOW

Spirometric records of infants during the first minutes after birth reveal single or multiple interruptions of the expiratory phase, with periods of zero flow of variable durations[11] (Fig. 9.2). This pattern is very common during the first hours, then it becomes progressively less frequent. Complete interruptions of the expiratory flow which have been observed in several newborn species[12,13] are not present after tracheostomy or during deep anaesthesia, and in rats, as in infants, they are much more frequent in the first minutes after birth than at one day of life (Fig. 9.3). During the periods of zero flow, with lung volume maintained above FRC, the diaphragm is not active and the pleural pressure is not more negative than at FRC, indicating that active inspiratory breath-holding is not the underlying mechanism[13]. The maintained augmented lung volume most likely reflects an increase in laryngeal resistance; the thyro-arytenoid muscle, a laryngeal adductor of the vocal cords, has been shown to be very active during the expiratory phase of the cycle in newborn lambs[14]. In infants,

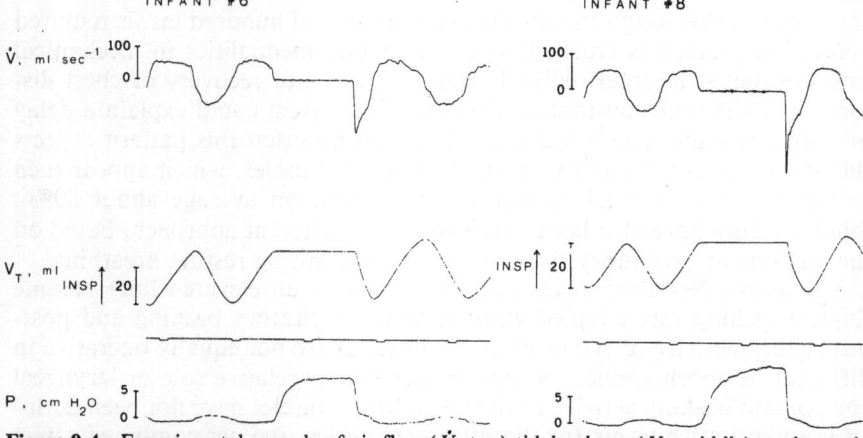

Figure 9.4 Experimental records of air flow ($\dot{V}$, top), tidal volume (V_T, middle), and mouth pressure (P, bottom) in two infants at a few days after birth. When the airways are occluded at end-inspiration P does not rise instantaneously, indicating the presence of post-inspiratory muscle activity. From Ref. 7, with permission

when the vocal cords are bypassed with an endotracheal tube, an end-expiratory pressure is commonly added to preserve blood gases within the normal range[15,16], a procedure which may be regarded as a replacement of the laryngeal function. The observation is also of interest that total closure of the larynx in expiration with maintained lung inflation is commonly adopted in snakes and other reptiles[17,18], while in adult mammals it seems to occur only in a few species, as in the seal resting ashore, in which the coupling between lung and chest does not favour a large V_T. After the first day of life periods of zero flow during expiration are less common, both in infants and in newborn animals. However, the phenomenon persists in the form of partial closure of the vocal cords, obviously aimed at prolonging the time required for expiration, i.e. the effective expiratory time constant of the respiratory system. In a few-days-old infant the partial narrowing of the glottis opening may be the source of perceivable noise, or grunting. In the adult this is much less pronounced, although some adduction of the vocal cords in expiration as a way to control the expiratory flow is well documented[19,20].

BRAKING ACTION OF THE INSPIRATORY MUSCLES

The second mechanism adopted by the infant to delay lung deflation, hence to maintain FRC elevated, is represented by the prolonged activity of the inspiratory muscles during expiration. The quantitative aspects of this mechanism can be estimated by occluding the airways of a spontaneously breathing infant exactly at end-inspiration. In fact, if all the inspiratory muscles ceased their activity precisely at end-inspiration, the pressure in the airways (and at the mouth, where it is actually recorded) should instantaneously rise to the value corresponding to the recoil pressure of the respiratory system. This is not the case (Fig. 9.4). On the contrary a rather long time, of the order of several hundred ms, is required before the plateau is reached; since peripheral inequalities in mechanical time constants, internal redistribution of air due to recovery of chest distortion or the time constant of the recording system could explain a delay of only a few ms, one is left with the conclusion that this pattern reflects the post-inspiratory activity of the inspiratory muscles, which appear then to last for a substantial portion of expiration, on average about 80%[7]. Similar values have also been obtained with a different approach, based on the analysis of expiratory flow–volume curves during resting breathing[7].

The above-described mechanisms to maintain an elevated lung volume (high breathing rate coupled with laryngeal expiratory braking and post-inspiratory activity of the inspiratory muscles) are not equally operative in different newborn species. Although the specific relative role of laryngeal control and braking activity of the inspiratory muscles have not been defined in quantitative terms for the different species, the net combined effect can be estimated through the analysis of the resting expiratory flow–volume curves[21]. The expiratory time constant, T_{exp}, is usually longer than the passive value T_{rs} in species breathing at relatively low rates as infants or lambs, while T_{exp} is more similar to T_{rs} in species breathing at high rates such as newborn rats or mice[21]. The difference in T_{exp} among species is so pronounced that it more than compensates their differences in T_E: hence the FRC-V_f difference tends to be less in smaller newborn species. In this respect it should be considered that an elevated FRC implies a prolongation of T_E through a vagally mediated pulmonary reflex, and some 'loss' of inspiratory muscle output at the beginning of the inspiratory phase in order to offset the internal recoil of the respiratory system. Neither aspect is probably desirable in newborns of the smallest species which have high oxygen consumption; hence their needs of high ventilatory rates. The observation[22] is relevant, however, that newborn rats resume the pattern of expiratory laryngeal braking in an obvious attempt to defend mean lung volume, when pressures tending to collapse the respiratory system are arti ficially applied. This indicates that the mechanisms controlling the expiratory flow are functionally developed even in these small fast-breathing animals. All these results suggest therefore that the control of FRC is an important aspect of the neonatal adaptation at birth, involving several controlling mechanisms; however, when metabolic and ventilatory requirements are very elevated, as in the smallest mammalian species, the control of FRC assumes a lower priority.

Acknowledgements

Supported by the Medical Research Council of Canada.

References

1. Stahl, W. R. (1967). Scaling of respiratory variables in mammals. *J. Appl. Physiol.*, **22**, 453–60
2. Karlberg, P., Cherry, R. B., Escardo, F. E. and Koch, G. (1962). Respiratory studies in newborn infants. II. Pulmonary ventilation and mechanics of breathing in the first minutes of life, including the onset of respiration. *Acta Paediatr.*, **51**, 121–36
3. Mortola, J. P., Fisher, J. T., Smith, J. B., Fox, G. S., Weeks, S. and Willis, D. (1982). Onset of respiration in infants delivered by cesarean section. *J. Appl. Physiol.*, **52**,716–24
4. Olinsky, A., Bryan, M. H. and Bryan, A. C. (1974). Influence of lung inflation on respiratory control in neonates. *J. Appl. Physiol.*, **36**, 426–9
5. Thach, B. T., Abroms, I. F., Frantz, I. D. III, Sotrel, A., Bruce, E. N. and Goldman, M. D. (1980). Intercostal muscle reflexes and sleep breathing patterns in the human infant. *J. Appl. Physiol.* **48**, 139–46
6. Mortola, J. P., Fisher, J. T., Smith, B., Fox, G. and Weeks, S. (1982). Dynamics of breathing in infants. *J. Appl. Physiol.*, **52**, 1209–15
7. Mortola, J. P., Milic-Emili, J., Noworaj, A., Smith, B., Fox, G. and Weeks, S. (1984). Muscle pressure and flow during expiration in infants. *Am. Rev. Resp. Dis.*, **129**, 49–53
8. Kosh, P. C. and Stark, A. R. (1984). Dynamic maintenance of end-expiratory lung volume in full-term infants. *J. Appl. Physiol.*, **52**, 1126–33
9. Brody, A. W. (1954). Mechanical compliance and resistance of the lung–thorax calculated from the flow recorded during passive expiration. *Am. J. Physiol.*, **178**, 189–96
10. Griffiths, G. B., Noworaj, A. and Mortola, J. P. (1983). End-expiratory level and breathing pattern in the newborn. *J. Appl. Physiol.*, **55**, 243–9
11. Fisher, J. T., Mortola, J. P., Smith, J. B., Fox, G. S. and Weeks, S. (1982). Respiration in newborns. Development of the control of breathing. *Am. Rev. Resp. Dis.*, **125**, 650–7
12. Farber, J. P. (1978). Laryngeal effects and respiration in the suckling opossum. *Respir. Physiol.*, **35**, 189–201
13. Mortola, J. P. (1984). Breathing pattern in newborns. *J. Appl. Physiol.*, **56**, 1533–40
14. Harding, R., Johnson, P. and McClelland, M. E. (1980). Respiratory function of the larynx in the developing sheep and the influence of sleep state. *Respir. Physiol.*, **40**, 165–79
15. Fox, W. W., Berman, L. S., Dinwiddie, R. and Shaffer, T. H. (1977). Tracheal extubation of the neonate at 2 to 3 cmH$_2$O continuous positive airway pressure. *Pediatrics*, **59**, 257–61
16. Berman, L. S., Fox, W. W., Raphaely, R. C. and Downes, J. D. Jr. (1976). Optimum level of CPAP for tracheal extubation of newborn infants. *J. Pediatr.*, **89**, 109–12
17. Naifeh, K. H., Huggins, S. E., Hoff, H. E., Hugg, T. W. and Norton, R. E. (1970). Respiratory patterns in crocodilian reptiles. *Respir. Physiol.*, **9**, 31–42
18. Rosenberg, H. I. (1973). Functional anatomy of pulmonary ventilation in the garter snake, *Thamnophis elegans*. *J. Morphol*, **140**, 171–84
19. Bartlett, D. Jr, Remmers, J. E. and Gautier, H. (1973). Laryngeal regulation of respiratory airflow. *Respir. Physiol.*, **18**, 194–204

20. England, S. J., Bartlett, D. Jr. and Daubenspeck, J. A. (1982). Influence of human vocal cord movements on airflow and resistance during eupnea. *J. Appl. Physiol.*, **52**, 773–9
21. Mortola, J. P., Magnante, D. and Saetta, M. (1985). Expiratory pattern of newborn mammals. *J. Appl. Physiol.*, **58**, 528–33
22. Marlot, D. and Mortola, J. P. (1984). Positive- and negative-pressure breathing in newborn rat before and after anaesthesia. *J. Appl. Physiol.*, **57**, 1454–61

Discussion

Dr A. C. Bryan It worries me that both the mechanisms you describe – thyroarytenoid activity and post-inspiratory diaphragmatic activity – are switched off in REM sleep, which is the predominant sleep state of the baby. So if the baby loses these mechanisms of maintaining FRC in REM sleep, what keeps his lungs inflated?

Dr J. P. Mortola You are right, both mechanisms decrease during rapid eye movement sleep, and in fact lung volume and Po_2 go down. There may be other priorities during REM sleep which require the abolition (or decrease effectiveness) of these mechanisms. Perhaps something else is required that cannot be achieved at the same time. It is certainly possible to breathe – many small newborn species do[1] – without keeping lung volume elevated. During REM sleep newborn infants behave just like certain small animals.

Bryan The fall in Po_2 in REM sleep is trivial really, so why are these mechanisms important?

Mortola As I mentioned before, perhaps there are other aspects of breathing which involve these mechanisms. For example, if I breathe in, close the larynx and relax, the pressure in the airways becomes positive, which may represent a 'useful' mechanism for reasons not directly related to gas exchange. In the very first hours after birth positive pressure may help in 'pushing' the fluid out of the lungs. This could be the function of the end-inspiratory pauses commonly observed in adult snakes, during which, just like in infants, alveolar pressure is positive[2]. Snakes have a high pulmonary artery pressure and low protein osmotic pressure, with a spontaneous tendency to fluid filtration in the alveoli, a fluid that must be reabsorbed during the expiratory phase. Their breathing strategy seems therefore very similar to that of newborn mammals during the first hours after birth.

Dr B. T. Smith As I understand it, you showed that the post-inspiratory braking mechanism is less effective in the premature infant than in later life. I have always thought of the grunt in respiratory distress syndrome as the sign of an airway closure mechanism which presumably protects lung volume. Would it be fair to assume that this mechanism is more primitive than the post-inspiratory braking mechanism?

Mortola I agree. Grunting is nothing but laryngeal narrowing (rather than complete closure). Post-inspiratory muscle activity is a more sophisticated way of keeping lung volume elevated, perhaps evolutionarily a more recent mechanism. It certainly requires more energy than just contracting the thyroarytenoid muscle.

Dr C. L. Gaultier Concerning the decrease in FRC during REM sleep, it has been reported that oxygen consumption is greater in REM sleep than in quiet sleep. Can you commend the strategy of the baby which decreases FRC at the same time as needing more O_2?

Mortola I am not aware of such a report for the newborn infant, which would indeed present a paradox. At the same time, though, it may indicate that there is no strict relationship between oxygen consumption and breathing pattern. At rest, the system has such a reserve of oxygen that one can afford to increase oxygen consumption despite an unfavourable

137

	pattern of breathing.
Dr C. J. Morley	From our mainly anecdotal experience it appears that the smaller the mammal and the more compliant its chest wall, the better its surfactant composition. When there is a very floppy chest wall, the only thing to hold the lung open is good surfactant. Another question: do you think all expiration in babies is passive or do you think that many expire actively? This is what we often observe.
Mortola	If active expiration means contraction of the expiratory muscles, I don't quite agree; but if you mean post-inspiratory activity of the inspiratory muscles, that is what I've shown.
Morley	I mean contraction of expiratory muscles.
Mortola	I don't think that active contraction of the expiratory muscles is common in the human baby at rest, except in the very first minutes after birth, as recorded by Karlberg and associates[3] and, later, by Milner and associates[4]. Both groups demonstrated positive oesophageal pressures during the expiratory phase of the first few breaths with small or no changes in lung volume, suggesting contraction of the expiratory muscles against closed upper airways.
Dr E. A. Egan	A number of papers suggest that it takes between 4 and 6 hours for the newborn lung to be completely cleared of liquid. Is there any continuing increase in FRC after the first minute or two of breathing showing that the FRC continues to climb as lung liquid is reabsorbed?
Mortola	We have not done the necessary measurements, but others have. With our type of measurement a small drift in the airflow integrated signal would alter the computation of a change in end-expiratory level. Klaus *et al.*[5] measured changes in FRC as a function of time and concluded that full aeration takes about 6 hours.
Egan	In my experiments it would seem that the FRC is independent of amount of lung liquid reabsorbed.
Mortola	If the matching between the amount of air entering and fluid leaving was not one-to-one, it would seem to me that the volume of the thoracic cage should change with time, which could be the case, but I do not think that it has ever been documented.
Dr W. Seeger	You mentioned that laryngeal narrowing controlling expiration is not present in adults. When we have patients with 'shock lung' being weaned from the respirator we often find that they improve immediately when we take the tube out. Hence we wonder if they too may use the larynx to maintain lung volume.
Mortola	I do not know to what extent the 'grunting pattern' is adopted in adults under special circumstances, but what you are saying could be a real possibility.

References

1. Mortola, J. P., Magnante, D. and Saetta, M. (1985). Expiratory pattern of newborn mammals. *J. Appl. Physiol.,* **58,** 528–33
2. Bartlett, D., Mortola, J. P. and Doll, E. J. (1986). Respiratory mechanisms and control of the ventilatory cycle in the garter snake. *Respir. Physiol.,* **64,** 13–27
3. Karlberg, P., Cherry, R. B., Escardo, F. E. and Koch, G. (1962). Respiratory studies in newborn infants. II. Pulmonary ventilation and mechanics of breathing in the first few minutes of life, including the onset of respiration. *Acta Paediat. Stockh.,* **51,** 121–36
4. Milner, A. D. and Saunders, R. A. (1977). Pressure and volume changes during the first breath of human neonates. *Arch. Dis. Child.,* **52,** 918–24
5. Klaus, M., Tooley, W. H., Weaver, K. H. and Clements, J. A. (1962). Lung volume in the newborn infant. *Pediatrics,* **30,** 111–16
6. Milner, A. D., Saunders, R. A. and Hopkin, I. E. (1978). Effects of delivery by caesarean section on lung mechanics and lung volume in the human neonate. *Arch. Dis. Child.,* **53,** 545–8

10
Postnatal Development of Lung Function

Cl. GAULTIER

Changes in pulmonary function during postnatal development are not yet very well understood. Most of the studies undertaken have concerned either neonates or children after the age of 6. The active period of postnatal lung growth occurs during the first years of life[1], and there is a lack of information about lung function development in this period due to limited cooperation of infants and young children. The present review summarizes the current knowledge on postnatal lung function development in humans.

CHEST WALL

The configuration of the rib cage in infants differs from that of adults[2,3]. In infants the rib cage is more circular than in the adult. This mechanical arrangement seems inefficient. In the adult the volume of the rib cage can be increased by raising the ribs. In infants, the ribs are already 'raised', and this may be one of the reasons why the motion of the rib cage contributes little to tidal volume. Moreover, the angle of insertion of the diaphragm is different: oblique in adults and almost horizontal in infants. This induces decreased efficiency of diaphragmatic contraction. This mechanical disadvantage is worsened in the supine posture which is the usual nursing position of babies in most modern societies. With age, changes in rib cage geometry occur[4]. Concurrently, there is progressive mineralization of the ribs. These changes in shape and structure are of major importance in improving the stiffness of the rib cage.

A large chest wall compliance (C_W) is an inherent characteristic of newborn mammals[5]. C_W has been measured in preterm and full-term newborns[6,7]. Whatever the methodology used, there is a tendency for C_W to decrease between preterm and term infants (Fig. 10.1)[7] and during the first 6 months of life[8]. After this age there is a gap in the literature until the age of 5. Total respiratory compliance of children between the ages of 5 and 16 was measured by Sharp et al.[9]. A progressive fall in compliance of total respiratory system (C_{rs}) with age was observed which was attributed to changes in C_W (Fig. 10.2).

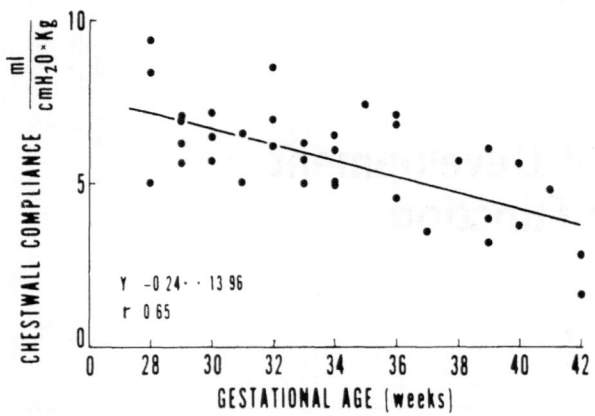

Figure 10.1 Relation between gestational age and chest wall compliance in 36 newborn infants. (From Ref. 7)

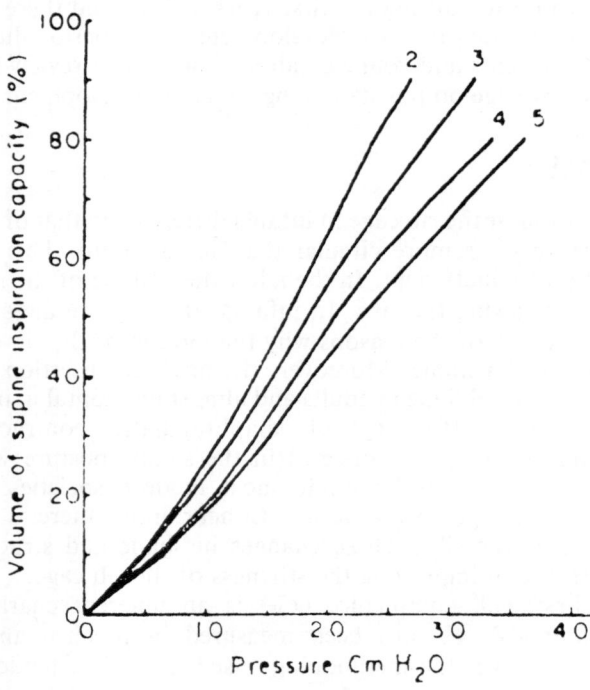

Figure 10.2 Changes in compliance of the total respiratory system with age. Group 2 had a mean age of 5 years; group 3, 8 years; group 4, 12 years; group 5, 16 years. (From Ref. 9)

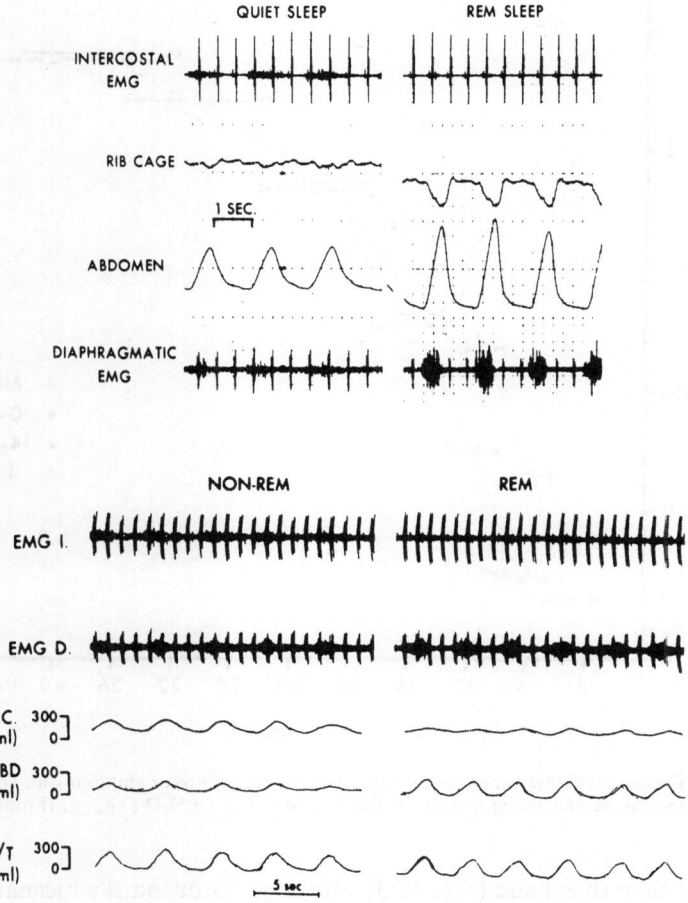

Figure 10.3 *Upper panel:* Changes in chest wall mechanics during REM sleep in an infant. Surface intercostal and diaphragmatic EMG and motion of rib cage and abdomen (magnetometers) in non-REM (quiet) and REM sleep (active). In REM sleep there is marked inhibition of intercostal muscle activity, significant increase in amplitude of diaphragmatic EMG and in excursion of abdominal magnetometer with paradoxical motion of the rib cage. (From Ref. 10). *Lower panel:* Changes in chest wall mechanics during REM sleep in normal adolescents: EMG I, intercostal electromyogram: EMG D, diaphragmatic EMG; RC: rib cage contribution to tidal volume (V_T); ABD: abdominal contribution to V_T. REM sleep is associated with decreased intercostal muscle activity. This is accompanied by a diminished RC contribution to tidal volume (V_T). V_T is maintained, however, because of a substantial increase in diaphragmatic muscle activity. No paradoxical movement of the rib cage was observed. (From Ref. 17)

The pliable rib cage of newborns and infants is therefore easily deformed under the effect of diaphragmatic contractions or when the stabilizing effect of the intercostal muscles is inhibited, such as during rapid eye movement (REM) sleep[10]. During REM the rib cage is deformed by the effect of phasic inspiratory diaphragmatic contraction, causing it to move in-

141

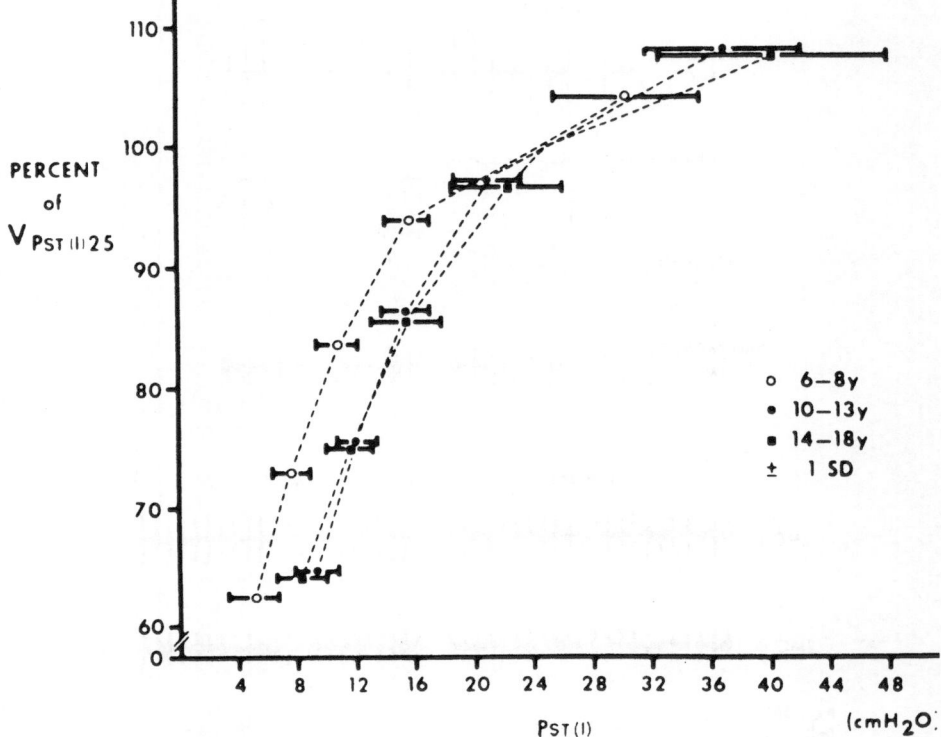

Figure 10.4 Pressure/volume curves of the lungs from three groups of children with volume expressed as percentage of volume at a distending pressue of 25 cmH₂O ($V_{Pst\,25}$). (From Ref. 26)

ward rather than to expand (Fig. 10.3). Rib cage distortion is a mechanical phenomenon which is unfavourable to sleep respiratory adaptation[11]. During REM, distortion is one of the factors responsible for the decrease in the end-expiratory lung volume[12] (Fig. 10.3); it is associated with a drop in transcutaneous partial pressure of oxygen[13]. In the distortion periods the efficiency of the diaphragm as a generator of pressure has been shown to diminish[14]. However, despite these disadvantages, it has been suggested that in infants the distorted breathing pattern may have an energetic advantage[15]. With age, periods of rib cage distortion during REM sleep get shorter[16] and disappear completely in adolescents because of their low C_W (Fig. 10.4)[17].

LUNG ELASTIC PROPERTIES

Little is known about the development of lung connective tissue. Emery[18] showed expansion of the elastic network in the peripheral pulmonary parenchyma with growth. More recently, Keely *et al.*[19] reported that true elastin expressed as a percentage of dry lung weight increases after full-term birth to reach adult proportions at about 6 months of postnatal age.

Functional studies of the elastic properties of the lung involve measurement of lung elastic recoil at the end expiratory level and static pressure–volume (P/V) curves. Absolute intraoesophageal pressure at the end-expiratory volume (PL_{FRC}) was found less negative in newborns and infants than in adults. Newborn PL_{FRC} values[20-22] range from -0.7 cmH$_2$O to -2.65 cmH$_2$O. The less negative absolute end-expiratory oesophageal pressure in infants when compared to that in adults can be explained by changes in lung elastic recoil, chest wall recoil, or a combination of these factors. Concerning P/V curves in newborns and infants, information can be obtained only from postmortem studies. Stigol et al.[23], using a maximal pressure of 20 cmH$_2$O, did not find any change in the overall shape of the P/V curves during infancy, while Fagan[24], using a 30 cmH$_2$O maximal pressure, observed a sharp drop in the proportion of volume retained at low pressure and then a shift to the right of the P/V curves during the first months of life. No *in vivo* studies are available in the young child. In older children and adolescents from 6 to 18 years old static P/V curves can be obtained. However, the problem is that of the comparison of P/V curves of different age groups. Volume used to be expressed as a percentage of total lung capacity (TLC)[25]. However, because the transpulmonary pressure at TLC increased with age[26], TLC is not measured at a fixed distending pressure. Bryan[26] therefore chose to use the volume at 25 cmH$_2$O, which is very close to the asymptote of the curve, and thus nearly independent of the shape. When the data are expressed in this way there is a progressive increase in lung elastic recoil with age at any lung volume and the shapes of the curves are quite comparable (Fig. 10.4), suggesting that there is no change in lung compliance between 6 and 18 years of age.

LUNG VOLUME

The end-expiratory lung volume, i.e. the functional residual capacity (FRC), is dependent upon several factors. As for any lung volume, FRC is influenced by alveolar growth. During the active period of postnatal alveolar multiplication[1] there is a significant relationship between increases in FRC and in alveolar number[27]. However, factors other than alveolar growth act on FRC: (1) the balance between elastic recoil of lung and chest wall, which implies lower passive FRC in newborns than in adults[5]; (2) neuromuscular control of the end-expiratory level, which explains why dynamic FRC is higher than passive FRC. Indeed, when infants become apnoeic their lung volumes fall to levels consistently lower than their end-tidal volumes[28]. The rise in dynamic FRC during normal breathing results from the parallel action of mechanisms that brake the expiratory flow: post-inspiratory muscle activity[29,30] and narrowing of the vocal cords[31]. These mechanisms which elevate FRC, are inefficient during REM sleep[11]. In full-term newborns, Henderson-Smart and Read[12] showed a decrease in FRC during REM sleep compared to NREM sleep (Fig. 10.5). The decrease in FRC during REM sleep is due to rib cage distortion, loss of tonic inspiratory diaphragmatic activity[29] and loss of the laryngeal break-

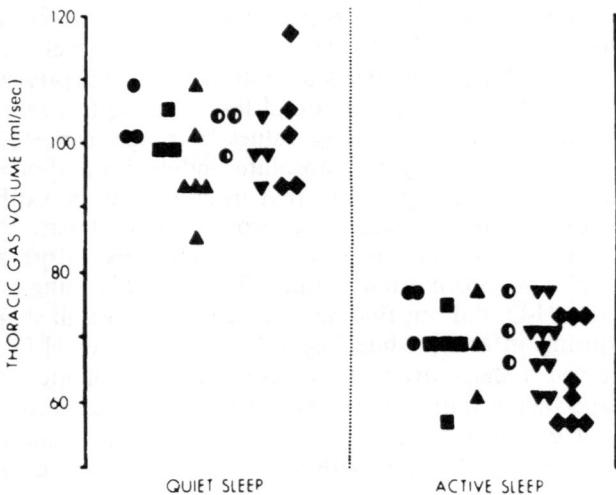

Figure 10.5 Thoracic gas volume in non-REM (quiet) and REM (active) sleep in seven infants, illustrating the approximately 30% fall in the end-expiratory lung volume in REM sleep. (From Ref. 12)

ing mechanism[31]. The changes in the dynamic control of FRC with growth and age are still unknown.

TLC is an effort-dependent measurement. The maximal pressures that children are capable of generating increase with age (see below). Therefore the increase in TLC with age reflects both the increase in lung volume and the increase in the strength of the child. FRC/TLC ratio does not change significantly between the age of 6 and adolescence[32] despite changes in the chest wall. However when FRC is related to a volume at a fixed distending pressure, there is a significant correlation with age[26]. Residual volume (RV/TLC) ratio decreases with age[33]. It is lower in males than in females, which can be explained by the greater increase in expiratory force in males[33].

AIRWAYS

Upper airways

The configuration of upper airways changes with age[34,35]. In the newborn the upper airways are narrow. The epiglottis is large and able to cover the soft palate. This forms the velo-epiglottic sphincter, favouring the obligatory 'nasal breathing' of the newborn. This configuration is associated with the horizontal position of the tongue and the elevated position of hyoid bone and laryngeal cartilage. In the course of the first 2 years of life the configuration changes, leading to a dynamic velo-lingual sphincter permitting buccal respiration and speech. The epiglottis, the larynx and the hyoid bone move down the posterior part of the tongue to take a vertical position during infancy. Despite the 'obligatory' nasal breathing newborns and infants can breathe through the mouth in cases of nasal obstruction[36]. Passive mechanical properties of the upper airways have been studied in newborn and adult animals[37]. In newborns nasal resistance was smaller than in adults, and mouth resistance similar to that found in adults. Thus the so-called obligatory nose breathing behaviour of newborns cannot be fully explained by the passive mechanical properties of the upper airways. The percentage contribution of nasal resistance (R_n) to airway resistance (R_{aw}) in sedated infants was assessed. R_n is equal to 49.2 ± 7.5 (SD)% of R_{aw} in Caucasian infants[38]. However, this percentage can be questioned because of the effect of sedation on upper airway resistance[39]. Furthermore, changes in upper airway resistance between wakefulness and the different stages of sleep are unknown in infants and children.

Intrathoracic airways

From morphometric studies it is known that conducting airways down to the terminal bronchioles are present at the sixteenth week of gestation, whereas respiratory bronchioles and alveolar ducts are present only at birth[40]. During growth airways increase in calibre. However, different results have been found concerning the proportional growth of central and peripheral airways. For Hislop et al.[40] the length and diameter of each branch appear to grow proportionately and to retain a constant relationship to the whole airways, while Hogg et al.[41] reported that peripheral airways are disproportionately narrow, suggesting that they grow at a delayed rate under 5 years of age.

Airway resistance and/or airway conductance have been assessed by plethysmographic measurement from birth to adolescence (Fig. 10.5)[42-45]. Specific airway conductance is primarily a measurement of central airways and is higher in infancy than in childhood. Thus growth of the lung is non-isotropic. Airways are present and relatively large in the newborn. Growth of lung volume occurs after birth and results in a dysanaptic process. For the same reasons there is a fall with age in size-corrected flows[22,25,46] and in specific upstream conductance[22].

In unsedated infants expiratory resistance is higher than inspiratory resistance[47]. This difference was not observed when infants were sedated, probably because of a marked reduction in thyroarythenoid muscle activity[39]. Lung tissue resistance appears to decrease with age[48,49].

Conflicting results have been reported concerning the dynamics of the peripheral airways. Hogg et al.[41] measured peripheral conductance per gram of lung tissue as a function of age, and found a sharp rise in peripheral conductance around the age of 5 years. This was in agreement with his pathological findings reported above. Other functional studies reported arguments in favour of high peripheral resistance in infants[50-52], while some studies suggested that central and peripheral airways may have a similar relationship in newborns and adults[22].

Finally, recent studies have shown sex differences in growth patterns of the airways and lung parenchyma. When corrected for lung size, young

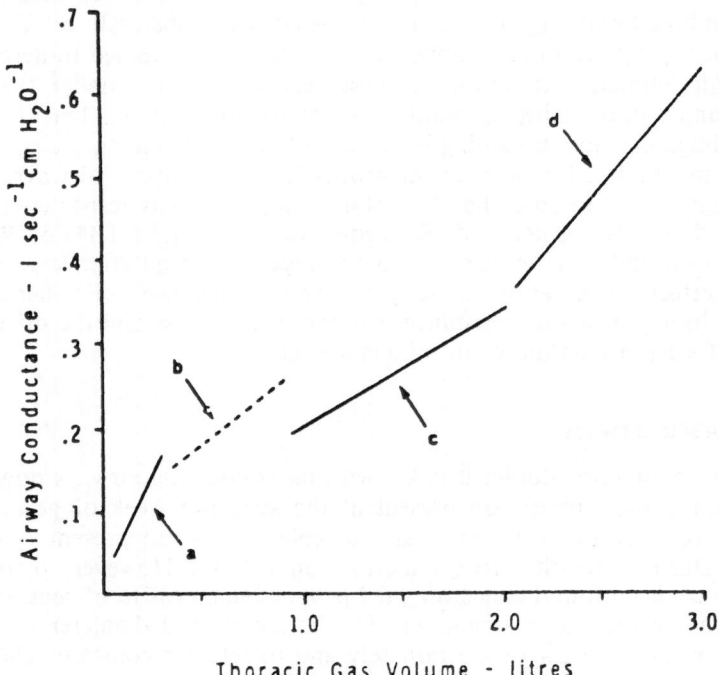

Figure 10.6 Comparison of regression lines of airway conductance (G_{aw}) during mouth breathing from infancy to adulthood. The regression lines have been obtained from the following studies: (a) Ref. 38; (b) Ref. 43 data on children 1 year to 5 years – this line was calculated from estimated G_{aw} by assuming 49% of R_{aw} to be due to nasal resistance; (c) Ref. 25; (d) Ref. 45 data on adult males. (From Ref. 38)

girls have higher flow rates than do boys of the same age[53]. The same results were found in older children and adolescents[54,55]. However the effects of puberty on the final process of development of airways and lung have yet to be completely described in both sexes[56].

In addition to the uncertainties surrounding the relationship between airways and lung parenchymal development, and thus airway dynamics, little is known about the role of genetic and postnatal environmental factors[57,58].

RESPIRATORY MUSCLES

With growth, there is a progressive increase in the bulk of the muscles of respiration. Coincident with this increase in muscle bulk, there is a progressive increase in the maximum inspiratory ($P_{I}max$) and expiratory pressures ($P_{E}max$) with substantial differences between sexes in all age groups[33,54,59] (Fig. 10.6). By 11–12 years of age adult values are attained in females for both $P_{I}max$ and $P_{E}max$, whereas this is true only for $P_{I}max$ in males. $P_{E}max$ in males continues to increase during adolescence (Fig.

146

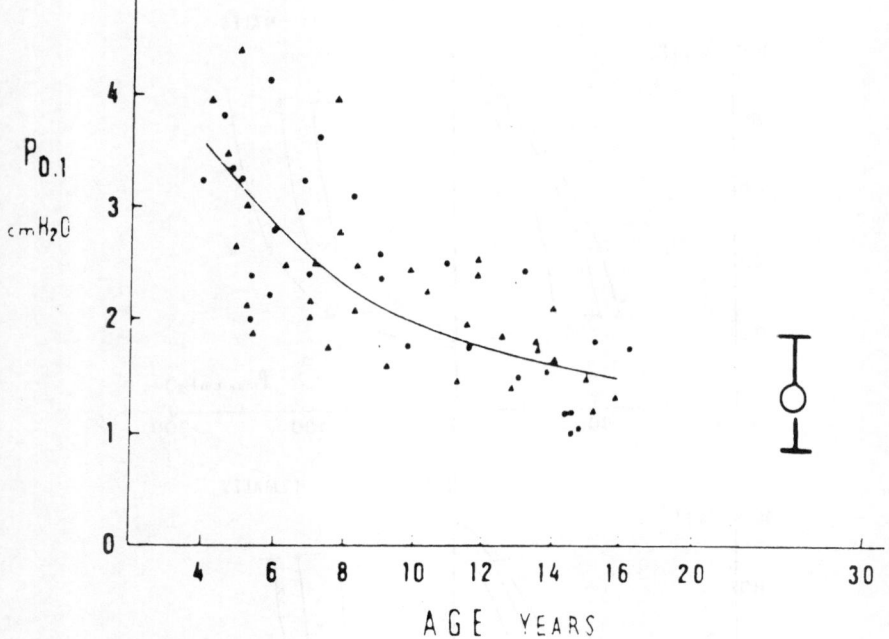

Figure 10.7 Relationship of $P_{0.1}$ (cmH$_2$0) and age (years) in 62 children aged 4 to 16 years. Circles: boys; triangles: girls. Average values ($\pm$ SD) for adults of both sexes aged from 18 to 32 years. (From Ref. 60)

10.6). However, the development of respiratory muscle force is only partly reflected by maximal pressure, since force is the product of pressure and surface area over which the pressure is applied, and both these parameters increase with growth. Indeed, when forces are determined the proportional increases in inspiratory and expiratory forces are greater than the corresponding increases in pressures[33].

Children have greater inspiratory pressure demands during breathing at rest than do adults[60], as assessed by measurement of the occlusion pressure ($P_{0.1}$) (Fig. 10.7). High inspiratory neuromuscular drive in children is explained by a higher metabolic rate. Thus inspiratory force reserve of the respiratory muscles in healthy children is reduced with respect to adults because the inspiratory pressure demands at rest are greater and $P_I$max is lower. Therefore the ratio : mean inspiratory pressure over $P_I$max ($\bar{P}_I/P_I$max) decreases with age (Fig. 10.8)[61]. In newborns and infants this ratio was estimated to be higher[62] than in the youngest children for whom results are available (Figs. 10.7 and 10.8).

Bellemare and Grassino[63] have shown in adults that the timing of the breathing cycle, as well as the pressure developed, both intervene in respiratory muscle fatigue. Depending on the ratio of inspiratory time over

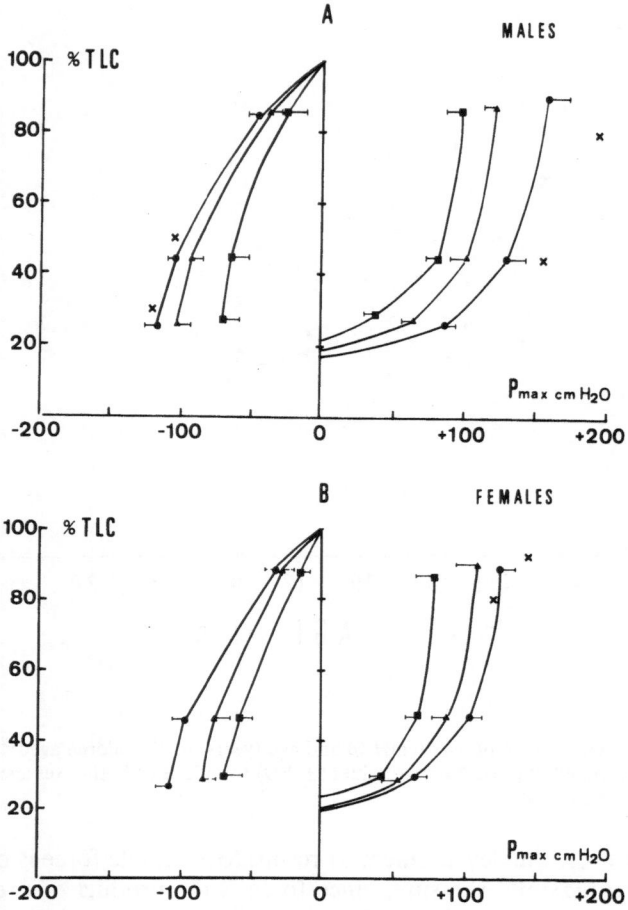

Figure 10.8 Maximal static pressures generated at different lung volumes in males (A) and females (B). Volume is plotted on the ordinate as percentage TLC, and pressures along the abscissa. The values are the means for 7–8 years (squares), 9–10 years (triangles), and 11–12 years (circles). The bars indicate 1 SD. The expiratory limb of the curves meets the volume axis at RV and the inspiratory limb at TLC. Crosses are values in healthy adults[59]. (From Ref. 33)

the total duration of the respiratory cycle (T_I/T_{tot}), there is a large spectrum of critical pressures above which fatigue occurs. In adults mean inspiratory pressure over maximal inspiratory pressure was assessed by transdiaphragmatic pressure ($\bar{P}_{di}/P_{di}max$) measurements[63]. In Fig. 10.9 it can be seen that adults during resting breathing conditions are far from the fatigue threshold of the respiratory muscles. When estimating $\bar{P}_{di}/P_{di}max$ ratio from $\bar{P}_I/P_Imax$[33,60] values, it appears that the younger the child is the nearer he is to the fatigue threshold of the respiratory muscles (Fig. 10.9)[64]. Presumably newborns and infants are even closer to this threshold. In newborns and infants the only easy approach to the diagnosis of respira-

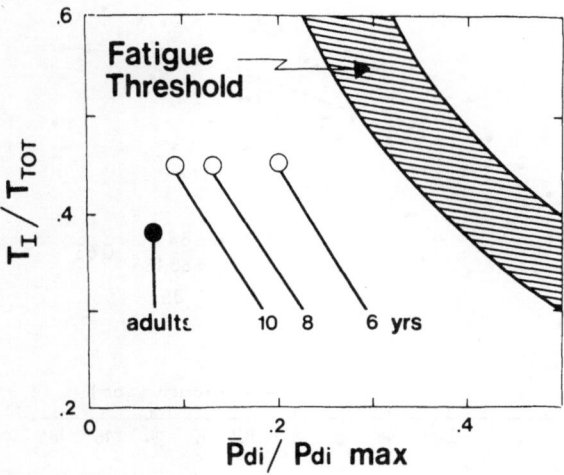

Figure 10.9 Relationship between T_i/T_{tot} and $\bar{P}_{di}/P_{di}$ max. The hatched area defines the diaphragmatic fatigue threshold. Filled circles: average value for adults during resting breathing[63]. Open values: estimated values for children aged 6, 8 and 10 years[33,60]. (From Ref. 64)

tory muscle fatigue is spectral analysis of the EMG of the respiratory muscles[10]. Using the ratio of low-frequency over high-frequency power of surface diaphragmatic EMG in preterm infants, Muller et al.[10] showed a decrease in this ratio during periods of marked chest wall distortion, suggesting diaphragmatic fatigue during resting breathing in REM sleep. One breathing strategy to cope with a fatiguing diaphragm is to shorten T_i and then to lower the T_i/T_{tot} ratio in order to breathe below the fatigue threshold. Such a breathing strategy, which can lead to apnoea, was observed in preterm infants resisting fatigue[10,65]. Children with an increase in elastic[66] or resistive[61] load behave in a similar way by shortening T_i and then decreasing the tension time of the diaphragm (i.e. $T_i/T_{tot} \times \bar{P}_{di}/P_{di}$ max).

Thus in infants and children the respiratory reserve in terms of diaphragmatic fatigue appears to be lower than in adults. Furthermore, there are considerable changes in the fibre composition of the respiratory muscles during the first year of life[67]. In preterm infants there are less than 10% type I fibres (slow-twitch high-oxidative fibres) in the diaphragmatic and intercostal muscles. The type I fibres increase rapidly to about 30% at term and continue to increase throughout the first year of life, when they reach adult values of about 50–60%[67]. A low proportion of type I fibres leads to a greater risk of respiratory muscle fatigue in preterms and during the first year of life.

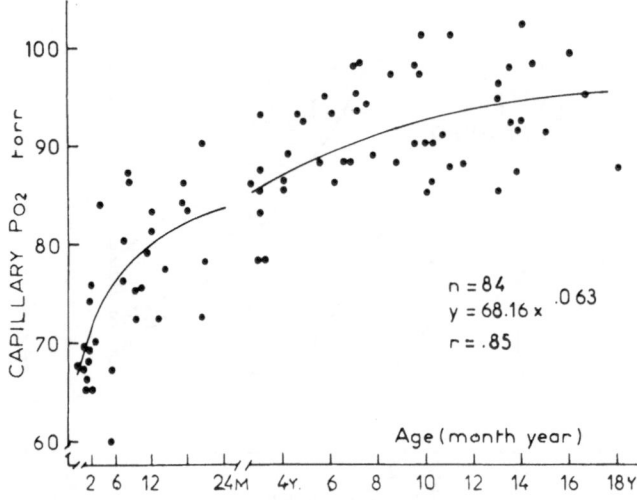

Figure 10.10 Capillary P_{O_2} in 84 children aged from 20 days to 18 years plotted against age. In the equation of the regression curve x is age expressed in months (From Ref. 70)

OXYGEN ARTERIAL TENSION

In the newborn the mean arterial oxygen pressure Pa_{O_2} equals 69.5 ± 0.86 torr[68]. The alveolo-arterial difference in partial pressure of O_2 (A-aP_{O_2}) is about 30 torr during air breathing and 120 torr during O_2 breathing. Anatomic R-L shunt and low ventilation–perfusion ratio account almost equally for the total venous admixture. In children after the age of 8, P ao$_2$ does not change with age and reaches adult values[69,70]. In this age range A-aP_{O_2} is equal to 9.4 ± 4.8 torr[69]. During infancy and childhood P ao$_2$ rises rapidly during the first 2 years of life and then slowly up to the age of 8 (Fig. 10.10) No A-aP_{O_2} measurements are available in the young child. The increase in P ao$_2$ with age results presumably from a reduction in the inequalities of the ventilation–perfusion ratio at the resting breathing level[71]. Children of 8 years of age have a higher closing volume (CV) compared to adolescents[72,73]. The closing capacity, i.e. CV plus RV, decreases with age. At 8 years the closing capacity is close to the FRC. Infants and young children may have closing capacities greater than FRC, and some areas of the lung may be closed throughout part or all of the tidal volume, with consequent impairment of gas exchange. However no results are available to confirm this assumption.

CONCLUSION

Despite two decades of important research many other studies are needed, especially in infants and young children, in order to fully describe the complexity of the development of lung function. We now know that newborns and infants risk respiratory failure when even minimal lung injury occurs. Futhermore, lung injury can induce abnormal lung development in structure and function[74], shown for example after bronchiolitis[75] and after severe viral infection[76]. Abnormal lung development presumably leads to respiratory diseases at the adult age. However, further studies of lung function follow-up in children with lung injury during growth are necessary to specify the dependence of lung function in adults on the individual's 'lung growth story'.

References

1. Thurlbeck, W. M. (1982). Postnatal lung growth. *Thorax*, **37**, 564–71
2. Muller, N. L. and Bryan, A. C. (1979). Chest wall mechanics and respiratory muscles in infants. *Pediatr. Clin. N. Am.*, **26**, 503–16
3. Bryan, A. C. and Gaultier, Cl. (1985). Chest wall mechanics in the newborns. In Roussos, C. and Macklem, P. T. (eds.) *The Thorax*. pp. 871–88. (New York: Marcel Dekker)
4. Openshaw, P., Edwards, S. and Helms, P. (1984). Changes in rib cage geometry during childhood. *Thorax.*, **39**, 624–7
5. Agostini, E. (1959). Volume–pressure relationship to the thorax and lungs in the newborn. *J. Appl. Physiol.*, **14**, 909–13
6. Reynolds, R. N. and Etstan, B. E. (1966). Mechanics for respiration in apneic anesthetized infants. *Anesthesiology*, **27**, 13–19
7. Gerhardt, T. and Bancalari, E. (1980). Chest wall compliance in full term and premature infants. *Acta. Paediatr. Scand.*, **69**, 359–64
8. Richards, C. C. and Blackman, L. (1961). Lung and chest wall compliance in apneic paralyzed infants. *J. Clin. Invest.*, **40**, 273–8
9. Sharp, M., Druz, W., Balgot, R., Baudelin, V. and Damon, J. (1970). Total respiratory compliance in infants and children. *J. Appl. Physiol.*, **2**, 775–9
10. Muller, N., Gulston, G., Cade, D., Whitton, J., Froese, A. B., Bryan, M. H. and Bryan, A. C. (1979). Diaphragmatic muscle fatigue in the newborn. *J. Appl. Physiol.*, **46**, 688–95
11. Gaultier, Cl. (1985). Breathing and sleep during growth: physiology and pathology. *Bull. Eur. Physiopath. Respir.*, **21**, 55–112
12. Henderson-Smart, D. J. and Read, D. J. (1979). Reduced lung volume during behavioural active sleep in the newborn. *J. Appl. Physiol.*, **46**, 1081–5
13. Martin, R. J., Okken, A. and Rubin, D. (1979). Arterial oxygen tension during active and quiet sleep. *J. Pediatr.*, **94**, 271–4
14. Lesoüef, P. N., Lopes, J. M., England, S. J., Bryan, M. H. and Bryan, A. C. (1983). Effect of chest wall distortion on occlusion pressure and the preterm diaphragm. *J. Appl. Physiol.*, **55**, 359–64
15. Mortola, J., Saetta, M., Fox, G., Smith, B. and Weeks, S. (1985). Mechanical aspects of chest wall distortion. *J. Appl. Physiol.*, **59**, 296–304
16. Gaultier, Cl., Praud, J. P., D'Allest, A. M. and Delaperche, M. F. (1986). Thoracoabdominal motion and diaphragmatic EMG activity during sleep in healthy infants. *Fed. Proc.* (In press)
17. Tabachnik, E., Muller, N. L., Bryan, A. C. and Levison, H. (1981). Changes in ventilation and chest wall mechanics during sleep in normal adolescents. *J. Appl. Physiol.*, **3**, 557–64
18. Emery, J. L. (1969). Connective tissue and lymphatics. In Emery, J. L. (ed.) *The Anatomy of the Developing Lung*. pp. 203–9. (London: Heinemann)
19. Keely, F. W., Fagan, D. G. and Webster, S. I. (1977). Quantity and character of elastin in developing lung parenchymal tissues of normal infants and infants with respiratory distress syndrome. *J. Lab. Clin. Med.*, **90**, 981–9
20. Senterre, J. and Geubelle, F. (1970). Measurement of endo-oesophageal pressure in the newborn. *Biol. Neonate.*, **16**, 47–53

21. Helms, P., Beadsmore, C. and Stocks, J. (1981). Absolute intraesophageal pressure at functional residual capacity in infancy. *J. Appl. Physiol.,* **51**, 270–5
22. Taussig, L. M., Landau, L. I., Godfrey, S. and Arad, I. (1982). Determinants of forced expiratory flows in newborn infants. *J. Appl. Physiol.,* **53**, 1220–7
23. Stigol, L. C., Vawter, G. F. and Mead, J. (1972). Studies on elastic recoil of the lung in a pediatric population. *Am. Rev. Respir. Dis.,* **105**, 552–63
24. Fagan, D. G. (1976). Post-mortem studies of the semistatic volume–pressure characteristics of the infant's lungs. *Thorax,* **31**, 534–43
25. Zapletal, A. E., Motoyama, K., Van de Woestijne, K., Hunt, V. and Bouhuys, A. (1969). Maximum expiratory flow–volume curves and airways conductance in children and adolescents. *J. Appl. Physiol.,* **26**, 308–16
26. Bryan, A. C., Mansell, A. L. and Levison, H. (1977). Development of the mechanical properties of the respiratory system. In Hodson, W. A. (ed.) *Development of the Lung.* pp. 445–68. (New York: Marcel Dekker)
27. Gaultier, Cl., Boulé, M., Allaire, Y., Clément, A. and Girard, F. (1979). Growth of lung volumes during the first three years of life. *Bull. Europ. Physiopathol. Respir.,* **15**, 1103–16
28. Olinsky, A., Bryan, M. H. and Bryan, A. C. (1974). Influence of lung inflation on respiratory control in neonates. *J. Appl. Physiol.,* **36**, 426–9
29. Lopes, J., Muller, N. L., Bryan, M. H. and Bryan, A. C. (1981). Importance of inspiratory muscle tone in maintenance of FRC in the newborn. *J. Appl. Physiol.,* **51**, 830–4
30. Mortola, J. P., Milic-Emili, J., Noworaj, A., Smith, B., Fox, G. and Weeks, S. (1984). Muscle pressure and flow during expiration in infants. *Am. Rev. Respir. Dis.,* **129**, 49–53
31. Harding, R., Johnson, P. and McClelland, M. E. (1980). Respiratory function of the larynx in developing sheep and the influence of sleep state. *Respir. Physiol.,* **40**, 165–79
32. Weng, T. R. and Levison, H. (1969). Standards of pulmonary function in children. *Am. Rev. Respir. Dis.,* **99**, 879–93
33. Gaultier, Cl. and Zinman, R. (1983). Maximal static pressures in healthy children. *Respir. Physiol.,* **51**, 45–61
34. Bosma, J. F. (1975). Introduction in the symposium. In Bosma, J. F. and Showacre, J. (eds.) *Development of Upper Respiratory Anatomy and Function.* pp. 5–49 (Washington: DHEW publication no. 75-941)
35. Moss, M. L. (1965). The veloepiglottic sphincter and obligate nose breathing in the neonate. *J. Pediatr.,* **67**, 330–1
36. Rodenstein, D. O., Perlemuter, N. and Stanescu, D. C. (1985). Infants are not obligatory nasal breathers. *Am. Rev. Respir. Dis.,* **131**, 343–7
37. Mortola, J. P. and Fisher, J. T. (1981). Mouth and nose resistance in newborn kittens and puppies. *J. Appl. Physiol.,* **51**, 641–5
38. Stocks, J. and Godfrey, S. (1978). Nasal resistance during infancy. *Respir. Physiol.,* **34**, 233–46
39. England, S. J., Lesoüef, P. N., Bryan, M. H. and Bryan, A. C. (1985). The role of upper airway in airway resistance in infants. *Am. Rev. Respir. Dis.,* **131**, A225
40. Hislop, A., Muir, D. C., Jacobson, M., Simon, G. and Reid, L. (1972). Postnatal growth and function of the pre-acinar airways. *Thorax,* **27**, 265–74
41. Hogg, J. C., Williams, J., Richardson, J. B., Macklem, P. T. and Thurlbeck, W. T. (1970). Age as a factor in the distribution of lower-airway conductance and in the pathologic anatomy of obstructive lung disease. *N. Engl. J. Med.,* **282**, 1283–7
42. Stocks, J. and Godfrey, S. (1977). Specific airway conductance in relation to postconceptional age during infancy. *J. Appl. Physiol.,* **43**, 144–54
43. Doershuk, C. F., Downs, T. D., Matthews, L. W. and Lough, M. D. (1970). A method for ventilatory measurements in subjects 1 month to 5 years of age: normal values and observation in disease. *Pediatr. Res.,* **4**, 165–77
44. Zapletal, A., Motoyame, E. K., Van de Woestijne, K. P., Hunt, J. R. and Bouhuys, A. (1969). Maximum expiratory flow volume curves and airway conductance in children and adolescents. *J. Appl. Physiol.,* **26**, 308–16
45. Briscoe, W. A. and Dubois, A. B. (1958). The relationship between airway resistance, airway conductance and lung volumes in subjects of different age and body size. *J. Clin. Invest.,* **37**, 1279–85

46. Taussig, L. M., Harris, T. R. and Labowitz, M. D. (1977). Functional residual capacity, tidal volume, and expiratory rate. Lung function in infants and young children. *Am. Rev. Respir. Dis.*, **116**, 233–9

47. Wohl, M. E., Stigol, L. C. and Mead, J. (1969). Resistance of total respiratory system in healthy infants and in infants with bronchiolitis. *Pediatrics*, **43**, 495–509

48. Polgar, G. and String, S. T. (1965). The viscous resistance of the lung tissues in newborn infants. *J. Pediatr.*, **69**, 787–92

49. Bachoffen, H. and Duc, G. (1968). Lung tissue resistance in healthy children. *Pediatr. Res.*, **2**, 119–24

50. Adler, S. M. and Wohl, M. E. (1978). Flow–volume relationship at low lung volumes in healthy term newborn infants. *Pediatrics*, **61**, 636–40

51. Williams, S. P., Pimmel, R. L., Fullton, J. M., Tsai, M. J. and Collier, A. M. (1979). Fractionating respiratory resistance in young children. *J. Appl. Physiol.*, **47**, 551–5

52. Stanescu, D., Moavero, N. E., Veriter, C. and Brasseur, L. (1979). Frequency dependence of respiratory resistance in healthy children. *J. Appl. Physiol.*, **47**, 268–72

53. Taussig, L. M. (1977). Maximal expiratory flows at functional residual capacity: A test of lung function for young children. *Am. Rev. Respir. Dis.*, **116**, 1031–8

54. Hibbert, M. E., Couriel, J. M. and Laudau, L. I. (1984). Changes in lung, airway and chest wall function in boys and girls between 10 to 12yr. *J. Appl. Physiol.*, **57**, 304–8

55. Pagtakhan, R. D., Bjelland, J. C., Laudau, L. I., Loghlin, G., Kaltenborn, W., Seeley, D. and Taussig, L. M. (1984). Sex differences in growth patterns of airways and lung parenchyma in children. *J. Appl. Physiol.*, **56**, 1204–10

56. Seely, J. E., Guzman, C. A. and Becklate, M. P. (1974). Heart and lung function at rest and during exercise in adolescence. *J. Appl. Physiol.*, **38**, 34–40

57. Brody, J. and Vaccaro, C. (1979). Postnatal formation of alveoli: interstitial events and physiologic consequences. *Federation Proc.*, **38**, 215–23

58. Gaultier, Cl. (1986). Influence de l'environnement sur la croissance du poumon. *Rev. Franc. Mal. Respir.*, 3, 233–234

59. Cook, C. D., Mead, J. and Orzalesi, M. M. (1964). Static volume–pressure characteristics of the respiratory system during maximal efforts. *J. Appl. Physiol.*, **19**, 1016–22

60. Gaultier, Cl., Perret, L., Boulé, M., Buvry, A. and Girard, F. (1981). Occlusion pressure and breathing pattern in healthy children. *Respir. Physiol.*, **46**, 71–80

61. Gaultier, Cl., Boulé, M., Tournier, G. and Girard, F. (1985). Inspiratory force reserve of the respiratory muscles in children with chronic obstructive pulmonary disease. *Am. Rev. Respir. Dis.*, **131**, 811–15

62. Milic-Emili, J. (1983). Respiratory muscle fatigue and its implications in RDS. In Cosmi, E. V., Scarpelli, E. M. (eds.) *Pulmonary Surfactant System.* pp. 135–41. (Amsterdam: Elsevier)

63. Bellemare, F. and Grassino, A. (1982). Effects of pressure and timing of contraction on the human diaphragm fatigue. *J. Appl. Physiol.*, **53**, 1190–5

64. Milic-Emili, J. (1984). Respiratory muscles fatigue in children. In Prakash, O. (ed.) *Critical Care of the Child.* pp. 87–94. (Dordrecht: Martinus Nijhoff).

65. Lopes, J., Muller, N. L., Bryan, M. H. and Bryan, A. C. (1981). Synergistic behaviour of inspiratory muscles after diaphragmatic fatigue in the newborn. *J. Appl. Physiol.*, **51**, 547–51

66. Gaultier, Cl., Peret, L., Boulé, M., Tournier, G. and Girard, F. (1982). Control of breathing in children with interstitial lung disease. *Pediatr. Res.*, **16**, 779–83

67. Keens, J. G., Bryan, A. C., Levison, H. and Ianuzzo, C. D. (1978). Developmental pattern of muscle fiber types in human ventilatory muscle. *J. Appl. Physiol.*, **44**, 909–13

68. Koch, G. (1968). Alveolar ventilation, diffusing capacity and the A-a PO_2 difference in the newborn infant. *Respir. Physiol.*, **4**, 168–92

69. Levison, H., Featherby, E. A. and Weng, T. R. (1969). Arterial blood gases, alveolar-arterial oxygen difference and physiologic dead space in children and young adults. *Am. Rev. Respir. Dis.*, **101**, 972–4

70. Gaultier, Cl., Boulé, M., Allaire, Y., Clément, A., Buvry, A. and Girard, F. (1978). Determination of capillary oxygen tension in infants and children. *Bull. Eur. Physiopathol. Resp.*, **14**, 287–97

71. Cooper, D. M., Mellins, R. B. and Mansell, A. L. (1981). Changes in distribution of ventilation with lung growth. *J. Appl. Physiol.*, **51**, 699–705

72. Mansell, A., Bryan, A. C., and Levison, H. (1972). Airway closure in children. *J. Appl. Physiol.*, **33**, 711–14
73. Gaultier, Cl., Allaire, Y., Pappo, A. and Girard, F. (1975). Etude du volume de fermeture chez l'enfant sain et atteint d'obstruction bronchique. In Hatzfeld, C. (ed.) *Distribution of Pulmonary Gas Exchange.* Colloque INSERM 51, pp. 365–72. (Paris, IN-SERM).
74. Gaultier, Cl. and Girard, F. (1980). Croissance pulmonaire normale et pathologique: relation structure–function. *Bull. Eur. Physiopathol. Respir.*, **16**, 791–842
75. Kattan, M., Keens, T., Lapierre, J. G., Levison, H., Bryan, A. C. and Reilly, B. J. (1977). Pulmonary function abnormalities in symptom free children after bronchiolitis. *Pediatrics*, **59**, 683–8
76. Gaultier, Cl. (1986). Abnormal development of lung function in children after severe viral infection. *Bull. Eur. Physiopathol. Respir.* (In press)

11
Alveolar Ventilation in Newborns and its Postnatal Development

D. LAGNEAUX AND F. GEUBELLE

Alveolar ventilation is that part of the total ventilation actually reaching the pulmonary structures where gases are exchanged with blood. For the other part of the total ventilation travelling through the bronchial tree, heat and water are exchanged in the so-called 'conducting airways', the volume of which corresponds to the anatomical dead space.

Evolution of these two parts in growing infants and young children depends on various factors. Firstly, tidal volume ($\dot{V}_T$) increases with body size, while respiratory rate decreases. Secondly, the morphological changes of the lung structures are actually specific in the first 8–10 postnatal weeks, and differ from changes observed later on.

Unfortunately, data are scarce, and without systematization in the morphological field. However, at least in a small age range – i.e. between birth and infancy – these data allow an estimation of gas displacement in the airways and its evolution with age.

Two sets of facts will be considered. Firstly, the relationship between pulmonary structures and their function. Secondly, the alveolar gas parameters estimated from available respiratory and metabolic data.

RELATION BETWEEN THE GROWING STRUCTURES AND THEIR FUNCTION

When analyzing ambient air flowing from the airway openings to exchanging structures, the most convenient approach is to refer to Weibel's A-model[1]. This symmetrical dichotomous system is useful but it does not take into account the asymmetry of branching and the dissimilarities between airways. Indeed, in adults the distance from the trachea and the respiratory bronchioles varies from 7 to 22 cm – i.e. a ratio of 1 to 3 for length and a ratio of 1 to 5 for gas transit time.

Nevertheless a lot of information can be obtained from a symmetrical branching system[1]. For the conducting airways, from the trachea to the respiratory bronchioles (16th generation) a similar type of branching system is already present before birth and will develop with body size, according to Hislop and Reid[2]. The bronchial tree should be a reduced model of the adult's one. Hofmann[3] fitted regression curves on the values collected from different published data. From these curves, anatomical – if not morphological – characteristics of conducting airways can be indirectly defined for postnatal growing lungs. These values will be used below in Weibel's model.

In the distal part of the airways (i.e. in the primary lobules) of adults, three generations of respiratory bronchioles, three generations of alveolar ducts and the terminal alveolar sacs are observed, corresponding to the respiratory zone with numerous alveoli. In newborns these distal parts of airways, beyond terminal bronchioles, are morphologically different and they will grow and develop extensively during the first 2 months. Anatomical data have been collected by Boyden and Tompsett[4] in a newborn, 1- and 2-month babies and a 7-year-old child. From their casts a schematic model has been derived by Hislop and Reid[2]. From a terminal bronchiole three generations of respiratory bronchioles are followed by short transitional ducts ending in a cluster of saccules. At birth no structures actually have the morphological characteristics of the alveolus, and gas exchange is probably performed through the capillaries of the saccule's epithelium. During the first 2 months after birth, explosive growth is observed, the terminal cluster growing from 1.1 to 1.75 mm. Moreover numerous alveolar structures develop, and their morphology then becomes similar to the usually described alveoli. Afterwards, during childhood, the number of alveoli increases, reaching about 300 million at 7–8 years, a figure which is also observed in the adult lung. The length between terminal bronchioles and the blind end of respiratory airways reaches 4 mm at 7 years and 8 mm in grown-ups. Total alveolar surface area is increased two-fold at 3 months, and two-fold again at 10 months. At the start this increase depends on identation of saccules and later on, on alveolar size increase.

What are the functional consequences of these morphological changes? Knowing the mean dimensions of the bronchial tree[3] and those of the terminal lobules[4], some classical data and their changes with growth can be calculated. They are illustrated (Fig. 11.1) for 2-day-, 2-month-, and 7-year-old children, and they are compared with data collected from adult's lung in Fig. 11.2. The classical 'trumpet model' of airways is drawn according to two dimensions: the length of the bronchial tree and its corresponding total cross-sectional area. After the trachea (generation number 0) there are 2^1 bronchi of first generation, 2^2 bronchi of second generation and so on, until 2^{16} terminal bronchioles. In successive generations the number of bronchioles increases far more rapidly than their section decreases, so that the total cross-sectional area increases greatly up to 600 cm^2 in the adult lung at the level of the terminal bronchioles. The same 'trumpet model' is illustrated for different ages (Fig. 11.1) with scales very different from those used for the adult lung model (Fig. 11.2). The cumulative volumes calculated from the successive generations up to the terminal bronchioles give a value for the anatomical dead space, the upper

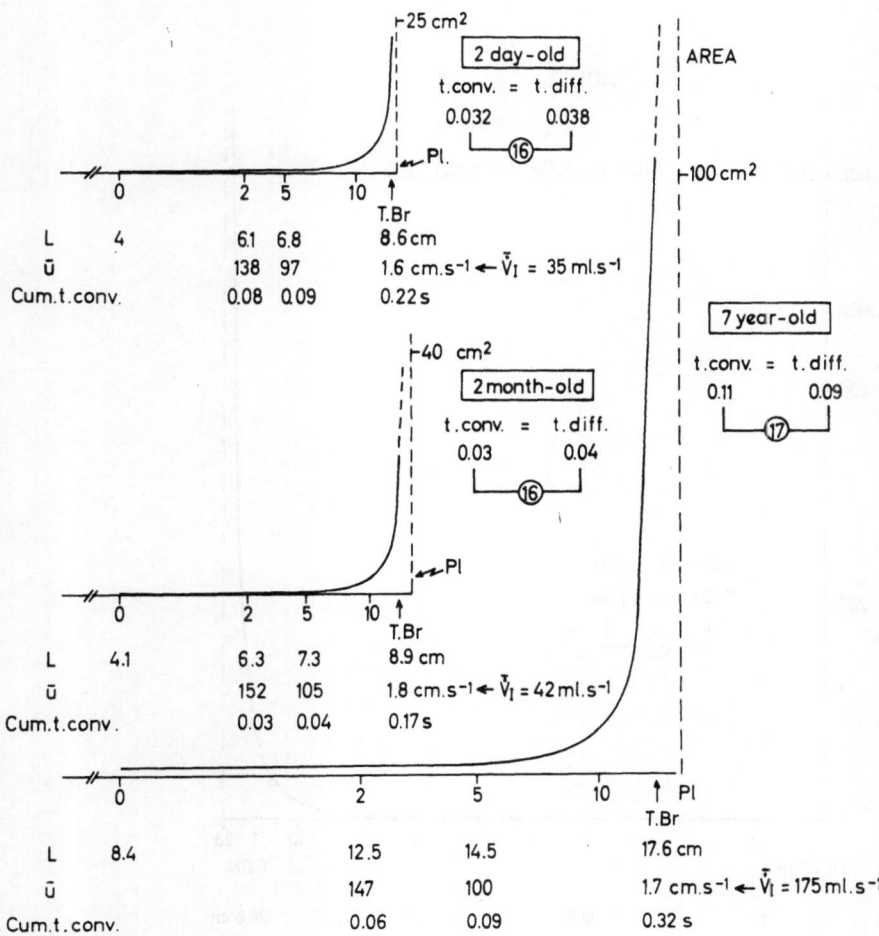

Figure 11.1 Relation between length and total cross-sectional area of the bronchial tree considered as a 'reduced model' of the adult's conducting airways for a newborn (2-day-old), 2-month-old and 7-year-old children. The starting point of the bronchial tree's length (L) is the distal part of trachea (generation 0) and the terminal bronchioles' situation (T.Br.) is indicated for the three ages considered. The vertical broken lines at the right locate the blind end of the airways (Pl = pleura). For a given mean inspiratory flow ($\bar{V}_I$) and considering the increase of the total cross-sectional area (A) in the latest generations, the mean axial velocity ($\bar{u} = \bar{V}_I/A$) falls considerably at the distal part of the airways. The segment of bronchial tree where the transit time by convection (t.conv.) is no longer different from the transit time by diffusion (t.diff.) (see text) is in the 16th generation for 2-day-old and 2-month-old children, and in the 17th generation for the 7-year-old. Above this 'transitional' generation O_2 (i.e.) travels by convection and its cumulative transit time (Cum.t.conv.) is indicated. Below this generation between this segment and the blind end of airways, gases are travelling by diffusion

airways being excluded since the trachea is the first section taken into account. This dead space volume is 6.3 ml in the newborn model, a figure which is at the upper limit of the values estimated *in vivo* by Koch[5] and 7.1 and 60 ml respectively for the 2-month-old and the 7-year-old children.

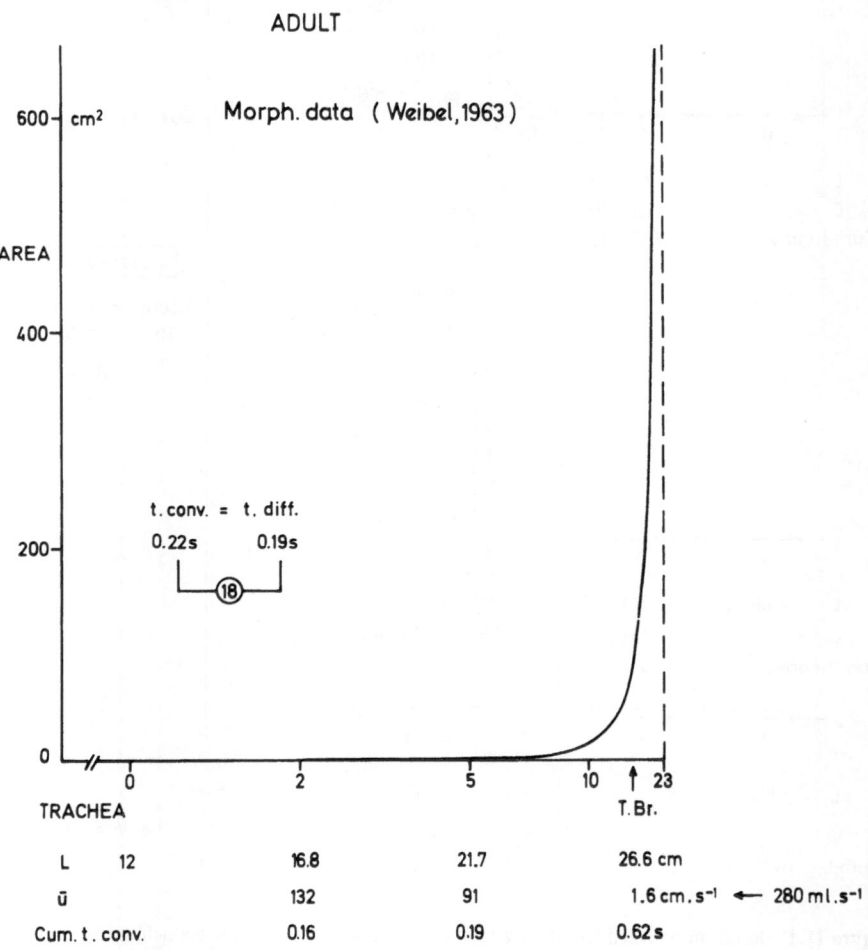

Figure 11.2 Relation between length and total cross sectional area in an adult's bronchial tree. The morphological data are obtained from Weibel[1]. For the derived values, see Fig. 11.1. The difference between the scales of Fig. 11.1 and of Fig. 11.2 must be emphasized

Broadly speaking, this kind of lung model gives an overestimation of the dead space volume, actually reaching 175 ml for the adult's model.

Other data are calculated from these models in the following way. The flow of ambient air from the airway opening to the gas exchange or respiratory zones is due partly to convection (mass movement of gas as a consequence of a total pressure gradient between two sites) and partly to diffusion depending on the thermokinetic movement of the molecules.

Conductive and diffusive transit times for each segment of the bronchial tree are calculated as follows:

1. mean transit time by convection (or: t.conv.): $L/\bar{u}$
2. mean transit time by diffusion (or: t.diff.): $\pi L^2/D$
   where L = the length of the segment,
   $\quad\quad u$ = the mean axial velocity at the level of the considered
   $\quad\quad\quad\quad$ segment = $\dot{V}/A$,
   $\quad\quad \dot{V}$ = flow rate of ventilation,
   $\quad\quad A$ = total cross-sectional area at the level of this segment,
   $\quad\quad D$ = gas diffusion constant in gas phase at 37 °C
   $\quad\quad\quad\quad (D_{O_2} = 0.222$ cm^2 s^{-1} and $D_{CO_2} = 0.200$ cm^2 s^{-1})

How do these derived values change during growth? Due to the increase of the total cross-sectional area with the successive generations, mean axial velocities, for a given mean inspiratory flow rate ($\bar{V}_I$) falls considerably. These values are indicated below the cumulative length of the airways in Figs. 11.1 and 11.2, the $\bar{V}_I$ values used being noted at the right-hand side. As the total cross-sectional area increases, the mean axial velocity for a given $\bar{V}_I$ falls and O_2 molecules are transported by convection in moving fluid only up to a given point. Indeed at this particular level travel time by convection through the segment is no longer different from the time needed for diffusion in the same segment. In adults, with a mean inspiratory flow of 280 ml s^{-1} at rest, and taking the largest morphological values observed by Weibel on lungs inflated to their maximal volumes, convection and diffusion transit times are equal in the 18th generation (Fig. 11.2). Above this so-called 'transitional' generation, the gas is transferred by convection and below it, by diffusion.

Taking the 'reduced model' of pre-acinar airways in newborns of Hislop and Reid[2], the Hofmann regression from dimensions of the structures and the resting ventilatory data at different ages compiled from the Geigy scientific tables[6] and from Hofmann's data[3], the mean axial velocities are also illustrated for children's models in Fig. 11.1. Convection transit time equals diffusion transit time in the 16th generation in 2-day-old and in 2-month-old infants, but in the 17th generation in 7-year-old children (Fig. 11.1).

This transitional point being determined, a total transit time for O_2 can be calculated. It is equal to cumulative convection times in the successive generations up to this transitional zone plus a diffusion transit time for the remaining length of the airways up to its blind end. The cumulative mean convection transit times (Cum.t.conv.) are indicated below the mean axial velocities in Figs. 11.1 and 11.2. For the different ages where the dimensions of the structures are known, the values for convection, diffusion and total transit times are summarized in Table 11.1.

The total transit time increases with age, this increase essentially depending on the diffusion time: from 0.17 to 2.2 seconds between newborns and adults respectively. The distance to be covered by diffusion is 1.1 mm in newborns versus 4.8 mm in adults (more than a four-fold increase).

Total transit time is also to be considered in relation to inspiratory time, T_I. T_I increases with age depending on the respiratory rate and the ratio T_I/T_{tot} (T_I/total breath time). As the increase of T_I is less than the increase

Table 11.1 Comparison between total transit time (total time) and inspiratory time from newborn to adult*

	t_{conv} +	t_{diff} =	Total time	Inspiratory time
Two-day-old	0.22	0.17	0.39	0.62 seconds
Two-month-old	0.17	0.42	0.59	0.66 seconds
Seven-year-old	0.41	1.38	1.79	1.25 seconds
Adult	0.62	2.20	2.82	2.13 seconds

*The total transit time equals cumulative convective times ($t._{conv}$.) from the trachea to the transitional generation plus the diffusive transit time ($t._{diff}$.) needed to travel from this generation to the blind end of airways. Total transit time increases with age, essentially depending on the larger distance to be travelled by diffusion. In comparison with the inspiratory time, this total transit time is shorter in 2-day - and 2-month-old children and larger later on, indicating that the stratified inhomogeneity present in a 7-year-old child and in an adult lung seems to be absent in very young babies

of the calculated total transit time, a stratified inhomogeneity may be present in the 7-year-old child, as in the adult (T_I being lesser than T_{tot}).

The diffusion transit time is calculated for an O_2 molecule travelling through the longest possible pathway. But alveoli can be observed in the 17th generation and can be reached earlier by radial diffusion within a reduced transit time. This radial diffusion increases the stratified inhomogeneity. However, as far as newborns are concerned, this inhomogeneity seems to be absent, at least during the first 2 months of life. Indeed, T_I values are usually longer than the calculated total transit times (Fig. 11.1).

In spite of, or because of, their 'reduced model' of conductive airways, newborns appear to be able to transfer O_2 molecules up to the capillarized epithelium of their immature lobules without diffusional inhomogeneity, the same also being true for CO_2 transfer. The expiratory time is longer than T_I and subsequently longer than total transit time. Thus no stratified inhomogeneity should be expected in alveolar gas.

ALVEOLAR GAS PARAMETERS

What is known about the alveolar gas formation and its changes during postnatal growth? The data to take into account include the changes of metabolic requirements and of the alveolar ventilation during growth.

All these variables are interdependent in the Bohr equation of mass conservation. For CO_2 i.e.:

$$\dot{V}_{CO_2} = FE_{CO_2} . \dot{V}_E - FI_{CO_2} . \dot{V}_I \tag{1}$$

and

$$\dot{V}_{CO_2} = FE_{CO_2} . \dot{V}_E = FA_{CO_2} . \dot{V}_A \tag{2}$$

with

$$\dot{V}_A = \dot{V}_E - f . VD$$

where V_{CO_2} = carbon dioxide production rate
F_{CO_2} = tractional concentration of CO_2 in mean expired (E),
inspired (I) or alveolar (A) gas
$\dot{V}_E$ = total expired ventilation
$\dot{V}_I$ = total inspired ventilation
$\dot{V}_A$ = alveolar ventilation
f = respiratory rate
VD = dead space volume

The amount of CO_2 which is produced during a given time can be measured at mouth level by measuring the net balance between CO_2 entering and leaving the airways (equation 1). No CO_2 being present in inspired air FI_{CO_2}. $\dot{V}_I$ = 0 and the equation for CO_2 production is simplified. CO_2 production measured at the airway opening is equal to the amount of CO_2 leaving the alveolar system in the same time (equation 2). This alveolar equation can be solved for FA_{CO_2} or more usually for PA_{CO_2} (the pressure of CO_2 in the mean alveolar gas).

$$PA_{CO_2} = k(\dot{V}_{CO_2}/\dot{V}_A) \tag{3}$$

This mean partial pressure of CO_2 in the alveolar gas depends on the ratio of CO_2 production rate to alveolar ventilation, with a coefficient (k) taking into account the transformation from fractional concentrations into partial pressures and the difference of gaseous states (STPD and BTPS) respectively used in numerator and denominator of the equation (3)

A similar equation can be derived for O_2 consumption ($\dot{V}_{O_2}$) in relation with $\dot{V}_A$, but the ratio $\dot{V}_{O_2}/\dot{V}_A$ with the same coefficient must be substracted from PI_{O_2} (partial pressure of O_2 in the inspired air).

$$PA_{O_2} = PI_{O_2} - k(\dot{V}_{O_2}/\dot{V}_A) \tag{4}$$

What is the postnatal change of the data used in the Bohr equation?

Only the metabolism at rest seems unquestionable: from Hill et al.[7], O_2 consumption increased as a function of body weight $(BW)^1$ between birth and 2 years, and according to the function $(BW)^{0.6}$ afterward. This value is also obtained from the data of Fleisch on metabolism in children[8]. From these data O_2 consumption per unit of BW at rest is maximal and stable at 7.2 ml/kg during the first 2 years, and decreases afterwards up to 4 ml/kg in young adults. The same change is observed for $\dot{V}_{CO_2}$/kg. The respiratory quotient (R) at rest is fixed at 0.8 all through life but in the first days R is 0.7.

The second factor to be considered is the relationship between alveolar ventilation, tidal volume (V_T), dead space volume (V_D) and respiratory rate. Published values are scarce and these relationships have to be deduced from indirect data. Generally, a V_D/V_T ratio around 0.3 in newborns as well as in adults seems to be the most reliable figure (the published data have been reviewed in Ref. 9). But the V_T data at rest are more questionable. If, as Gaultier and Girard[9] do, we consider (Table 11.2) that

V_T/BW is constant from 4-year-old children to adults, with a V_D/V_T ratio of about 0.3, the fall of respiratory rate from 23 to 10/min leads to a fall in alveolar ventilation values from 163 ml/kg in 4-year-old children to 71 ml/kg in young adults. Considering now the O_2 consumption data given above, corresponding $\dot{V}_{O_2}/\dot{V}_A$ ratio would be different (about one unit in Table 11.2 where the ratio is multiplied by 100 to avoid decimals) in childhood and in adults leading to a 10 torr PA_{O_2} difference, with relative hyperoxia in children. While this difference may be acceptable for O_2, the same argument when applied to the P_{CO_2} equation would indicate that the children are unexpectedly hypocapnic. As such a hypocapnia is not actually observed, one may suggest that $\dot{V}_A$ is overestimated and consequently that the $\dot{V}_T$/kg is not constant from early in life up to adulthood.

As a matter of fact, other figures of V_T (7.7 ml/kg) have been observed in 5- and 12-year-old children[10]. Using these values in the below equations (Table 11.3), more reliable values of P_{O_2} and P_{CO_2} are obtained. They also agree with alveolar values usually considered as normal and with the published arterial P_{CO_2} values, no alveolo-arterial P_{CO_2} difference being observed in healthy subjects.

As the P_{CO_2} is constant in this period, the $\dot{V}_{CO_2}/\dot{V}_A$ ratio must also be similar whatever the age. Thus alveolar ventilation is adapted to the metabolic requirements. Since the V_D/V_T ratio is constant and the respiratory rate decreases between 4 years and adulthood, V_T/kg actually changes during childhood.

As far as newborns are concerned, the published data are more scattered in all studies except in the observations of Koch[5]. All his alveolar data were

Table 11.2 Alveolar data calculated from Hill's O_2 consumption data ($\dot{V}_{O_2}$) and using a respiratory quotient of 0.8, a constant tidal volume (V_T) per unit of body weight[9] and a constant dead space/tidal volume ratio (V_D/V_T)

	Four-year-old	Adult
V_T (ml kg^{-1})	10	10
V_D/V_T	0.29	0.29
f (min^{-1})	23	10
V_A (ml min^{-1} kg^{-1})	163	71
$\dot{V}_{O_2}/\dot{V}_A$ ($\times$ 100)	4.5	5.8
$\downarrow$		
PA_{O_2} (torr) calc.	111	100
$\dot{V}_{CO_2}/\dot{V}_A$		
$\downarrow$		
PA_{CO_2} (torr) calc.	31	40

f: Respiratory rate. V_A: minute alveolar ventilation. PA_{O_2}: calculated alveolar O_2 tension. PA_{CO_2}: calculated alveolar CO_2 tension. $\dot{V}_{CO_2}$: CO_2 production

Table 11.3 Alveolar data calculated as in Table 11.2 considering that V_T/kg should be different in children and in adults[10]

	4–5 years	12 years	Adult
V_T (ml kg^{-1})	7.75	7.72	10
$\dot{V}_{O_2}/\dot{V}_A$ (ml min^{-1} kg^{-1})	5.7	5.5	5.8
P_{AO_2} (torr) calc.	100	105	100
P_{ACO_2} (torr) calc.	40	38	40

estimated from alveolar equations in which arterial P_{CO_2} is assumed to be equal to the mean alveolar P_{CO_2} according to Riley et al.[11]. But in the first day of life (Table 11.4) metabolism is different and the respiratory quotient is 0.7[5,12]. The $\dot{V}_{O_2}$/kg values observed by Koch[5] are similar to the figures collected by Hill[7], and the V_T/kg is at the lower limit of the figures published up to now[13], but the derived values for P_{CO_2} suggest a relative hyperventilation which is demonstrated by the measured arterial P_{CO_2}.

In the 7-day-old baby (Table 11.4) recently published data are more scattered from 4.7 to 6.4 ml/kg for V_T, from 6.4 to 8.1 for $\dot{V}_{O_2}$/kg, from 0.8 to 0.94 for R. Assuming a V_D/V_T of 0.3, alveolar ventilation calculated from total ventilation by Schulze et al.[14] or by Stark et al.[15] is higher than the values obtained by Koch[5]. Derived P_{O_2} and P_{CO_2} once more suggest a relative hyperventilation as confirmed by measured end-tidal P_{CO_2} by Stark[15].

Thus in the first week of life, alveolar hyperventilation seems to exist. In 1-day newborns this can be explained by the metabolic acidosis due mainly to fatty metabolism. In older babies this acidosis regresses, and as the persistent hypoxaemia depending on large shunt does not seem to be a respiratory stimulus in newborns, an alternative explanation may be found in an important reticular activity with numerous new stimulations: gravitational stresses, ambient temperature and humidity – all new sensory stimuli acting on an immature brainstem.

It is not known at what age this hyperventilation disappears. More longitudinal studies including all the alveolar parameters during the first months of life are needed in order to obtain more accurate values. Such research would be difficult not only from a technical point of view, but also in pediatric practice.

To follow up healthy babies longitudinally over a period of months is the most difficult problem to be faced. It is also difficult to perform systematic morphometric data studies in order to draw theoretical lung models for children.

Table 11.4 Alveolar data published for 1- and 7-day-old newborns by Koch[5], Cross[13], Schultze et al.[14], Stark et al.[15]

	24 hours		7 days		
	Koch[5]	Cross[13]	Koch[5]	Stark et al.[15]	Schulze et al.[14]
V_T (ml kg^{-1})	4.5	5.9	4.7	6.4	—
$\dot{V}_{O_2}$ (ml kg^{-1})	6.8	—	6.4	—	8.1
$\dot{V}_A$ (ml kg^{-1})	123	(127)	120	(200)	(200)
$\dot{V}_{O_2}/\dot{V}_A$ ($\times$ 100)	5.5	—	5.3	—	4.1
$P_{A_{O_2}}$ (torr) calc.	103	—	104	—	115
$\bar{R}$	0.7	—	0.78	—	0.94
$P_{A_{CO_2}}$ (torr) calc.	34	—	36	—	33
P_{CO_2} (torr) mes.	(a) 34.7	—	(a) 36.7	(ET) 33.2	—

P_{CO_2} is measured in arterial blood (a) or in the end-tidal gases (ET). $P_{A_{CO_2}}$ and $P_{A_{O_2}}$ are calculated from the alveolar equations (see text)

References

1. Weibel, E. (1963). *Morphometry of the Human Lung.* (Berlin: Springer)
2. Hislop, A. and Reid, L. (1974). Development of the acinus in the human lung. *Thorax,* **29**, 90–4
3. Hofmann, W. (1982). Mathematical model for the postnatal growth of the human lung. *Respir. Physiol.,* **49**, 115–29
4. Boyden, E. A. and Tompsett, D. H. (1965). The changing patterns in the developing lungs of infants. *Acta Anat.,* **61**, 164–92
5. Koch, G. (1968). Alveolar ventilation, diffusing capacity and the A–a PO$_2$ difference in the newborn infant. *Respir. Physiol.,* **4**, 115–29
6. Geigy: *Tables Scientifiques* (1972), 7th edn. (Basle: Ciba-Geigy)
7. Hill, J. R. and Rahimtulla, K. A. (1965). Heat balance and the metabolic rate of newborn babies in relation to environmental temperature and the effect of age and of weight on basal metabolism rate. *J. Physiol. (Lond.),* **180**, 239–65
8. Fleich, A. (1954). *Nouvelles méthodes d'étude des échanges gazeux et da la fonction pulmonaire.* (Basle: Schwabe)
9. Gaultier, C. and Girard, F. (1980). Croissance pulmonaire normale et pathologique: relation structure–fonction. *Bull. Physiopathol. Respir.,* **16**, 791–842
10. Blomer, A. and Hahn, N. (1963). Atemwerte der neugeborenen Saüglinge und Kinder bis 0 zu 6 Jahren. *Z. Kinderheilk,* **87**, 466
11. Riley, R. L., Lilienthal, J. R., Proemmel, D. D. and Franke, R. E. (1946). On the determination of the physiologically effective pressures of oxygen and carbon dioxide in alveolar air. *Am. J. Physiol.,* **147**, 191–8
12. Senterre, J. and Karlberg, P. (1970). Respiratory quotient and metabolic rate in normal full term and small-for-date newborn infants. *Acta Paediat. Scand.,* **59**, 653–8
13. Cross, K. W. (1949). The respiratory rate and ventilation in newborn baby. *J. Physiol. (Lond.),* **109**, 459–74

14. Schulze, K., Kairam, R., Stephansky, M., Sciacca, R. and James, L. S. (1981). Continuous measurement of minute ventilation and gaseous metabolism in newborn infants. *J. Appl. Physiol.: Respir. Environ. Exercice Physiol.*, **50**, 1098–103
15. Stark, A. R., Waggener, T. B., Frantz, I. D. III, Cohlan, B. A., Feldman, H. A. and Kosch, P. C. (1984). Effect on ventilation of change to the upright posture in newborn infants. *J. Appl. Physiol.: Respir. Environ. Exercice Physiol.*, **56**, 64–71

Discussion

Dr J. P. Mortola	If inspiratory pressure is higher in infants than in the older child or adult, is this because their muscle generates more force, or is it because the area of the surface to which the force is applied is smaller?
Dr C. L. Gaultier	In infants the mean inspiratory pressure during resting breathing conditions is higher than in the older child because of a higher metabolic rate. There is no available measurement of static maximal inspiratory pressure in infants, but data in children showed that static maximal inspiratory pressure increased with age. The increase in force was suggested by the estimation of inspiratory force computed as the product of static maximal pressure and estimated surface area over which the pressure is applied[2].
Dr A. C. Bryan	I would like to make a point about the evolution of metabolic needs. The use of a constant RQ of 0.8 may be a trap because it depends on feeding. A diet high in carbohydrate, as compared to an isocaloric fat diet, may increase CO_2 production by 25%, so one of the difficulties in your computations is what figure to use for RQ.
Dr D. Lagneaux	At rest the respiratory gradient reflects the metabolic rate and is thus dependent on the foodstuffs; in practical terms, physiological values around 0.8 to 0.85 are found during childhood, indicating a customary diet.
Bryan	You have mentioned, Dr Lagneaux, that from the first day of life you used an R value of 0.7 because at this age the infant is mainly burning its own fat. The changes observed between birth and a week of age could very well be due to a change in the diet yielding higher RQ values.
Lagneaux	0.7 for R seems well documented for the immediate neonatal period with a progressive rise to 0.8 afterwards when the babies received breast milk. Effectively different kinds of diet can explain the discrepancies found in published data.
Gaultier	You said that convection time plus diffusion time was less during the first 2 months of life than inspiratory time. What is the extra inspiratory time used for?
Lagneaux	I wanted to say that inspiratory time is large enough to obtain theoretical equilibration for P_{CO_2} and P_{O_2}. As CO_2 and O_2 continuously flow through the alveolar surface, steady-state conditions are never effectively reached.
Dr L. B. Strang	A number of people would like Dr Mortola to clarify the importance of a positive airway pressure for liquid absorption.
Mortola	Transpulmonary pressure is always positive in the vital capacity range, which means that the pressure inside the lung must be higher than the pressure outside it. This difference increases the higher the lung volume, and whether the subject exhales actively (by contracting the expiratory muscles) or not, is not going to change this gradient at any given lung volume. During active expiration, in fact, pleural pressure rises; but so

	does airway pressure, and the difference between the two remains constant. Hence whenever lung volume is maintained elevated against an upper airway obstruction (like in the infant during the first minutes after birth) the transpulmonary pressure is higher than at FRC and airway pressure is positive. This represents a 'back-force' for the clearing of the pulmonary fluid from the lung, and could be an important factor in shifting the Starling equilibrium in the direction of absorption.
Strang	Perhaps Dr Egan might like to comment on the variation in the solute permeability of the pulmonary epithelium as a function of lung expansion.
Dr E. A. Egan	The normal epithelium effectively sieves even very small solutes like sodium chloride. If you hyperinflate areas of the lung, you can increase solute permeability, and if you hyperinflate enough you can make the pulmonary epithelium a non-sieving pathway[1]. The increase in solute permeability should certainly facilitate reabsorption of liquid down a pressure gradient.
Strang	We are happy to accept Dr Mortola's suggestion that expansion of the lungs provides a pressure gradient causing reabsorption of liquid, particularly when allied to an increase in the diameter of the pathways for solute absorption across the pulmonary epithelium[1]. Dr Walters produced data earlier to show that there is another mechanism for fluid reabsorption from the lungs which is dependent on β-adrenergic stimulation of Na transport but independent of lung expansion. There is nothing mutually exclusive about these two mechanisms. The mechanism dependent on Na transport is probably the most important prenatally, during labour, and the two mechanisms probably work in tandem in the post-delivery period.

Reference

1. Egan, E. A., Olver, R. E. and Strang, L. B. (1975). Changes in non-electrolyte permeability of alveoli and the absorption of lung liquid at the start of breathing in the lamb. *J. Physiol.*, **244**, 161–79
2. Gaultier, C. and Zinman, R. (1983). Maximal static pressures in healthy children. *Respir. Physiol.*, **51**, 45–61

12
Some Relationships Among Structure, Composition, and Functional Characteristics of Lung Surfactant

J. A. CLEMENTS

It is a truism that the functional characteristics of a complex biological material such as lung surfactant are inherent in its structure and ultimately in its molecular composition. Several recent advances in our knowledge of lung surfactant underscore this principle. The purpose of this article is to show how these results deepen our understanding of surfactant function. No attempt is made in this brief review to cover the assigned topic completely, to repeat many observations that have already been described repeatedly, or to reference every assertion. What is presented here is mainly a commentary on the work of other investigators.

During its life cycle lung surfactant passes through several recognizable forms, and probably through some that have not been recognized. Within the type II alveolar epithelial cells that are thought to carry out its *de novo* synthesis, surfactant components have been associated by immunocytochemical and autoradiographic methods with endoplasmic reticulum, Golgi apparatus, multivesicular bodies, and lamellar bodies. The latter appear to function as accumulators and storage granules for this glycoprotein–lipid complex. It is not evident at present whether the components of the complex are ordered in a specific arrangement in lamellar body lamellae. Its behaviour subsequent to secretion into the alveolar liquid could imply a prior ordering. However, as shown in Fig. 12.1A, ultrarapid freeze–fracture images reveal smooth-surfaced lamellae rather than the pebbled, pitted, or ridged appearances characteristic of protein-rich, cellular membranes. Thus, the M_r 32 kilodalton apoprotein (apo 32) of surfactant that has been localized in lamellar bodies by immunocytochemical techniques may be buried in aqueous and/or lipid phases of the multilamellar structure, or may be too small to be seen by the freeze–fracture method. Aggregation of apo 32 in a particle that can be seen in or against the lipid layer may require an extracellular environment, with calcium ion concentrations of the order of 10^{-3} mol/l.

Freeze–fracture images also suggest that the average repeat distance in the lamellar stack is normally about 100 Å, of which the lipid might

169

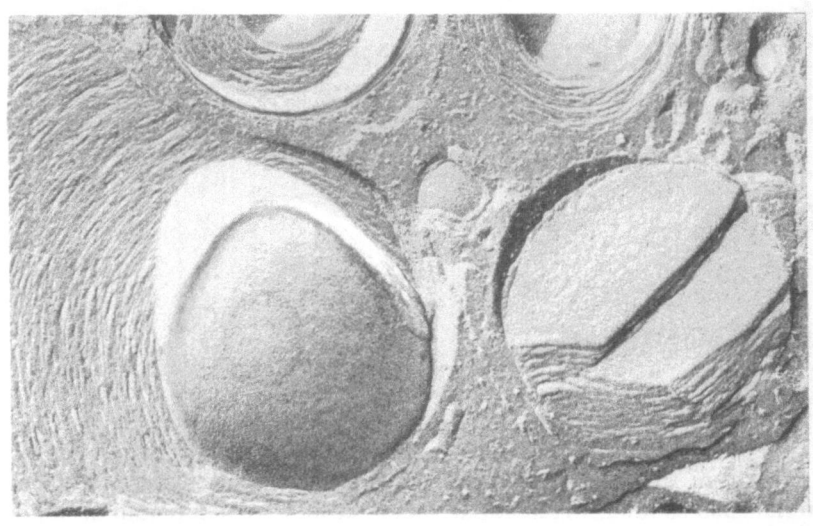

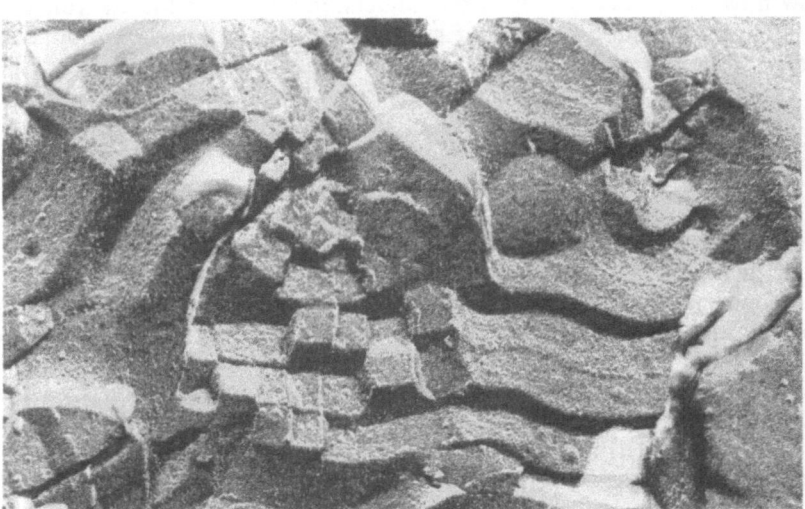

Figure 12.1 Freeze–fracture electron micrographs of lamellar bodies and tubular myelin in adult rat lung tissue prepared by the ultrarapid freezing method of Heuser *et al.*[48]. **A:** Lamellar bodies (× 55 000). Note the lack of particles on the faces of the lamellae. **B:** Tubular myelin, (× 88 000). Particles can be seen in longitudinal rows at the corners of adjacent tubules and in the corners of cross-fractured tubules. Courtesy of M. C. Williams, Department of Anatomy, University of California, San Francisco

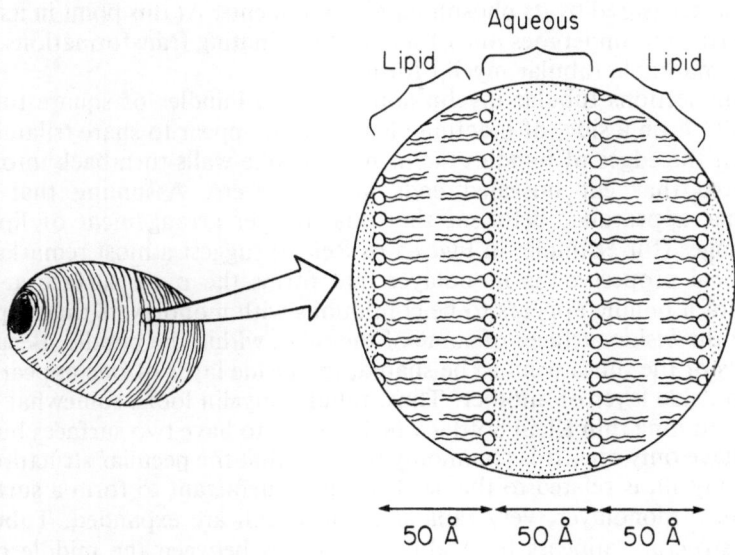

Figure 12.2 Idealized scheme of the multilamellar structure of a lamellar body, showing the alternating lipid bilayers and aqueous layers. The location of apo 32 is not shown

reasonably constitute 50 Å. When lung tissue is prepared for transmission electron microscopy with severely dehydrating methods, however, the repeat distance falls[1] to about 50 Å, indicating that the aqueous layers account for about half of the thickness of the stack. Thus, normal lamellar bodies are apparently about 50% water, a conclusion at odds with proton magnetic resonance measurements made on lamellar body fractions isolated using hypertonic sucrose[2].

The composition of isolated lamellar bodies (summarized in Ref. 3) is consistent with their appearance in tissue, and the phospholipid proportions are approximately the same as in surfactant isolated by lung lavage. These conclusions are subject to the caveat that none of the published methods for isolating lamellar bodies can be expected to yield highly pure, completely intact lamellar bodies. Some components, therefore, are likely to have been gained or lost. As of this writing the quantification of surfactant apoproteins in lamellar bodies has not been reported, though antibody to apo 32 clearly binds to lamellar bodies in lung tissue[4,5]. What we know at this moment about lamellar bodies is concordant with the postulate that lamellar bodies store surfactant components and that these are in the multilamellar arrangement schematized in Fig. 12.2. One would like to say much more about the details of the relationships between apoproteins, lipid, and water in this structure, but current information does not justify doing so.

There is abundant evidence, on the other hand, that when stimulated adequately type II cells release lamellar body contents into the alveolar lining liquid, and that this secretion correlates with the arrival of surfactant, at least as measured by its phospholipid components. At this point in its life cycle surfactant undergoes one of its most fascinating transformations, into the remarkable tubular myelin form[6].

In thin sections tubular myelin appears to be bundles of square tubes, about 420 Å on a side, of indefinite length, that appear to share trilaminar walls. At the edges of bundles the membrane-like walls turn back into the lattice, so that cut unsealed ends are not seen[6]. Assuming that the trilaminar appearance betokens the usual bilayer arrangement of lipids, such images (for example, in Fig. 8a of Ref. 6) suggest a most remarkable topological property: the monolayer that forms the *outer* surface at the surface of a bundle appears to be continuous with monolayers that appear to form the *inside* surfaces of some of the tubes within the bundle. Because the walls of the tubes seem to be shared, the inside layer of one appears to be the outside layer of another. Thus, tubular myelin looks somewhat like an array of long thin Klein bottles which appear to have two surfaces but in reality have only one. It is commonly believed that the peculiar structure of tubular myelin is related to the need for lung surfactant to form a surface film, i.e. a monolayer, very rapidly when alveoli are expanded. Tubular myelin structure appears to establish pathways between the middle of a particle of surfactant and the outer surface, from which alveolar surface films must be generated. This description is only geometric, of course. It does not purport to explain the molecular details of the process of rapid film formation. Nor does it explain at the molecular level how the lipid bilayers can meet at sharp angles, predominantly 90°, in tubular myelin. What fills the centres of the 'intersections'[7]?

Particles, presumably aggregates of protein, are associated with the corners[6-8]. Ultrarapid freeze fracture shows this association clearly (Fig. 12.1B). The particles are lined up in rows where the corners of adjacent tubes meet. In thin sections the particles look filament-like, often appearing to meet in the centre of the tube and forming a diagonal X[8]. Since ultrarapid freeze–fracture images do not reveal particles on the stacked bilayers of lamellar bodies but show them clearly in tubular myelin, aggregation of protein, possibly induced by calcium ions[9], may result in structures that can fill the centres of the 'intersections'. In a geometric sense this would mean that the lipid bilayers of tubular myelin do not actually intersect, but only touch, at the corners of the tubes. In other words the bilayers are not fused at the corners in the usual sense, and this is compatible with the ready reversibility of the lamellar–tubular conversion[11].

A simple calculation, taking the bilayer thickness as 46 Å and the side of a tube as 420 Å , shows that the aqueous phase constitutes about 80% of tubular myelin volume, and that the void in the corners would be 6.2% of the volume of the lipid phase. Is it reasonable to postulate that this void could be filled by part of an apoprotein that also extends to the centre of a tube? Would both apo 32 and apo 10 groups of proteins be involved?

Table 12.1 shows that the abundance of apo 32 correlates better than that of apo 10 with the amount of tubular myelin structure in several surfactant fractions. Both the amount and the pattern of distribution of apo

Table 12.1

	Apo 32 (% wt)	Apo 10 (% wt)	Area of TM (%)‡
'Tubular myelin' (TM)*	24	<2	95
P3+	11	10	25
P4+	4	1	8
S4 vesicles †	0.5	0.3	0

* Calculated from unpublished data of B. J. Benson, M. W. Williams, and K. Sueishi
†Data from Ref. 10
‡Area of TM estimated by point counting of electron micrographs. Vesicles examined by negative staining

10 argue against a significant role for it in tubular myelin formation. In the nearly pure tubular myelin fraction, apo 32 accounts for 24% of the lipid and protein mass. Assuming its density to be 1.3 and that of the hydrated lipid 1.04, about one-quarter of the apo 32 could be accommodated in the corner void, the other three-quarters being in the aqueous phase.

Before carrying this analysis further, it would be in order to ask whether tubular myelin contains the postulated components. Assay of the lipids suggests normal phospholipid-rich surfactant composition[11,12] and immuno-cytochemical staining for the apoprotein heavily labels tubular myelin, especially in the corners[13]. It has been clearly shown that calcium ions are required for tubular myelin formation[11]. Thus, the expected components are present. In addition the surface activity correlates with the presence of the tubular myelin structure and is also calcium-dependent[11].

Is it possible for apo 32 to stretch from the corner to the centre of the tubular myelin tubule, a distance of some 264 Å? Is it likely? Just recently the complete 231 and 228 amino acid sequences of the canine[14] and human[15] apoproteins have been determined and they show very high homology with each other (73%). They are unusual in containing a collagen-like (Gly–X–Y) sequence of 24 triplets near the amino terminus. This is preceded by 7 or 10 rather hydrophilic residues and followed by another relatively hydrophilic stretch of 17 residues. If these regions were in an alpha-helical conformation (with a pitch of 1.5 Å per residue) and the Gly–X–Y triplets were in their usual collagen-like triple helix (with a pitch of 2.9 Å per residue) the length of the chains would be about 252 Å, that is, approximately one-half the length of the aqueous phase diagonal of tubular myelin. It seems possible, therefore, that the X seen in thin sections of tubular myelin[8] could represent the filamentous portions of four apoprotein trimers, linked together at or near their amino termini, perhaps by calcium ions. Presumably the rod-like character of the triple helix[16] would help to stabilize the diagonal dimension of tubular myelin and through symmetry enforce a square pattern on the structure in cross-section.

In the rest of the amino acid sequence there are six hydrophobic regions of 6 to 10 residues each, totalling 46, or about 25% of the protein. These are separated by rather hydrophilic regions, including the putative site (Asn 190) of glycosylation. Since these hydrophobic regions are calculated to have a high potential for alpha-helix formation[17], it seems possible that, properly folded, they occupy the void in the lipids at the corners of tubular myelin. The hydrophobic segments are only half the typical length of lipid bilayer-spanning alpha helices[18], and it is difficult to arrange them in sensible patterns that would span both layers of the lipid. Whatever the fine details of the protein-folding and association may eventually prove to be, it seems clear that apo 32 contains enough hydrophobic residues to fill the lipid voids in the corners of tubular myelin. The rest of the more hydrophilic regions probably remain exposed to the aqueous phase, especially the glycosylated segment, where they can be recognized by ligands, such as concanavalin A[19] or, one might suppose, surface membrane protein of alveolar epithelial cells after tubular myelin has disaggregated. Thus the dimensions of the apoprotein are consistent with those of the tubular myelin structure, and the protein/lipid mass ratio is correct if one-quarter of the protein is buried in the corners.

Figure 12.3 shows these ideas in a highly speculative model, using average dimensions for tubular myelin. Viewing the schema along a diagonal makes it obvious that the dimensions of the protein determine the size and shape of the tubular myelin lattice, provided of course that the model is correct. If specific protein–protein interactions occur in the corners, these would presumably help to keep tubules in register laterally while permitting them to slide longitudinally against each other. Figure 12.3 does not attempt to depict any superstructure that the apoprotein molecules may form. Molecules containing collagen-like sequences such as collagen[16], C1q[20], and acetylcholinesterase of *Torpedo*[21] form supercoils that are apparently critical to their functions. Plotting the collagen-like sequence of apo 32 on a triple helix net reveals hydrophobic periodicities that could facilitate superhelix formation[22]. Whether apo 32 forms such structures is not known. Its amino acid sequence and susceptibility to bacterial collagenase suggest that it may[14].

Despite the simplicity of Fig. 12.3, it does not really explain the functions of tubular myelin. Perhaps the interaction of apo 32 and lipids results in a secondary annulus of disordered lipids around the protein[23] that can generate monolayers more rapidly than neat lipids. Possibly apo 32 binds specifically to certain of the lipids in surfactant and organizes them into a substructure that facilitates film formation[24,26]. The observation that the abundance of apo 10 does not correlate well with the amount of tubular myelin in surfactant subfractions does not rule out an important role for apo 10 in speeding surface film formation. It is apparently the major (or only) protein in an artificial surfactant that has excellent adsorption properties[27]. Evidence has been presented that the positive effect of apo 10 on adsorption rate is further enhanced by addition of apo 32[28]. The meaning of these results is not yet clear.

From the general perspective of energetics the structure of tubular myelin is very improbable. The negentropy it implies must be compensated

420 Å

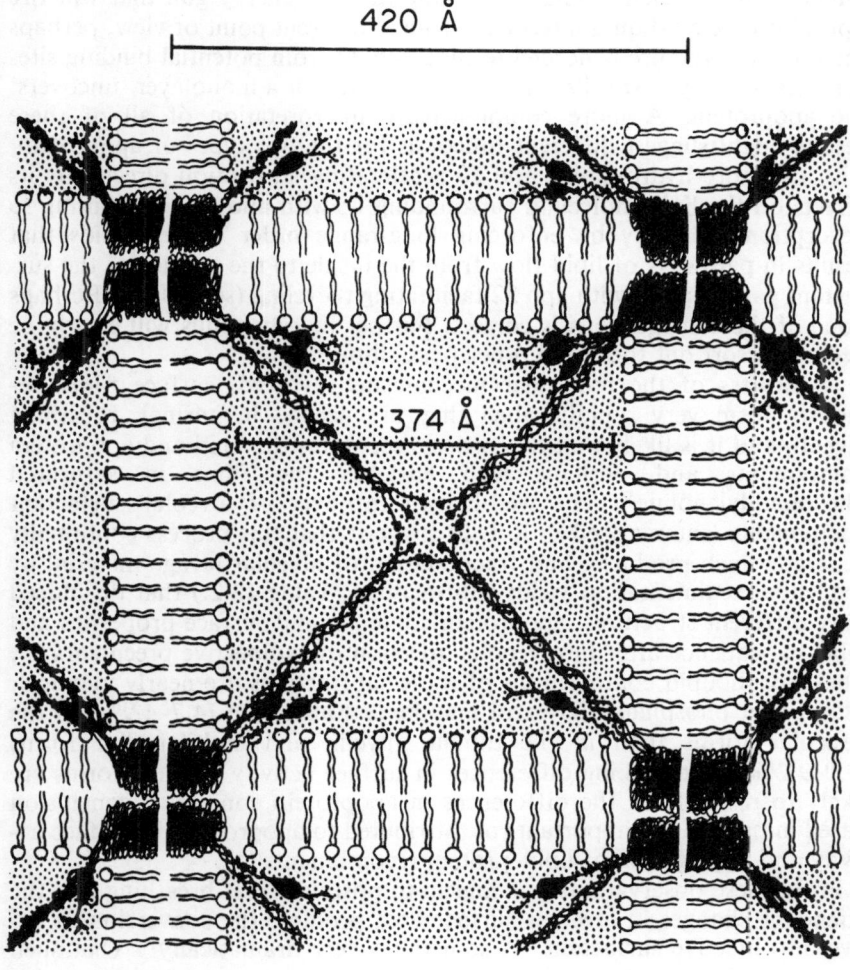

374 Å

Figure 12.3 Speculative model of tubular myelin structure, emphasizing the role of apo 32. The filamentous amino terminal parts of the postulated triple helices are indicated by intertwined spirals stretching from the corners to the centre of the tube. The hydrophobic regions are shown packed into the corner voids of the lipid layers. The (presumably globular) carboxy terminal glycosylated ends of the three associated chains are shown as cobra-like projections into the corners of the aqueous phases, the forked tongues representing the branched carbohydrate chains[49]. The location of apo 10 is not known

in some way. Presumably, uptake of water (80% in tubular myelin vs. 50% in lamellar bodies) and binding of calcium ions during tubular myelin formation pay the free energy bill, including that of curving the lipids in the corners[29,30]. Both long- and short-range intermolecular forces must be involved[31], and summation of all of these for the lamellar body to tubular myelin change would seem unattainable at present. In a crude sense one might think of calcium ions as cocking the free energy gun that will fire lipids into the air–liquid interface. From a different point of view, perhaps the tubular structure is needed to hide apo 32 from potential binding sites for uptake on type II cells[32] until the formation of a monolayer 'uncovers' the apoprotein. A more comprehensive interpretation of all of these results might suggest different functions for the two types of apoprotein, with the more hydrophobic apo 10 accelerating adsorption directly by its effects on the lipid molecules surrounding it; with apo 32 contributing to adsorption indirectly by enforcing long-range order on the lipids that results in pathways of lipid flow from the inside to the surface of the surfactant particle; and with apo 32 facilitating recycling (see below). Perhaps none of these suggestions is correct. Further investigations will clearly be needed to sort out these and other possibilities.

Regardless of the molecular mechanisms involved, surface films obviously form very rapidly when they are needed in normal, breathing alveoli, and it is likely that this process separates the lipid and apoprotein components and perhaps also enriches the films in saturated phosphatidylcholine[33]. The well-known turnover of alveolar surfactant components (summarized in Ref. 3) suggests that this process continually generates such products, and fractionation of alveolar lavage material by sequential sedimentation yields subfractions (Table 12.2.) that do indeed have different structures, apoprotein contents, and surface properties and label in sequence after intravenous injection of radioactive precursors[10,34]. The phospholipid compositions of these subfractions are nearly identical, except that phosphatidylglycerol may be less abundant (4.7-4.9%) in the vesicular forms than in the tubular myelin and multilamellar forms (9.0-9.2%). The striking differences in surface activity of these forms are likely to result from the differences in apoprotein content, a conclusion based in part on the important role attributed to apoproteins in surface activity and aggregation of lipid–protein recombinants[24-28].

From these observations it is logical to postulate that breathing and the attendant changes in alveolar surface area promote the conversion of active into inactive surfactant[35,36], sometimes very dramatically[37]. That such changes are more than laboratory artifacts is suggested by the major decreases in sedimentable surfactant phospholipid that occur in newborn rabbits (fetuses—79%; 2 hours of breathing—62%; 4 days—37%)[38]. In adult rat lungs the sedimentable fraction can be decreased from 36% to 18% by a deep breath given after a period of underventilation[36]. Thus it appears that the balance between the active and the inactive fractions of surfactant may vary from 4 : 1 to 1 : 4 in normal lungs, depending upon age and ventilatory status. The exact mechanisms that effect these interconversions are not known in detail yet, but it is clearly important to understand them and how they are controlled. Besides mechanical forces, enzymatic and cellular reactions might be involved, or a combination of processes.

The final step in the life cycle of lung surfactant is removal from the alveolar lumen. In some ways this is the most mysterious aspect of surfactant turnover. Only occasional deposits of tubular myelin or multilamellar material are seen normally in alveolar macrophages and only minor

Table 12.2 Properties of subfractions of alveolar surfactant

	P3	P4	P5
Minimum surface tension (mN m^{-1})	4	3	12
Adsorption rate $\dfrac{\text{ml} \times \text{min}}{\mu\text{mol phospholipid}}$	1010	510	0.30
Apoprotein 28–36 kDa (%)	26	24	6
Apoprotein 10–14 kDa (%)	23	5	3

Abundance of apoproteins is given as percentage of total protein. Data are taken from Refs. 10 and 34

amounts of phospholipid appear in the airways[39]. Some apoprotein is found in the macrophages by immunocytochemical staining[13], but type I cells appear to take up trivial amounts. Electron micrographs fail to show distinct images of phospholipid structures in transit into type II cells. Yet tracer studies with instillation of surfactant clearly demonstrate prompt movement of label from alveoli into lamellar bodies[40–42]. While the form in which the components normally travel into type II cells is not evident, the main pathway is probably an endocytotic vesicular one that leads through multivesicular bodies to lamellar bodies[32,43,44]. Recent evidence from tracer studies in rabbits has been interpreted as showing that mechanical ventilation may shift the uptake away from lamellar bodies to a 'lysosomal compartment'[45]. The authors postulate that disaggregated surfactant may be recognized differently by type II cells. The possibility that apo 32 acts as a ligand in receptor-mediated endocytosis is supported by very recent experiments in which the uptakes into lamellar bodies of instilled alveolar surfactant subfractions were compared. The apo 32-rich fractions were taken up 2 to 3 times faster than the apo 32-poor fraction[42]. In other studies incorporation of low molecular weight hydrophobic proteins isolated from alveolar lavage material into liposomes enhanced their uptake by isolated type II cells[46]. At present the relative importance of the two types of protein in stimulating uptake is not clear. It seems possible that they could act at separate sites and affect type II cell metabolism differently, as indeed may lipid components of surfactant[47]. Information on these effects is fragmentary at present. Much additional investigation of all aspects of surfactant recycling is needed before the interrelationships between protein composition, lipid composition, ultrastructure of the particles, cellular binding sites, internalization processes, and intracellular handling of the component molecules will become clear. It is obvious that such information is essential if we are to understand properly the interactions between the cellular processing of surfactant components, the physicochemical states of alveolar surfactant, and the mechanical properties of the lungs.

Acknowledgements

I thank Drs B. J. Benson, J. Goerke, S. Hawgood, M. C. Williams, and J. R. Wright for helpful discussions of several of the topics in this paper and for their generosity in sharing unpublished data. I am grateful to B. A. Ehrlich and S. Fox for preparation of the manuscript. This work was supported by NIH Program Project Grant HL-24075. The author is a Career Investigator of the American Heart Association.

References

1. Douglas, W. H. J., Redding, R. A. and Stein, M. (1975). The lamellar substructure of osmiophilic inclusion bodies present in rat type II alveolar pneumonocytes. *Tissue and Cell*, **7**, 137–42
2. Grathwohl, C., Newman, G. E., Phizackerley, P. J. R. and Town, M. H. (1979). Structural studies on lamellated osmiophilic bodies isolated from pig lung. ^{31}P NMR results and water content. *Biochim. Biophys. Acta*, **552**, 509–18
3. King, R. J. and Clements, J. A. (1985). Lipid synthesis and surfactant turnover in the lungs. In Fishman, A. P. and Fisher, A. B. (eds.) *Handbook of Physiology. Vol. I*, pp. 309–36. (Washington, DC: Am. Physiol. Soc.)
4. Coalson, J. J. and King, R. J. (1984). Immunocytochemical localization of rat surfactant using a gold immunocolloid marker. *Am. Rev. Respir. Dis.*, **129**, 295A
5. Walker, S. R., Williams, M. C. and Benson, B. J. (1984). Immunocytochemical localization of a major surfactant-specific apoprotein on ultrathin frozen sections of rat lung. *Am. Rev. Respir. Dis.*, **129**, 295A
6. Williams, M. C. (1977). Conversion of lamellar body membranes into tubular myelin in alveoli of fetal rat lungs. *J. Cell Biol.*, **72**, 260–77
7. Chi, E. Y. and Lagunoff, D. (1978). Linear arrays of intramembranous particles in pulmonary tubular myelin. *Proc. Natl. Acad. Sci.*, **75**, 6225–9
8. Williams, M. C. (1982). Ultrastructure of tubular myelin and lamellar bodies in fast-frozen adult rat lung. *Exp. Lung Res.*, **4**, 37–46
9. Sanders, R. L., Hassett, R. J. and Vatter, A. E. (1980). Isolation of lung lamellar bodies and their conversion to tubular myelin figures in vitro. *Anat. Rec.*, **198**, 485–501
10. Wright, J. R., Benson, B. J., Williams, M. C., Goerke, J. and Clements, J. A. (1984). Protein composition of rabbit alveolar surfactant subfractions. *Biochim. Biophys. Acta*, **791**, 320–32
11. Benson, B. J., Williams, M. C., Sueishi, K., Goerke, J. and Sargeant, T. (1984). Role of calcium ions in the structure and function of pulmonary surfactant. *Biochim. Biophys. Acta*, **793**, 18–27
12. Gil, J. and Reiss, O. K. (1978). Isolation and characterization of lamellar bodies and tubular myelin from rat lung homogenates. *J. Cell Biol.*, **58**, 152–71
13. Williams, M. C. and Benson, B. J. (1981). Immunocytochemical localization and identification of the major surfactant protein in adult rat lung. *J. Histochem. Cytochem.*, **29**, 291–305
14. Benson, B., Hawgood, S., Schilling, J., Clements, J. A., Damn, D., Cordell, B., and White, R. T. (1985). Structure of canine pulmonary surfactant apoprotein: cDNA and complete amino acid sequence. *Proc. Natl. Acad. Sci.*, **82**, 6379–83
15. White, R. T., Damm, D., Miller, J., Spratt, K., Schilling, J., Hawgood, S., Benson, B. and Cordell, B. (1985). Isolation and expression of the human pulmonary surfactant apoprotein gene. *Nature*, **317**, 361–3
16. Piez, K. A. (1984). Hierarchical structure and assembly of type I collagen: In Wetlaufer, D. B. (ed.) *The Protein Folding Problem*. pp. 47–63 (Boulder, Colorado: Westview Press)
17. Chou, P. Y. and Fasman, G. D. (1978). Empirical predictions of protein conformation. *Ann. Rev. Biochem.*, **47**, 251–76

18. Kyte, J. and Doolittle, R. F., (1982). A simple method for displaying the hydropathic character of a protein. *J. Mol. Biol.*, **157**, 105-32

19. Nir, I. and Pease, D. C. (1977). Polysaccharides in lung alveoli. *Am. J. Anat.*, **147**, 457-70

20. Reid, K. B. M. (1982). Proteins containing collagen sequences. In Weiss, J. B. and Jayson, M. I. V. (eds.) *Collagen in Health and Disease.* pp. 18-27. (Edinburgh: Churchill Livingstone)

21. Lee, S. L. and Taylor, P. (1982). Structural characterization of the asymmetric (17 + 13) Species of acetylcholinesterase from Torpedo. II. Component peptides obtained by selective proteolysis and disulfide bond reduction. *J. Biol. Chem.*, **257**, 12292-301

22. Bear, R. S., Adams, J. B. and Poulton, J. W. (1978). Disclosure by Fourier methods of a long-range pattern of non-polar residues in the alpha 1 (I) sequence of collagen. *J. Mol. Biol.*, **118**, 123-6

23. Lentz, B. R., Clubb, K. W., Barrow, D. A. and Meissner, G. (1983). Ordered and disordered phospholipid domains coexist in membranes containing the calcium pump protein of sarcoplasmic reticulum. *Proc. Natl. Acad. Sci.*, **80**, 2917-21

24. King, R. J., Carmichael, M. C. and Horowitz, P. M. (1983). Reassembly of lipid–protein complexes of pulmonary surfactant. Proposed mechanism of interaction. *J. Biol. Chem.*, **258**, 10672-80

25. Hawgood, S., Benson, B. J. and Hamilton, R. L. (1985). Effects of a surfactant-associated protein and calcium ions on the structure and surface activity of lung surfactant lipids. *Biochemistry*, **24**, 184-90

26. Notter, R. H., Finkelstein, J. N. and Taubold, R. D. (1983). Comparative adsorption of natural lung surfactant, extracted phospholipids, and artificial phospholipid mixture to the air–water interface. *Chem. Phys. Lipids*, **33**, 67-80

27. Tanaka, Y., Takei, T. and Kanazawa, Y. (1983). Lung surfactants. II. Effects of fatty acids, triacylglycerols, and protein on the activity of lung surfactant. *Chem. Pharm. Bull.*, **31**, 4100-9

28. Suzuki, Y. (1982). Effect of protein, cholesterol, and phosphatidylglycerol on the surface activity of the lipid–protein complex reconstituted from pig pulmonary surfactant. *J. Lipid Res.*, **23**, 62-9

29. Rand, R. P. (1981). Interacting phospholipid bilayers: measured forces and induced structural changes. *Ann. Rev. Biophys. Bioeng.*, **10**, 277-314

30. Gruner, S. M. (1985). Intrinsic curvature hypothesis for biomembrane lipid composition: a role for nonbilayer lipids. *Proc. Natl. Acad. Sci.*, **82**, 3665-9

31. Israelachvili, J. N. and Ninham, B. W. (1977). Intermolecular forces – the long and short of it. *J. Colloid Interface Sci.*, **58**, 14-25

32. Williams, M. C. (1984). Endocytosis in alveolar type II cells: effects of charge and size of tracers. *Proc. Natl. Acad. Sci.*, **81**, 6054-8

33. Clements, J. A. Functions of alveolar lining. *Am. Rev. Respir. Dis.*, **115**, (part 2), 67-71

34. Magoon, M. W., Wright, J. R., Baritussio, A., Williams, M. C., Goerke, J., Benson B. J., Hamilton, R. L. and Clements, J. A. (1983). Subfractionation of lung surfactant. Implications for metabolism and surface activity. *Biochim. Biophys. Acta*, **750**, 18-31

35. Wyszogrodski, I., Kyei-Aboagye, K., Taeusch, H. W. and Avery, M. E. (1975). Surfactant inactivation by hyperventilation: conservation by end-expiratory pressure. *J. Appl. Physiol.*, **38**, 461-6

36. Thet, L. A., Clerch, L., Massaro, G. D. and Massaro, D. (1979). Changes in sedimentation of surfactant in ventilated excised rat lungs. Physical alterations in surfactant associated with the development and reversal of atelectasis. *J. Clin. Invest.*, **64**, 600-8

37. Clements, J. A., Goerke, J., Wright, J. R. and Beppu, O. (1984). Turnover of lung surfactant. In Herzog, H. (ed.) *Progress in Respiration Research.* pp. 133-42. (Basel: Karger)

38. Moxley, M. A., Harlow, R. D., and Kotas, R. V. (1982). Sedimentation characteristics of new born rabbit surfactant. *Fed. Proc.*, **41**, 1602A

39. Baritussio, A. G., Magoon, M. W., Goerke, J. and Clements, J. A. (1981). Precursor–product relationship between rabbit type II cell lamellar bodies and alveolar surface-active material. Surfactant turnover time. *Biochim. Biophys. Acta*, **666**, 382-93

40. Hallman, M., Epstein, B. L. and Gluck, L. (1981). Analysis of labeling and clearance of lung surfactant phospholipids in rabbit. Evidence of bidirectional surfactant flux between lamellar bodies and alveolar lavage. *J. Clin. Invest.*, **68**, 742-51

41. Jacobs, H. C., Jobe, A. H., Ikegami, M. and Jones, S. (1985). Reutilization of phosphatidylglycerol and phosphatidylethanolamine by the pulmonary surfactant system in 3-day-old rabbits. *Biochim. Biophys. Acta.*, **834**, 172-9

42. Wright, J. R., Wager, R. E., Huang, M. and Clements, J. A. (1985). Differential uptake of surfactant subfractions from alveoli into lamellar bodies of adult rabbit lungs. *Fed. Proc.*, **44**, 1023A

43. Williams, M. C. (1984). Uptake of lectins by pulmonary alveolar type II cells: subsequent deposition into lamellar bodies. *Proc. Natl. Acad. Sci.*, **81**, 6383-7

44. Moxley, M. A., Corpus, V. M., Westrich, D., Lawson, E., Mumm, S. and Longmore, W. J. (1985) Evidence of the direct incorporation of pulmonary surfactant into alveolar type II epithelial cells in primary culture. *Fed. Proc.*, **44**, 1606A

45. Ennema, J. J., Reijngoud, D. J., Wildevuur, C. R. H. and Egberts, J. (1984). Effects of artificial ventilation on surfactant phospholipid metabolism in rabbits. *Respir. Physiol.*, **58**, 15-23

46. Claypool, W. D., Wang, D. L., Chander, A. and Fisher, A. B. (1984). An ethanol/ether soluble apoprotein from rat lung surfactant augments liposome uptake by isolated granular pneumocytes. *J. Clin. Invest.*, **74**, 677-84

47. Miles, P. R., Wright, J. R., Bowman, L. and Castranova, V. (1983). Incorporation of [^{3}H] palmitate into disaturated phosphatidylcholines in alveolar type II cells isolated by centrifugal elutriation. *Biochim. Biophys. Acta*, **753**, 107-18

48. Heuser, J. E., Reese, T. S. and Landis, D. M. D. (1976). Preservation of synaptic structure by rapid freezing. *Cold Spring Harbor Symp. Quant. Biol.*, **40**, 17-24

49. Munakata, H., Nimberg, R. D., Snider, G. L., Robsin, A. G., Van Halbeek, H., Vliegenthart, J. F. G. and Schmid, K. (1982). The structure of the carbohydrate units of the 36K glycoprotein derived from the lung lavage of a patient with alveolar proteinosis by high resolution ^{1}H-NMR spectroscopy. *Biochem. Biophys. Res. Commun.*, **108**, 1401-5

Discussion

Dr B. T. Smith	I was fascinated by your speculation on the structure of the protein and how it might interact functionally with the tubular myelin structure. You considered the potential role of the amino terminus in calcium binding and of the hydrophilic portion in determining the right angle in the structure of tubular myelin; the hydrophobic portion was seen as interacting with the lipid, but you didn't say very much about the final hydrophylic portion and its glycosylated area.
Dr J. A. Clements	It is still too early to say, but it appears that removal of the sialic acid terminus of the carbohydrate tree does not modify the surface activity of the material. Comparable experiments have not been done on uptake but we would like to think that – as with many other secreted proteins – glycosylation provides an address which may be important in guiding the protein through intracellular pathways and which may, in this particular case, allow recognition by the surface of the type II cells – presumably an essential step in endocytic uptake.
Dr J. J. Batenburg	Is it possible from the freeze–fracture studies to quantitate the amount of material (presumably protein) in the corners of the tubular myelin? Is the 8% protein in the lamellar bodies enough to account for all the fuzzy material we can see in the corners of the myelin tubes?
Clements	The 8% refers to 'whole' surfactant, but analysis of a tubular myelin-rich fraction (approximately 95% tubular myelin) shows it to contain 24% protein, and this with the remaining 76% phospholipid will space-fill the array proposed in my speculative diagram.
Dr L. M. G. Van Golde	It appears that the percentage reutilization is less in the adult lung. You suggest it could be more than 90% in the newborn whereas it has been estimated at only 23% in adult rabbits[1]. Do you have any evidence at what age during fetal development this reutilization might start?
Clements	No. We have no data on that and I think, possibly, the story is not completely known on whether or not there are really such large differences in reutilization. One difficulty in interpreting the published experiments[1,2] is that the quantities of surfactant in the alveoli of the newborn and adult were so very different (per unit of body weight), which complicates the measuring of turnover rates. I am more impressed by the similarities in the surfactant tracer data for adult and newborn animals than by the differences. I think that further analysis may suggest a high proportion of reutilization of the phospholipid components in adult as well as newborn animals.
Van Golde	In view of the structure of the surfactant apoprotein is it possible that it could penetrate the surfactant monolayer?
Clements	That's a difficult question to answer. By analogy with earlier studies on the penetration of surface films by proteins[3], I would expect even the most hydrophobic of proteins to be squeezed out of a monolayer at film pressures above 35 mN/m. If the surfactant apoprotein is in some way special we could not immediately extrapolate from these earlier results, but I would still be quite surprised if a protein which is one-quarter hydrophobic and three-quarters hydrophilic would penetrate the lipids in

	a monomolecular layer at a film pressure of 65 to 70 mN/m – the value at FRC. Under such conditions I would assume that the protein hangs in festoons beneath the surface and that little if any penetrates the surface film.
Dr G. Enhorning	At what gestation do you think the protein is synthesized in the fetal lung?
Clements	Gikas *et al.*[4] took fetal lung fluid from lambs at various gestational ages from 102 days to 147 days and showed by immunoassay that the 32 000 dalton apoprotein appeared at about 115–125 days. At that age there is essentially none of the 10 000 dalton protein. Then at 135–145 days, when there is a great increase in surfactant production, the 10 000 dalton protein appeared.
Dr M. Hallman	To return to reutilization, I think the present data[5] indicate that if you compare the newborn and adult rabbit, the fluxes due to reutilization are practically the same. Why adults have a lower *percentage* reutilization is that the biological half-life of surfactant is faster in the adult rabbit. Do your data suggest that the protein-rich fraction of surfactant is taken up much more quickly than the rest?
Clements	Much more quickly[6]. As you know Williams[7] has shown a vesicular pathway for uptake of lectins which specifically bind to the surface of type II cells, and her experiments with ferritin-labelled lectins show a pathway likely to be followed by surface-active material when it is internalized. Williams is also doing autoradiographic studies with labelled surface-active material. She will try to get more direct evidence on whether surfactant components travel that same vesicular pathway.

References

1. Jacobs, H. C., Ikegami, M., Jobe, A. H., Berry, D. D. and Jones, S. (1985). Reutilization of surfactant phosphatidycholine in adult rabbits. *Biochim. Biophys. Acta.*, **837**, 77–84
2. Jacobs, H., Jobe, A. and Jones, A. (1982). Surfactant phosphatidylcholine source, fluxes, and turnover times in 3-day-old, 10-day-old and adult rabbits. *J. Biol. Chem.*, **257**, 1805–10
3. Kaiser, E. T. and Kezdy, F. J. (1983). Secondary structures of proteins and peptides in ampiphilic environments (a review). *Proc. Natl. Acad. Sci. USA.*, **80**, 1137–43
4. Gikas, E. G., King, R. J., Mescher, E. J., Platzker, A. C. G., Kitterman, J. A., Ballard, P. L., Benson, B. J., Tooley, W. H. and Clements, J. A. (1977). Radioimmunoassay of pulmonary surface-active material in the tracheal fluid of the fetal lamb. *Am. Rev. Respir. Dis.*, **115**, 587–93
5. Jacobs, H., Jobe, A., Ikegami, M., Conaway, D. (1983). Significance of reutilization of surfactant phosphatidylcholine. *J. Biol. Chem.* **258**, 4159–65
6. Wright, J. R., Wager, R. E., Hamilton, R. L., Huang, M. and Clements, J. A. (1986). Uptake of lung surfactant subfractions into lamellar bodies of adult rabbit lungs. *J. Appl. Physiol.*, **60**, 817–25
7. Williams, M. C. (1984). Uptake of lectins by pulmonary alveolar type II cells: subsequent deposition into lamellar bodies. *Proc. Natl. Acad. Sci. USA*, **81**,6383–7

13
Aspects of Surfactant Metabolism in the Adult and Perinatal Lung

L. M. G. VAN GOLDE, R. BURKHARDT, A. C. J. DE VRIES AND J. J. BATENBURG

INTRODUCTION: COMPOSITION OF PULMONARY SURFACTANT

Pulmonary surfactant is a highly surface-active material which lines the alveolar surfaces. Its major function is to prevent collapse of the alveoli by decreasing the surface tension at low lung volumes[1]. The composition of extracellular surfactant isolated from bronchoalveolar lavage fluid has been characterized for a variety of mammalian species[2]. The following general picture emerges from these studies. The majority of pulmonary surfactant (approx. 90%) consists of lipids. About 85% of the surfactant lipid is phospholipid with the fully saturated dipalmitoylphosphatidylcholine (DPPC) as the most abundant single component. There is general agreement that DPPC, which comprises almost half of the total surfactant lipids, is the principal surface-active component of pulmonary surfactant[3]. The other surfactant lipids may play an important role in ensuring a rapid adsorption and spreading of surfactant at the air–liquid boundary[4]. Another general conclusion from investigations with various mammalian species appears to be the striking similarity between the lipid composition of extracellular surfactant and that of lamellar bodies[2]. This endorses the generally accepted view that the lamellar bodies are the type II cell vehicles for the secretion of surfactant into the liquid layer lining the alveoli.

In addition to lipids, pulmonary surfactant contains 8–10% proteins and a small amount of carbohydrate. Studies with purified canine surfactant showed the presence of at least two surfactant-specific proteins, with molecular masses of about 34 kilodaltons (kDa) and 10 kDa, respectively. Proteins with a molecular mass of 28–40 kDa, similar to the 34 kDa protein of canine lung surfactant, were subsequently identified in surfactant preparations from a number of different mammalian species (see King[5] for a review of these studies). In the alveolar lining these proteins appear to be associated primarily with the tubular myelin fraction, which is believed to be the immediate precursor of the monolayer at the air/water interface[6]. In this respect it is interesting that the 34 kDa protein of canine surfactant associates readily with surfactant lipids, and that it promotes extremely rapid formation of phospholipid surface films if calcium ions are present[7].

BIOSYNTHESIS OF DIPALMITOYLPHOSPHATIDYLCHOLINE IN ALVEOLAR TYPE II PNEUMOCYTES

The heterogeneity of lung tissue, which may contain as many as 40 different cell types, has long been a serious handicap for studies on surfactant lipid synthesis. As there is no doubt from careful radioautographic/electron micrographic studies[8] that the production of alveolar surfactant is limited to the alveolar epithelial type II cell, results of biochemical experiments with preparations from whole lung should always be interpreted with caution. However, in recent years methods have been developed to isolate virtually pure preparations of type II pneumocytes from adult lung tissue[9]. Efforts to obtain similarly pure preparations of type II cells from fetal lung tissue have so far been somewhat less successful, although Post et al.[10] recently reported a method that yielded a relatively pure (83%) preparation of type II cells from fetal rat lung. It is obvious that isolated type II cells should be the model of choice for investigations on the pathways of surfactant lipid synthesis. It is not surprising that most of the investigations on the pathways involved in the biosynthesis of surfactant lipids have been focused on DPPC, the principal component of surfactant.

Our current ideas about the pathways leading to the production of DPPC in the alveolar type II cells are summarized in Fig. 13.1. Several investigations[11] have provided evidence that DPPC can be synthesized in this cell type by direct synthesis de novo via the CDPcholine pathway. This direct pathway starts with the formation of 1-palmitoyl-sn -glycerol-3-phosphate by acylation of sn -glycerol-3-phosphate with palmitoyl-CoA. The sn-glycerol-3-phosphate which is required for this reaction is formed in the type II cell predominantly by reduction of glucose-derived dihydroxy-yacetonephosphate. 1-Palmitoyl-sn -glycerol-3-phosphate can also be synthesized by acylation of dihydroxyacetonephosphate with palmitoyl-CoA, followed by reduction of the resulting 1-palmitoyldihydroxyacetone-phosphate in the presence of NADPH (Fig. 13.1). It has been estimated by Mason[12] that this latter so-called acyldihydroxyacetonephosphate pathway may contribute for up to 60% to the synthesis of phosphatidic acid in the type II cell. We reported recently[13] that the glycerolphosphate acyltransferase system of type II cells has the potential to synthesize phosphatidic acid with a substantial proportion of the dipalmitoyl species. In view of the earlier evidence that phosphatidic acid phosphatase[14] and cholinephosphotransferase[15] of type II cells do not discriminate against disaturated substrates, dipalmitoylphosphatidic acid can be converted into 1,2-dipalmitoyl-sn-glycerol and, subsequently, into DPPC. The CDPcholine which is required as second substrate for the latter reaction is synthesized in the type II cell from choline, which is taken up from blood. The

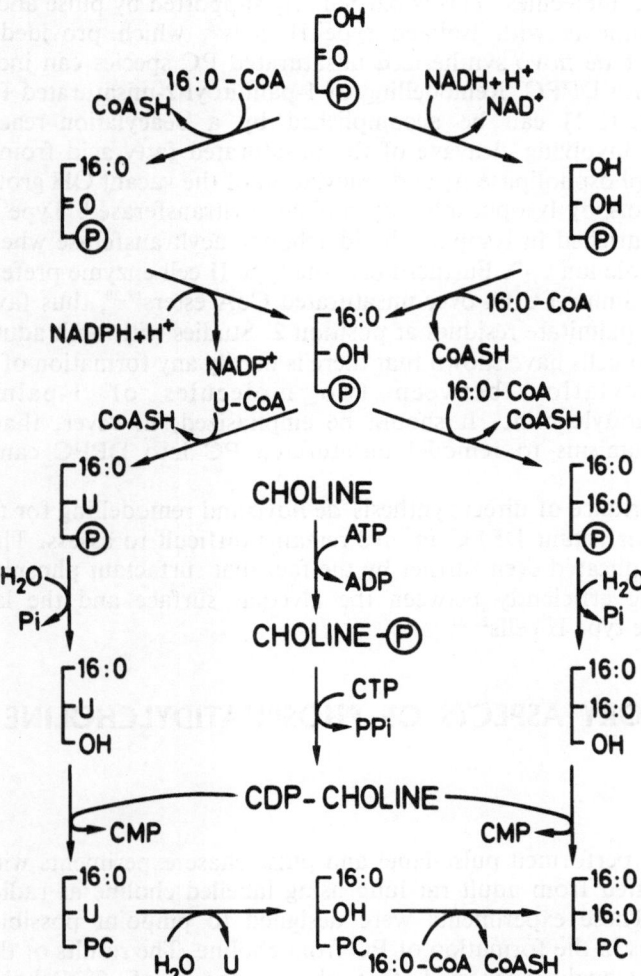

Figure 13.1 Formation of dipalmitoylphosphatidylcholine (DPPC) in alveolar type II cells by direct synthesis *de novo* and by deacylation–reacylation of phosphatidylcholines containing an unsaturated fatty-acyl constituent at postition 2. Substrates, intermediates and products are presented in short-hand formulas. 16:0 = palmitate; U = unsaturated fatty-acyl constituent

choline is converted into CDPcholine by the subsequent action of choline kinase and cholinephosphate cytidylyltransferase. As will be described in a following section, the latter enzyme catalyses in the type II cell a rate-regulatory step in the formation of phosphatidylcholine (PC) from choline.

Recent experiments with isolated type II cells[15,16] endorsed earlier studies with whole lung[17] that DPPC is not only produced by direct synthesis *de novo* via the pathway outlined above, but also by remodelling of unsaturated PC molecules. This is particularly supported by pulse and pulse-chase experiments with isolated type II cells[16], which provided direct evidence that *de novo* synthesized unsaturated PC species can indeed be converted into DPPC. Remodelling of 1-palmitoyl-2-unsaturated PC into DPPC (Fig. 13.1) can be accomplished by a deacylation–reacylation mechanism, involving cleavage of the unsaturated fatty acid from the 2-position by phospholipase A_2 and reacylation of the vacant OH group with palmitoyl-CoA by lysophosphatidylcholine acyltransferase[11]. Type II cells are highly enriched in lysophosphatidylcholine acyltransferase when compared to whole lung[18,19]. Furthermore, the type II cell enzyme preferentially utilizes palmitoyl-CoA over unsaturated CoA esters[18,20], thus favouring the entry of palmitate residues at position 2. Studies with both adult[18] and fetal[21] type II cells have shown that there is hardly any formation of DPPC by transacylation between two molecules of 1-palmitoyl-lysophosphatidylcholine. It should be emphasized, however, that alternative mechanisms to remodel unsaturated PC into DPPC cannot be excluded.

The importance of direct synthesis *de novo* and remodelling for the formation of surfactant DPPC *in vivo* remains difficult to assess. This problem is complicated even further by the fact that surfactant phospholipids are recycling efficiently between the alveolar surface and the lamellar bodies in the type II cells[22,23].

REGULATORY ASPECTS OF PHOSPHATIDYLCHOLINE SYNTHESIS

Adult lung

Post *et al.*[24] performed pulse-label and pulse-chase experiments with type II cells isolated from adult rat lung using labelled choline as radioactive precursor. These experiments were designed to pinpoint possible rate-limiting steps in the formation of PC from choline. The results of their experiments strongly suggested that the synthesis of CDPcholine by cholinephosphate cytidylyltransferase represents such a rate-controlling step in the CDPcholine pathway. This suggestion was strengthened by measurement of the pool sizes of choline and its metabolites in isolated adult rat type II cells. The pool size of cholinephosphate appeared indeed to be much larger than that of choline and CDPcholine[25], which corroborates the concept that the formation of CDPcholine is rate-limiting in the sequence of reactions from choline to PC.

Cholinephosphate cytidylyltransferase shows a bimodal subcellular distribution, as has been demonstrated for a variety of mammalian cell types[26], including type II cells from adult rat lung (R. Burkhardt, J. J. Batenburg and L. M. G. van Golde, unpublished data). The enzyme is found both in the microsomal and in the cytosolic fraction. Vance and Pelech[26] proposed, on the basis of experiments with cultured rat hepatocytes and established cell lines, that the biosynthesis of PC is regulated by translocation of inactive cholinephosphate cytidylyltransferase from the cytosol to the endoplasmic reticulum, where the enzyme becomes activated. They suggested that this translocation is regulated both by reversible phosphorylation of the enzyme and by a direct effect of long-chain fatty acids or acylCoAs on the enzyme.

We recently investigated the effect of increasing concentrations of palmitate on the formation of PC by adult type II cells isolated from rat lung. The type II cells were pulse-labelled with radioactive choline, and subsequently transferred to a chase medium containing unlabelled choline and varying concentrations of palmitate. It is clear from the results shown in Fig. 13.2 that the addition of palmitate exerts a dose-dependent stimulatory effect on PC synthesis. The accelerated appearance of label in PC (Fig 13.2, upper panel) is paralleled by an accelerated disappearance of label from cholinephosphate (Fig. 13.2, lower panel).

In a similar pulse-chase experiment we compared the stimulatory effect on PC synthesis by equal concentrations of palmitate, oleate and linoleate, respectively. Fig. 13.3. shows that palmitate exhibits a larger accelerating effect on the appearance of label into PC (Fig. 13.3, lower panel) and on the disappearance of label from cholinephosphate (Fig. 13.3., upper panel) than either oleate or linoleate. At the beginning of the chase period the radioactivity of CDPcholine in the control cells (without exogenous fatty acids) appeared to be about a factor 50 lower than that of cholinephosphate (data not shown). During the chase period the radioactivity of CDPcholine decreased further. However, this loss of label from CDPcholine was delayed in the presence of fatty acids, most notably by the unsaturated fatty acids.

The findings described above could be explained by a direct effect of fatty acids on the activity of cholinephosphate cytidylyltransferase, possibly by promoting the translocation of the enzyme from the cytosol to the endoplasmic reticulum of the type II cell. We are currently investigating this intriguing possibility.

On the other hand, it should be emphasized that there may be additional enzymes that catalyse rate-regulatory steps in the formation of surfactant PC. These may include glycerolphosphate acyltransferase, the enzyme that commits glycerol-3-phosphate to glycerolipid synthesis, and phosphatidic-acid phosphatase, which may control the rate at which diacylglycerols are produced as substrates for the cholinephosphotransferase reaction. The stimulatory effect of exogenous fatty acids on PC synthesis in type II cells (Figs. 13.2 and 13.3.) could, in principle, also be explained by enhanced production of diacylglycerols. In this light it is important to mention that phosphatidic-acid phosphatase, which controls the production of diacylglycerols, also appears to be a ubiquitous enzyme. Studies with hepatocytes[27] have provided evidence that phosphatidic-acid phosphatase, like cholinephosphate cytidylyltransferase, can be activated by translocation from the cytosol to the endoplasmic reticulum, and that this translocation is enhanced in the presence of fatty acids. On the other hand, if the stimulatory effect of fatty acids on PC synthesis from choline (Figs 13.2 and

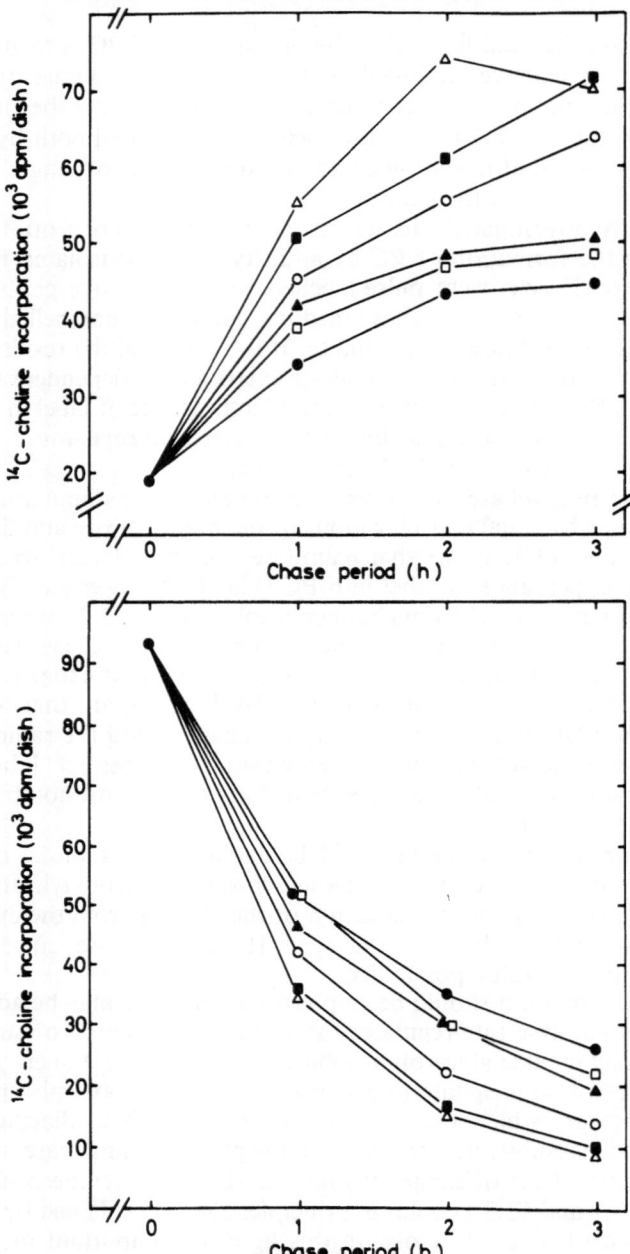

Figure 13.2 Effects of various concentrations of palmitate on the metabolism of [Me -¹⁴C] choline in type II cells isolated from adult rat lung. Type II cells in primary culture were labelled for 1 h with [Me -¹⁴C] choline (spec. act. 59 200 dpm/nmol) as described by Post *et al.*[24]. Subsequently the cells were exposed to fresh medium containing unlabelled choline in the same concentration as during the pulse period[24]. Palmitate (complexed to bovine serum albumin, molar ratio 5.3 : 1) was added to the chase medium in the following concentrations: 0.002 mmol/l (□—□), 0.01 mmol/l (▲—▲), 0.05 mmol/l (O—O), 0.2 mmol/l (■—■) and 1.0 mmol/l (△—△). Controls (●—●) contained no palmitate in the chase medium. After the indicated periods the radioactivity incorporated into phosphatidylcholine (upper panel) and cholinephosphate (lower panel) was determined as reported earlier[24]

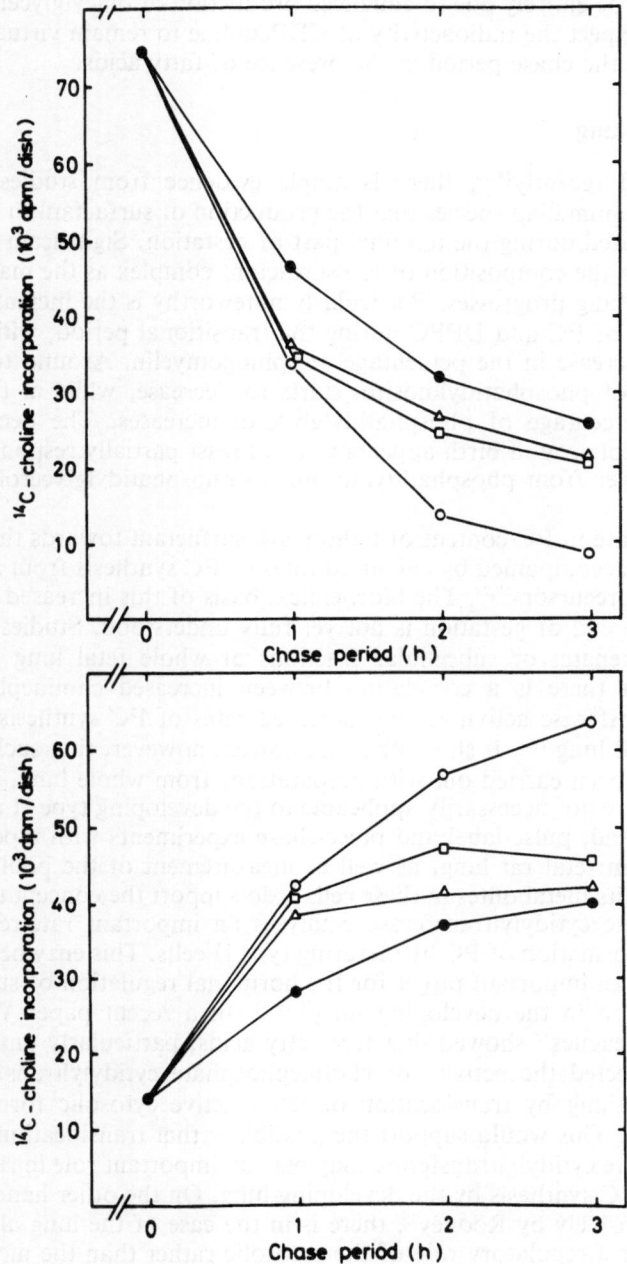

Figure 13.3 Effects of equal concentrations of palmitate, oleate and linoleate on the metabolism of [*Me*-¹⁴C] choline in type II cells isolated from adult rat lung. O——O: 0.2 mmol/l palmitate in the chase medium; □——□ : 0.2 mmol/l oleate; △——△ : 0.2 mmol/l linoleate; ●——● : no fatty acids in the chase medium. For other incubation conditions see legend to Fig. 13.2. Upper panel: cholinephosphate; lower panel: phosphatidylcholine

13.3) would be entirely due to enhanced production of diacylglycerols, one would not expect the radioactivity of CDPcholine to remain virtually constant during the chase period in the presence of fatty acids.

Developing lung

As reviewed recently[28,29], there is ample evidence from studies with a variety of mammalian species that the production of surfactant in the fetal lung is initiated during the terminal part of gestation. Significant changes take place in the composition of the surfactant complex as the maturation of the fetal lung progresses. Particularly noteworthy is the increase in the proportions of PC and DPPC during the transitional period, with a concomitant decrease in the percentage of sphingomyelin. Around term, the proportion of phosphatidylinositol starts to decrease, while at the same time the percentage of phosphatidylglycerol increases. The decrease in serum inositol around birth appears to be at least partially responsible for the switchover from phosphatidylinositol to phosphatidylglycerol synthesis[30].

The increase in PC content of pulmonary surfactant towards the end of gestation is accompanied by enhanced rates of PC synthesis from a variety of labelled precursors[28,29]. The biochemical basis of this increased PC synthesis at the end of gestation is not yet fully understood. Studies *in vitro* with homogenates or subcellular fractions of whole fetal lung have indicated that there is a correlation between increased cholinephosphate cytidylyltransferase activities and increased rates of PC synthesis in fetal and neonatal lung[28,29]. It should be emphasized, however, that such studies have so far been carried out with preparations from whole lung, and that the results are not necessarily applicable to the developing type II cells. On the other hand, pulse-label and pulse-chase experiments with type II cells isolated from fetal rat lung, as well as measurement of the pool sizes of choline and its metabolites in these cells[31], do support the concept that cholinephosphate cytidylyltransferase catalyses an important rate-regulatory step in the formation of PC by maturing type II cells. This enzyme also appears to be an important target for the hormonal regulation of surfactant PC formation in the developing lung[28,29,32]. In a recent paper Weinhold and his colleagues[33] showed that free fatty acids, particularly unsaturated species, affected the activity of cholinephosphate cytidylyltransferase in whole fetal lung by translocation of the inactive cytosolic form to the microsomes. This would support the possibility that translocation of cholinephosphate cytidylyltransferase may play an important role in regulating surfactant PC synthesis by the developing lung. On the other hand, as discussed extensively by Rooney[29], there is in the case of the lung also much evidence for a regulatory role of the cytosolic rather than the membrane-bound cholinephosphate cytidylyltransferase.

It has been suggested that glycogen may constitute an important source of substrate for the production of DPPC and other surfactant lipids in the fetal lung. This is supported by the temporal relationship between the disappearance of glycogen from fetal lung epithelial cells and the onset of surfactant PC synthesis during the terminal period of gestation, that has been observed for several mammalian spcies[28]. In addition, radioactivity from prelabelled endogenous glycogen in explants of fetal lung is incorporated into DPPC and phosphatidylglycerol[34]. Glycogen can provide the glycerol backbone for surfactant lipids and serve as carbon and NADPH source for the *de novo* synthesis of the fatty-acyl constituents of surfactant lipids. In a recent study[35] we investigated the developmental profile of various glycolytic enzymes during perinatal development of fetal rat lung. Phosphofructokinase is the only regulator enzyme of glycolysis located between glycogen-derived glucose-6-phosphate and the formation of dihydroxyacetonephosphate, which is the direct glycolytic precursor of the glycerol backbone of surfactant lipids (Fig. 13.1). Interestingly, the developmental profile of phosphofructokinase coincided with those of enzymes for glycogenolysis[36] and phospholipid synthesis[28]. Although these studies have so far been carried out with whole fetal lung preparations, the results do suggest that phosphofructokinase may play a regulatory role linking glycogen catabolism and surfactant lipid synthesis.

INTRACELLULAR STORAGE OF SURFACTANT IN LAMELLAR BODIES: A SPECIFIC MARKER ENZYME FOR THESE ORGANELLES

Both biochemical and autoradiographic[8] studies have shown that the surfactant components are synthesized predominantly, if not entirely, at the endoplasmic reticulum of the type II cell. The surfactant components are then transferred through the Golgi complex and, most likely via multivesicular bodies, packaged into 'growing' lamellar bodies. These organelles are considered to be the intracellular storage sites of surfactant. The contents of mature lamellar bodies can be secreted by the type II cells into the alveolar lining layer. After secretion the lamellae can transform into the characteristic lattice-like structure that is known as tubular myelin[37]. As discussed in an earlier section, this tubular myelin is probably the direct precursor of the monolayer film that stabilizes the alveoli.

The lack of a specific marker enzyme for lamellar bodies has seriously hampered biochemical studies on the metabolism and biogenesis of these organelles. Positive identification of isolated lamellar bodies had to rely mainly on morphologic appearance and on rather non-specific biochemical parameters such as a high phospholipid/protein ratio. In a recent study on lysosomal-type hydrolases in preparations of lamellar bodies isolated from adult human lung tissue, we discovered the presence of two α-glucosidases with an acid pH optimum[38]. One of the acid α-glucosidases in the lamellar body fraction was similar to the acid α-glucosidase in a lysosomal fraction of human lung: it could be precipitated by the lectin Concanavalin-A immobilized to Sepharose 4B, and showed a high affinity to specific antibodies against lysosomal α-glucosidase from human placenta. The second acid α-glucosidase in the lamellar body fraction could, unlike the lysosomal α-glucosidase, not be precipitated by the immobilized Concanavalin-A and

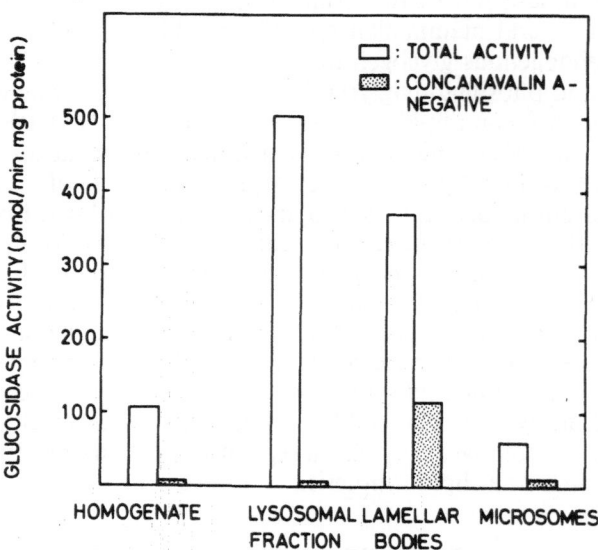

Figure 13.4 Total α-glucosidase activity and α-glucosidase activity without binding affinity to immobilized Concanavalin-A in preparations from adult human lung. The α-glucosidase activity was determined with 4-methylumbelliferyl-α-D-glucoside at pH 4.5. For further details see Ref. 38

showed a very low affinity towards the anti-α-glucosidase. Figure 13.4 shows the distribution of the total acid α-glucosidase activity and that of the Concanavalin-A-negative acid α-glucosidase activity among subcellular fractions of adult human lung. In whole lung homogenate, and in the lysosome-enriched and microsomal lung fractions, the specific activities of the Concanavalin-A-negative α-glucosidase were below 10 pmol min^{-1} mg protein^{-1}. The specific activity of this enzyme in the lamellar body fraction was at least an order of magnitude higher (115.8 $\pm$ 12.0 pmol min^{-1} mg protein^{-1}; $n=4$). In addition, the small amount of Concanavalin-A-negative α-glucosidase in the microsomal fraction has no acid pH optimum and, in contrast to the lamellar body-specific enzyme, has no affinity towards glycogen as substrate (data not shown).

Very recently (A. C. J. de Vries, A. W. Schram, J. M. Tager, J. J. Batenburg and L. M. G. van Golde, unpublished observation) we measured the activity of the lamellar body-specific α-glucosidase and that of lysosomal α-glucosidase in a patient affected by a lysosomal α-glucosidase deficiency. The activity of the lamellar body-specific α-glucosidase was not affected in the patient, whereas the lysosomal α-glucosidase activity was strongly depressed. These results suggest the intriguing possibility that the lysosomal and lamellar body-specific α-glucosidases do not arise from the same gene.

Although nothing is known about the function of specific lysosomal-type enzymes in lamellar bodies, this lamellar body-specific α-glucosidase should prove useful as a lamellar body-specific marker enzyme in future studies on the metabolism and biogenesis of these organelles.

Acknowledgements

Studies by the authors described in this review were supported in part by the Netherlands Foundation for Chemical Research (SON) with financial aid from the Netherlands Organization for the Advancement of Pure Research (ZWO) and by the Dutch Asthma Foundation (Nederlands Astma Fonds). One of the authors (R. Burkhardt) was recipient of a Postdoctoral Fellowship from the Deutsche Forschungsgemeinschaft. The authors are indebted to Mrs J. A. H. Verweij for preparing the manuscript.

References

1. Goerke, J. (1974). Lung surfactant. *Biochim. Biophys. Acta,* **344,** 241-61
2. King, R. J. (1984). Isolation and chemical composition of pulmonary surfactant. In Robertson, B., Van Golde, L. M. G. and Batenburg, J. J. (eds.) *Pulmonary Surfactant.* pp. 1-16. (Amsterdam: Elsevier)
3. King, R. J. and Clements, J. A. (1972). Surface active materials from dog lung. II. Composition and physiological correlations. *Am. J. Physiol.,* **223,** 715-26
4. King, R. J. (1982). Pulmonary surfactant. *J. Appl. Physiol.,* **53,** 1-8
5. King, R. J. (1985). Composition and metabolism of the apolipoproteins of pulmonary surfactant. *Ann. Rev. Physiol.,* **47,** 775-88
6. Clements, J. A., Goerke, J., Wright, J. R. and Beppu, O. (1984). Turnover of lung surfactant. *Prog. Respir. Res.,* **18,** 133-42
7. Hawgood, S., Benson, B. J. and Hamilton, R. J. (1985). Effects of a surfactant-associated protein and calcium ions on the structure and surface activity of lung surfactant lipids. *Biochemistry,* **24,** 184-90
8. Chevalier, G. and Collet, A. J. (1972). In vivo incorporation of choline-^{3}H, leucine-^{3}H, and galactose-^{3}H in alveolar type II pneumonocytes in relation to surfactant synthesis. A quantitative radioautographic study in mouse by electron microscopy. *Anat. Rec.,* **174,** 289-310
9. Mason, R. J. (1982). Isolation of alveolar type II cells. In Farrell, P. M. (ed.) *Lung Development: Biological and Clinical Perspectives.* Vol. 1, pp. 135-150. (New York: Academic Press)
10. Post, M., Torday, J. S. and Smith, B. T. (1984). Alveolar type II cells isolated from fetal rat lung organotypic cultures synthesize and secrete surfactant-associated phospholipids and respond to fibroblast-pneumonocyte factor. *Exp. Lung Res.,* **7,** 53-65
11. Van Golde, L. M. G. (1985). Synthesis of surfactant lipids in the adult lung. *Ann. Rev. Physiol.,* **47,** 765-74
12. Mason, R. J. (1978). Importance of the acyl dihydroxyacetone phosphate pathway in the synthesis of phosphatidylglycerol and phosphatidylcholine in alveolar type II cells. *J. Biol. Chem.,* **253,** 3367-70
13. Van Golde, L. M. G., Den Breejen, J. N. and Batenburg, J. J. (1985). Isolated alveolar type II cells: A model for studies on the formation of surfactant dipalmitoylphosphatidylcholine. *Biochem. Soc. Trans.,* **13,** 1087-9
14. Crecelius, C. A. and Longmore, W. J. (1983). Phosphatidic acid phosphatase activity in subcellular fractions derived from adult rat type II pneumocytes in primary culture. *Biochim. Biophys. Acta,* **750,** 447-56
15. Post, M., Schuurmans, E. A. J. M., Batenburg, J. J. and Van Golde, L. M. G. (1983). Mechanisms involved in the synthesis of disaturated phosphatidylcholine by alveolar type II cells isolated from adult rat lung. *Biochim. Biophys. Acta,* **750,** 68-77

16. Mason, R. J. and Nellenbogen, J. (1984). Synthesis of saturated phosphatidylcholine and phosphatidylglycerol by freshly isolated rat alveolar type II cells. *Biochim. Biophys. Acta*, **794**, 392-402

17. Van Golde, L. M. G. (1976). Metabolism of phospholipids in the lung. *Am. Rev. Respir. Dis.*, **114**, 977-1000

18. Batenburg, J. J., Longmore, W. J., Klazinga, W. and Van Golde, L. M. G. (1979). Lysolecithin acyltransferase and lysolecithin:lysolecithin acyltransferase in adult rat lung alveolar type II epithelial cells. *Biochim. Biophys. Acta*, **573**, 136-144

19. Finkelstein, J. N., Maniscalco, W. M. and Shapiro, D. L. (1983). Properties of freshly isolated type II alveolar epithelial cells. *Biochim. Biophys. Acta*, **762**, 398-404

20. Finkelstein, J. N. and Kramer, C. (1982). Acyltransferase activities in isolated type II alveolar epithelial cells. *Fed. Proc.*, **41**, 668 (Abstract)

21. De Vries, A. C. J., Batenburg, J. J. and Van Golde, L. M. G. (1985). Lysophosphatidylcholine acyltransferase and lysophosphatidylcholine:lysophosphatidylcholine acyltransferase in alveolar type II cells from fetal rat lung. *Biochim. Biophys. Acta*, **833**, 93-9

22. Hallman, M., Epstein, B. L. and Gluck, L. (1981). Analysis of labeling and clearance of lung surfactant phospholipids in rabbit. Evidence of bidirectional surfactant flux between lamellar bodies and alveolar lavage. *J. Clin. Invest.*, **68**, 742-51

23. Jacobs, H., Jobe, A., Ikegami, M. and Conaway, D. (1983). The significance of reutilization of surfactant phosphatidylcholine. *J. Biol. Chem.*, **258**, 4156-65

24. Post, M., Batenburg, J. J., Schuurmans, E. A. J. M. and Van Golde, L. M. G. (1982). The rate-limiting step in the biosynthesis of phosphatidylcholine by alveolar type II cells from adult rat lung. *Biochim. Biophys. Acta*, **712**, 390-4

25. Post, M., Batenburg, J. J., Smith, B. T. and Van Golde, L. M. G. (1984). Pool sizes of precursors for phosphatidylcholine formation in adult rat lung type II cells. *Biochim. Biophys. Acta*, **795**, 552-7

26. Vance, D. E. and Pelech, S. L. (1984). Enzyme translocation in the regulation of phosphatidylcholine biosynthesis. *Trends Biochem. Sci.*, **9**, 17-20

27. Brindley, D. N. (1984). Intracellular translocation of phosphatidate phosphohydrolase and its possible role in the control of glycerolipid synthesis. *Prog. Lipid. Res.*, **23**, 115-33

28. Rooney, S. A. (1983). Biochemical development of the lung. In Warshaw, J. B. (ed.) *The Biological Basis of Reproductive and Developmental Medicine*. pp. 239-287. (New York: Elsevier Biomedical)

29. Rooney, S. A. (1985). The surfactant system and lung phospholipid biochemistry. *Am. Rev. Respir. Dis.*, **113**, 439-60

30. Hallman, M. and Epstein, B. L. (1980). Role of myo-inositol in the synthesis of phosphatidylglycerol and phosphatidylinositol in the lung. *Biochem. Biophys. Res. Commun.*, **92**, 1151-9

31. Post, M., Batenburg, J. J., Van Golde, L. M. G. and Smith, B. T. (1984). The rate-limiting reaction in phosphatidylcholine synthesis by alveolar type II cells isolated from fetal rat lung. *Biochim. Biophys. Acta*, **795**, 558-63

32. Smith, B. T. (1984). Pulmonary surfactant during fetal development and neonatal adaptation: hormonal control. In Robertson, B., Van Golde, L. M. G. and Batenburg, J. J. (eds.) *Pulmonary Surfactant*. pp. 357-82. (Amsterdam: Elsevier)

33. Weinhold, P. A., Rounsifer, M. E., Williams, S. E., Brubaker, P. G. and Feldman, D. A. (1984). CTP: phosphorylcholine cytidylyltransferase in rat lung. The effect of free fatty acids on the translocation of activity between microsomes and cytosol. *J. Biol. Chem.*, **259**, 10315-21

34. Bourbon, J. R., Rieutort, M., Engle, M. J. and Farrell, P. M. (1982). Utilization of glycogen for phospholipid synthesis in fetal rat lung. *Biochim. Biophys. Acta*, **712**, 382-9

35. Rijksen, G., Staal, G. E. J., Streefkerk, M., De Vries, A. C. J., Batenburg, J. J. Heesbeen, E. C. and Van Golde, L. M. G. (1985). Activity and isoenzyme patterns of glycolytic enzymes during perinatal development of rat lung. *Biochim. Biophys. Acta*, **838**, 114-21

36. Maniscalco, W. M., Wilson, C. M., Gross, I., Gobran, L., Rooney, S. A. and Warshaw, J. B. (1978). Development of glycogen and phospholipid metabolism in fetal and newborn rat lung. *Biochim. Biophys. Acta*, **530**, 333-46

37. Williams, M. C. (1977). Conversion of lamellar body membranes into tubular myelin in alveoli of fetal rat lungs. *J. Cell. Biol.,* **72,** 260–77

38. De Vries, A. C. J., Schram, A. W., Tager, J. M., Batenburg, J. J. and Van Golde, L. M. G. (1985). A specific acid α-glucosidase in lamellar bodies of the human lung. *Biochim. Biophys. Acta,* **837,** 230–8

Discussion

Dr B. T. Smith   Have you looked for the α-glucosidase in airways or in amniotic fluid?

Dr L. M. G. Van Golde   We are planning to look to see whether the enzyme is secreted into the airways, which I would expect.

Dr J. A. Clements   What do you think are the natural substrates of this enzyme?

Van Golde   I have to answer that we just don't know. I may say, however, that the enzyme can use glycogen as a substrate. Until now we focused our attention on proving that the enzyme may be specific for the lamellar body.

Dr C. A. R. Boyd   In relation to the synthesis of phosphatidylcholine and other lipids, is it known how choline gets into these cells? Is there a choline transport system and if so is it electrogenic?

Van Golde   I don't know if it is electrogenic but I think that there is evidence for a system for active uptake of choline.

Clements   Remodelling of phosphatidylcholine seems to be a wasteful process because the cell has to make phosphatidylcholine twice to get the product. Why can't the cell make up its mind in the first place how much saturated PC it wants and just go ahead and make it, or is there some advantage in the remodelling process? Have you conducted your experiments at different temperatures to find out whether the saturation ratios (saturated/unsaturated) are temperature-dependent?

Van Golde   We haven't looked at the effect of temperature but I think it is a very interesting suggestion. Remodelling always requires one extra high energy bond, and that may be the price the type II cell has to pay to produce such an enormously high proportion of disaturated phosphatidylcholine. I don't expect there is much difference in the substrate specificity of the glycerolphosphate acyltransferase in type II cells as compared to other cells. In the type II cell, however, there may be much more palmitate around than in other cell types, providing more dipalmitoyl phosphatidic acid than in other cells, but I don't think it would ever be enough without remodelling to produce 60% or 70% disaturated PC.

14
myo-Inositol and Perinatal Development of Surfactant

M. HALLMAN

ABSTRACT

myo-Inositol (henceforth called inositol) increases surfactant phosphatidy-linositol (PI) synthesis and decreases phosphatidylglycerol (PGl). Additionally, it potentiates the glucocorticoid and thyroid hormone-induced increase in surfactant phosphatidylcholine (PC) in the fetus. In the present study the mechanisms of inositol–surfactant interaction were investigated. The availability of inositol for surfactant synthesis in type II cells decreased during perinatal development by two mechanisms: (1) decrease in serum inositol, and (2) decrease in inositol permeability of type II cells. To study the development of surfactant PC fetal lung explants were grown in serum-free medium in the presence of dexamethasone and thyroxine. In explants from 20–21-day-old fetal rabbits, the hormones increased surfactant PC first in the presence of inositol excess. There was no increase in PGl in the absence of inositol. Inositol increased de novo synthesis of fatty acids destined to become surfactant phospholipids, stimulated incorporation of acetate into microsomal and lamellar body-associated PI, and increased the rate-limiting cholinephosphate cytidylyltransferase activity. These effects of inositol decreased from 20 to 28 fetal days. In explants from 24-day-old fetuses, the hormones increased surfactant PC and PGl even in the absence of inositol. We propose that inositol–PI pair serves as a 'tertiary messenger' of glucocorticoid and thyroid hormones in immature lung. Later, both PGl and PI promote the synthesis and surface activity of surfactant PC.

INTRODUCTION

Glucocorticoids and thyroid hormones accelerate the increase in synthesis and secretion of surfactant during the perinatal period[1]. However, the hormones often do not prevent RDS and produce a barely detectable increase in surfactant[2]. This is not surprising, since there may be a number of poorly understood interactions, not necessarily always hormonal, that affect the

197

development of surfactant secretion. In the present report we discuss the role of *myo* - inositol (henceforth called inositol) as a regulatory substrate.

Gluck *et al.*[3] showed the correlation between lung maturity and the amniotic fluid phospholipids. However, the hypothesis that the perinatal development of the major surfactant phospholipid takes place according to successive activation of the methylation and choline incorporation pathways of surfactant phosphatidylcholine (PC) synthesis[4] was proven to be untenable. This evidence came from two sources: (1) investigation of the biosynthesis of PC in the lung and in type II cells revealed that the choline incorporation pathway is the major if not the exclusive pathway for surfactant PC; (2) the minor surfactant phospholipid was proven to be phosphatidylglycerol (PGl), instead of dimethyl phosphatidylethanolamine, an intermediate of the methylation pathway of PC synthesis[5].

Further study of surfactant revealed a striking trend in the acidic phospholipids: normal surfactant contained a uniquely high PGl (6–13% of total surfactant phospholipids), whereas surfactant from immature fetuses and newborn had no detectable PGl. Interestingly, PGl-poor surfactant had prominent amounts of phosphatidylinositol (PI), instead[6]. In RDS, PGl was specifically lacking among lung effluent phospholipids, whereas PGl was present in surfactant of a healthy newborn[7].

According to Van Golde *et al.*[8] there is a specific intracellular soluble protein that binds PGl in the lung. There are no data on its ontogeny. King and MacBeth[9] have described the surfactant-associated apoprotein A that specifically binds PGl but not, for instance, PI. Although surfactant apoprotein A increases during perinatal development, the increase does not necessarily take place similarly to that of PGl[10].

Enzymes or substrates involved in biosynthesis of PGl or PI may control the composition of the acidic phospholipids[11]. According to Bleasdale *et al.*[12] high CMP (as a result of active PC synthesis), reverses or decreases PI synthesis, and therefore the limited amount of CDP-diacylglycerol is utilized for PGl. Others have failed to substantiate the role of CMP[13].

Inositol increases surfactant PI and correspondingly decreases surfactant PGl in adults[14]. This inositol effect was evident *in vivo* and *in vitro* using lung microsomes[14], or type II alveolar cells[13]. The suppressive effect of inositol on PGl synthesis seems to depend upon rate-limiting CDP-diacylglycerol and the dominating activity of CDP-diacylglycerol inositol transferase (PI synthesis) that is about one order of magnitude higher than that of microsomal glycerophosphate phosphatidyltransferase (PG synthesis)[14]. Although serum inositol decreases during perinatal development, the following arguments are against the regulatory role of this sugar alcohol:

1. Tissues, including the lung[15], take up inositol by an active, energy-dependent transport, and synthesize inositol glucose 6-phosphate.
2. The concentration of inositol in the whole lung is 2–4 μmol/g wet wt. It does not tend to be higher in the fetus than in the adult.
3. The concentration of inositol required to suppress PGl in isolated type II cells, 0.5–5 mmol/l, is almost two orders of magnitude *higher* than

the suppressive concentration of inositol[13,14] in a microsomal preparation, 1–100 μmol/l.

Teleologically PGl should be advantageous during postnatal life and/or PI during prenatal development. Indeed, PI-surfactant from the fetus did not have all the desirable surface-active properties present in postnatal PGl-surfactant[6]. However, when PGl-rich and PGl-devoid (produced by dietary inositol excess) surfactants from adult animals were compared, there were no detectable differences[16,17], suggesting that PGl does not improve surfactant function. It may still be argued that the presence of PGl provides an as yet unrecognized advantage, or that PI is indispensable for fetal surfactant.

The period of prenatal development, during which PI-surfactant prevails, is characterized by a striking increase in the pool size of surfactant. In order to evaluate further the importance of inositol, fetal rabbits *in vivo* and fetal lung explants *in vitro* were exposed to inositol and hormones known to accelerate the lung maturity. It was found that inositol *potentiated* the glucocorticoid and/or thyroid hormone-induced increase in surfactant[18]. The present report deals with the mechanisms by which inositol influences the ontogeny of surfactant PC.

MATERIALS AND METHODS

Organ culture

The lungs for the organ culture[18] were obtained from 23-day-old rabbit fetuses. The lung parenchyma was chopped into 0.3–0.8 mm^3 cubes, and 20–30 explants were placed on a plastic culture dish, diameter 35 mm. The culture medium (0.6 ml a dish) contained 100 U penicillin, 100 μg streptomycin/ml and, when indicated, hormones, inositol and/or choline. The explants were kept at 37 °C in humidified atmosphere of 20% O_2/5% CO_2. The culture dish was rotated at a rate of 9 cycles/min allowing the explants to be cyclically exposed to the air and to the culture medium. After 4 days in culture the medium was removed and the subcellular fractions isolated, or a new medium containing radiolabelled precursors was added.

Isolation of type II cells

Type II cells were isolated from the lungs of adult and 30-day-old fetal rabbits[19]. Pulmonary vessels of the heparinized rabbits were perfused through a catheter placed in the pulmonary artery. until the lungs appeared bloodless. The perfusion medium contained 135 mmol/l NaCl, 4 mmol/l KCl, 2 mmol/l sodium phosphate, 10 mmol/l HEPES, and 5 mmol/l glucose (pH 7.4). The trachea were cannulated and the airways lavaged five times with isotonic saline. Thereafter, the lung parenchyma was minced with scissors into 1 mm^3 pieces. A medium containing 3 mg trypsin, 30 μg DNA:se/ml, was added (10 ml/g of tissue). The dispersion was incubated at 37 °C for 35 min in a water bath reciprocating at 60 cycles/min.

Thereafter fetal calf serum was added, and the suspenson filtered through 150 μm and 20 μm nylon mesh. The filtrate was layered on the top of a discontinuous gradient containing 10 ml of albumin, density 1.088, and 10 ml of albumin, density 1.040. After centrifugation at 200g for 20 min the cells in between the two albumin layers were recovered, and type II cells further purified by differential adherence in primary culture[19]. More than 90% of the cells that adhered to the culture dish during 20 h excluded the vital dye, and electron microscopy revealed that 75–85% of the cells resembled type II alveolar cells.

Other methods

The lamellar body fraction and the microsomes were isolated as described previously[11,18]. Cholinephosphate cytidylyltransferase activity was assayed by measuring the rate of incorporation of methyl-^{14}C phosphorylcholine into CDP-choline[20]. The phospholipids were isolated and analysed as described previously[11].

RESULTS

The availability of inositol in type II cells during perinatal development

The vectorial transport of inositol into tissues requires Na^+ and energy. In theory, a high serum inositol concentration potentiates the tissue uptake, since the apparent K_m for the inositol transport (60–90 μm) is similar or higher than serum inositol concentration in the adult. However, there were no significant differences either in saturable inositol uptake into lung cells or in concentrations of inositol between the fetal and adult lungs.

Some cells take up inositol by an energy-independent, non-saturable mechanism. A similar uptake of inositol is also present in the lung. In contrast to the energy-dependent uptake, the non-saturable uptake decreased during fetal development, or following glucocorticoid treatment (data not shown).

Figure 14.1 shows the intracellular inositol uptake into the isolated type II cells from adult and fetal lung. The uptake takes place preferentially by the non-saturable mechanism. An additional finding of interest was that the uptake per cell was higher in the fetus than in the adult. The adult cells required a higher inositol concentration than the fetal cells for suppression of PGl synthesis (data not shown).

The mechanism of inositol in potentiating the hormone-induced increase in surfactant PC *in vitro*

The phospholipids were analysed in the subcellular fractions of lung explants. In 20–21-day-old fetuses glucocorticoid/and thyroid hormone had a barely detectable effect on incorporation of acetate into saturated PC from lamellar bodies (Table 14.1). However, the effect of hormones became evident in the presence of inositol excess. In explants from older

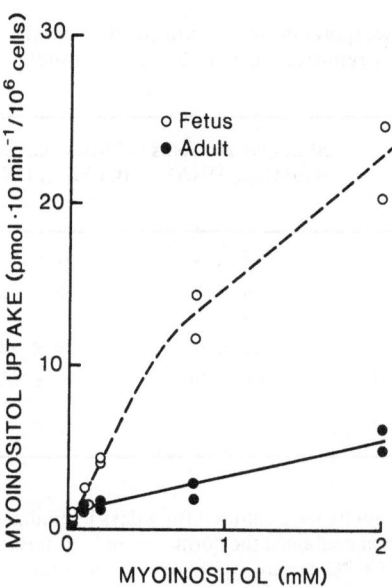

Figure 14.1 Inositol uptake into type II alveolar cells, isolated from 31-day-old fetus and adult. The suspension, containing $1.5-2 \times 10^6$ type II cells in 0.5 ml serum-free minimal essential medium was incubated in the presence of 2 - [³H]inositol, and 10 μm [¹⁴C-]mannitol for 15 min in 95% O_2–5% CO_2. After the incubation the suspension was washed on Millipore filters, and the radioactivity associated with the filter was counted. The amount of inositol taken up into the cells was calculated as follows: 2-[³H]inositol in filter – [¹⁴C]mannitol in filter × total 2-[³H]inositol/total [¹⁴C]mannitol (Reproduced from Hallman, M. et al. (1986). *Pediatr. Res.*, **20**, 179–85 by kind permission of the International Pediatric Research Foundation.)

fetuses, the hormones stimulated the incorporation of surfactant PC regardless of inositol.

The pool sizes of the lamellar body-associated saturated PCs were measured. Saturated PC was undetectable (i.e. <0.4 nmol/μg DNA) in explants from 20–21-day-old fetuses, *except* when excess of inositol and the hormones were present (1.2 ± 0.2 nmol/μg DNA, $n= 3$).

Table 14.2 shows the incorporation of acetate into PI and PGl from lung microsomes. Inositol stimulated PI incorporation. The effect tended to decrease and become less hormone-dependent in more mature lung. There was no detectable PGl incorporation in microsomes from 20-day-old rabbit fetuses regardless of inositol concentration. The hormones induced PGl incorporation in explants from 24-day-old fetuses, whereas in explants from 28-day-old fetuses PGl incorporation was present without exogenous hormones. Inositol always suppressed PGl incorporation. Inositol and the hormones similarly affected the labelling of both microsomal and lamellar body-associated phospholipids (data not shown).

Cholinephosphate cytidylyltransferase is considered to be a rate-limiting enzyme for PC synthesis. As shown in Table 14.3 inositol and hormones together always increased the activity, whereas the hormones alone signi-

Table 14.1 ^{14}C-acetate incorporation into saturated PC from the lamellar body fraction of lung explants, cultured in serum-free medium. Effect of inositol and the hormones

	20–21-day-old fetus (CPM/μg DNA)	24-day-old fetus (CPM/μg DNA)	28-day-old fetus (CPM/μg DNA)
No addition	8 ± 3	61 ± 8	371 ± 22
Dexamethasone, 10^{-7} mol/l; thyroxine, 10^{-7} mol/l	14 ± 5	355 ± 42	528 ± 41
Inositol, 1.5 mmol/l	22 ± 6	189 ± 18	413 ± 17
Dexamethasone, 10^{-7} mol/l; thyroxine, 10^{-7} mol/l; inositol, 1.5 mmol/l	519 ± 29	605 ± 25	806 ± 39

Lung explants from fetal rabbits were cultured for 4 days in minimal essential medium. When indicated the culture medium contained the hormones and/or inositol. On day 4 a new culture medium, containing 1.0 μCi ^{14}C-acetate (spec. act. 58 mCi/mmol) was added, and the culture was continued for another 20 h. The results are expressed as means SE of three to five analyses

Table 14.2 ^{14}C-acetate incorporation into PGl and PI from the microsomal fraction of lung explants, cultured in serum-free medium. Effect of inositol and the hormones

	20-21-day-old fetus		24-day-old fetus		28-day-old fetus	
	PGl	PI	PGl	PI	PGl	PI
No addition	0.2±0.0	0.5±0.1	0.7±0.1	2.2±0.2	5.9±0.4	3.5±0.2
Dexamethasone, 10^{-7} mol/l thyroxine, 10^{-7} mol/l	0.4±0.1	0.0±0.0	3.7±0.2	5.3±0.4	4.4±0.9	2.7±0.3
Inositol, 1.5 mmol/l	0.0±0.0	1.6±0.2	0.4±0.0	7.7±0.5	0.4±0.1	5.3±0.4
Dexamethasone, 10^{-7} mol/l thyroxine, 10^{-7} mol/l inositol, 1.5 mmol/l	0.0±0.0	5.9±0.3	0.7±0.1	9.9±1.0	0.6±0.1	6.2±0.3

Lung explants from fetal rabbits were cultured for 4 days in minimal essential medium. When indicated the culture medium contained the hormones and/or inositol. On day 4 a new culture medium, containing 1.0 μCi of ^{14}C-acetate (spec. act. 58 mCi/mmol) was added, and the culture was continued for another 20 h. The microsomes were isolated as previously described[11] using discontinuous gradient, containing 0.55 and 1.3 mol/l sucrose. The material that sedimented in between the two sucrose layers was collected. The results are the means SE of three to five analyses. They are expressed as CPM/μg total lung DNA

Table 14.3 Cholinephosphate cytidylyltransferase activity in lung explants from fetal rabbits. Effects of inosital and/or the hormones

	20–21-day-old fetus		24-day-old fetus	
	Specific activity	Total protein	Specific activity	Total protein
No addition	0.21 ± 0.03	0.12 ± 0.02	1.04 ± 0.07	0.20 ± 0.02
Dexamethasone, 10^{-7} mol/l, thyroxine, 10^{-7} mol/l	0.18 ± 0.05	0.10 ± 0.01	1.47 ± 0.09	0.22 ± 0.01
Inositol, 1.5 mmol/l	0.34 ± 0.03	0.15 ± 0.02	1.29 ± 0.14	0.23 ± 0.03
Dexamethasone, 10^{-7} mol/l, thyroxine, 10^{-7} mol/l, inositol, 1.5 mmol/l	0.83 ± 0.06	0.13 ± 0.01	2.20 ± 0.17	0.27 ± 0.01

The fetal lung explants were cultured for 4 days. Thereafter cholinephosphate cytidylyltransferase activity (nmol CDP-choline min^{-1} mg $protein^{-1}$), and the protein content (mg protein/dish) of the homogenized explants were analysed. The results were expressed as means ± SE of six to eight analyses. The protein content cannot be compared between the two age groups, because the number of explants/dish was not always constant

ficantly increased the enzyme activity only in explants from 24-day-old fetuses. The increase in cholinephosphate cytidylyltransferase activity took place concomitant with activation of surfactant PC synthesis, and with increase in PI and/or PGl incorporation. Choline (1.9 mmol/l) had an additive effect on inositol-induced increase in surfactant PC (data not shown).

DISCUSSION

Binding of many hormones and other agonists onto plasma membrane receptors induces a rapid turnover of phosphoinositides. As a result of a change in the phospholipid structure of the membrane, the hormone or neurotransmitter binding is amplified often within a fraction of seconds. The turnover of phosphoinositides may precede, follow, or enforce changes in the commonly accepted 'second messengers', cAMP and/or Ca^{2+}. An incomplete list of the targets includes exocrine and endocrine pancreas, adrenal cortex and medulla, some pituitary cells, parotid gland, intestinal smooth muscle, platelets, neutrophils, and adipose tissue[21].

We have tentatively identified the inositol–monophosphoinositide pair as an intermediate required for expression of the glucocorticoid and thyroid hormone-induced effects on surfactant PC synthesis in immature lung. The mechanism of the interaction between inositol and these hormones is poorly understood. For instance, there are no data as to whether or not inositol influences synthesis, secretion or membrane binding of the fibroblast pneumonocyte factor (see Chapter 2). According to preliminary data, lung fibroblasts concentrate inositol by energy-dependent uptake, and synthesize inositol from glucose-6-phosphate (data not shown), similar to most lung cells[15]. However, the type II cells, at least the site of the acidic surfactant phospholipid synthesis, require exogenous inositol for maintenance of the PI synthesis[13].

The function of inositol–PI pair in surfactant synthesis is different from other systems involving inositide-mediated hormone action. The following features may be pointed out:

1. The distribution of PI in surfactant may increase or decrease, depending on hormones, nutrients, or on developmental stage. However, there is little evidence on induced *catabolism* of surfactant PI but rather a switch from PI to PGl synthesis or vice-versa. In the adrenal cortex, too, ACTH induces net synthesis of triphosphoinositide. This phospholipid is able to stimulate steroid synthesis, in a similar way to ACTH[21]. It is unknown (and unlikely) whether PI alone stimulates the differentiation of type II cells, as do glucocorticoid and thyroid hormones.

2. Phosphoinositide-messenger is physically close to the binding site of the agonist at the surface of the cell[22]. In contrast, glucocorticoid and thyroid hormones bind to cytoplasmic and nuclear receptors in lung fibroblasts, although type II cells may have hormone binding, too. According to present data inositol–PI pair directly affects the phospholipid metabolism in type II cells. It is unknown whether inositol–PI pair responds only to specific hormones, or to other agonists that stimulate the supply of precursors (CDP-diacylglycerol?), as well.

3. In the liver and the lung, the rate-limiting enzyme activity in PC synthesis is cholinephosphate cytidylyltransferase[23]. The present study demonstrated that inositol-induced stimulation of surfactant PC synthesis is associated with increase in cholinephosphate cytidylyltransferase activity. According to Feldman *et al.*[24] PI is second to PGl in its ability to activate cholinephosphate cytidylyltransferase in cytosol from the fetal lung. However, microsomal, rather than the cytosolic, enzyme catalyzes PC synthesis[23]. A major mechanism responsible for the membrane binding involves long chain fatty acids. They increase the affinity of cholinephosphate cytidylyltransferase to membranes which contain phospholipids, which in turn activate the cytidylyltransferase[23]. Inositol increased incorporation of both PI and *de novo* fatty acid destined for surfactant[18]. Therefore the mechanism of activation of surfactant PC synthesis may involve activation of cholinephosphate cytidylyltransferase enzyme.

4. The magnitude of the effect of inositol on surfactant PC synthesis depends on maturity and on exogenous hormone stimulus. In mature lung PGl synthesis proceeds maximally in the absence of inositol. It may be argued that PI (and inositol) is superfluous or even harmful in mature lung. On the other hand, in a very immature lung there was very little microsome- or lamellar body-associated PGl incorporation, regardless of the extracellular inositol concentration, and the ability of the hormones to stimulate surfactant PC synthesis was poor (Tables

14.1 and 14.2). It is proposed that PGl does not amplify a hormonal response in very immature lung, whereas inositol–PI pair is active in this respect. The cause of the absence of extramitochondrial PGl synthesis, despite the low serum/medium inositol, is unknown[18]. It is intriguing that the coupling between inositol and PGl is absent both in immature and in severely damaged lung.

Do the present findings on inositol have any practical importance? Some of the preterm infants (<32 weeks gestation) are born with exceptionally low serum inositol, especially after prolonged rupture of fetal membranes (lack of recirculation of urinary inositol), or following severe maternal pre-eclampsia. Secondly, many of the sick preterm infants will fail to maintain the high serum inositol concentration, since inositol-rich breast milk feeding is withheld. Despite low serum inositol there is often no PGl in lung effluent and the infants have a severe respiratory failure. On the other hand, small preterm infants often recover from RDS despite high serum inositol, prominent PI and low PGl[25]. The present results justify further evaluation on the role of inositol as a regulatory substrate in immature fetuses and infants.

Acknowledgements

This research was supported by grants from the Finnish Academy, The Sigrid Juselius Foundation and the Paulo Foundation. I thank Mrs H. Ahola and Mrs E. Riihela for excellent technical assistance.

References

1. Rooney, S. A. (1985). The surfactant system and lung phospholipid biochemistry. *Am. Rev. Respir. Dis.*, **131**, 439–60
2. Avery, M. E. (1984). Prevention of neonatal RDS by pharmacological methods. In Robertson, B., Van Golde, L. M. G. and Batenburg, J. (eds.) *Pulmonary Surfactant.* pp. 449–57 (Amsterdam: Elsevier)
3. Gluck, L., Kulovich, M. V., Borer, R. C., Brenner, P. H., Anderson, G. G. and Spellacy, W. N. (1971). Diagnosis of the respiratory distress syndrome by amniocentesis. *Am. J. Obstet. Gynecol.*, **109**, 440–5
4. Gluck, L. and Kulovich, M. (1973). Fetal lung development. *Pediatr. Clin. N. Am.* **20**, 367–79
5. Van Golde, L. M. G. (1976). Metabolism of phospholipids in the lung. *Am. Rev. Respir. Dis.*, **113**, 977–1000
6. Hallman, M., and Gluck, L. (1976). Phosphatidylglycerol in lung surfactant. III. Possible modifier of surfactant function. *J. Lipid Res.*, **17**, 257–62
7. Hallman, M., Feldman, B. H., Kirkpatrick, E., and Gluck, L. (1977). Absence of phosphatidylglycerol in respiratory distress syndrome in the newborn. *Pediatr. Res.*, **11**, 714–20
8. Van Golde, L. M. G., Oldenborg, V., Post, M., and Batenburg, J. J. (1980). Phospholipid transfer proteins in rat lung. *J. Biol. Chem.*, **255**, 6011–13
9. King, R. and MacBeth, M. C. (1981). Interaction of the lipid and protein components of pulmonary surfactant. Role of phosphatidylglycerol and calcium. *Biochim. Biophys. Acta,* **647**, 159–68
10. Katyal, S. L., and Singh, G. (1983). An enzyme-linked immunoassay of surfactant apoproteins. Its application to the study of fetal lung development in the rat. *Pediatr. Res.*, **17**, 439–43

11. Hallman, M. and Gluck, L. (1980). Formation of acidic phospholipids in rabbit lung during perinatal development. *Pediatr. Res.*, **14**, 1250-9

12. Bleasdale, J. E. and Johnston, J. M. (1982). CMP-dependent incorporation of 14-C glycerol 3-phosphate into phosphatidylglycerol and phosphatidylglycerol phosphate by rabbit lung microsomes. *Biochim. Biophys. Acta*, **710**, 377-90

13. Batenburg, J. J., Klazinga, W., and Van Golde, L. M. G. (1982). Regulation of phosphatidylglycerol and phosphatidylinositol synthesis in alveolar type II cells isolated from adult rat lung. *FEBS Lett.*, **147**, 171-4

14. Hallman, M. and Epstein, B. L. (1980). Role of myo-inositol in the synthesis of phosphatidylglycerol and phosphatidylinositol in the lung. *Biochem. Biophys. Res. Commun.*, **92**, 1151-9

15. Bleasdale, J. E., Maberry, M. C., and Quirk, J. G. (1982). myo-Inositol homeostasis in foetal rabbit lung. *Biochem. J.*, **206**, 43-52

16. Beppu, O. S., Clements, J. A. and Goerke, J. (1983). Phosphatidylglycerol-deficient lung surfactant has normal properties. *J. Appl. Physiol.*, **55**, 496-502

17. Hallman, M., Enhorning, G. and Possmayer, F. (1985). Composition and surface activity of normal and phosphatidylglycerol-deficient lung surfactant *Pediatr. Res.*, **19**, 286-92

18. Hallman, M. (1984). Effect of extracellular myo-inositol on surfactant phospholipid synthesis in the fetal rabbit lung. *Biochim. Biophys. Acta*, **795**, 67-78

19. Mason, R. J., Williams, M. C., Greenleaf, R. D., and Clements, J. A. (1976). Isolation and properties of type II alveolar cells from rat lung. *Am. Rev. Respir. Dis.*, **115**, 1015-26

20. Freese, W. B. and Hallman, M. (1983). The effect of betamethasone and fetal sex on the synthesis and maturation of lung surfactant phospholipids in rabbits. *Biochim. Biophys. Acta*, **750**, 47-59

21. Farese, R. V. (1983). Phosphoinositide metabolism and hormone action. *Endocrine Rev.*, **4**, 78-95

22. Michell, R. H. (1975). Inositol phospholipids and cell surface receptor function. *Biochim. Biophys. Acta*, **415**, 81-147

23. Vance, D. E. and Pelech, S. L. (1984). Enzyme translocation in the regulation of PC biosynthesis. *Trends Biochem. Sci.*, **9**, 17-20

24. Feldman, D. A., Kovac, C. R., Dranginis, P. L. and Weinhold, P. A. (1978). The role of phosphatidylglycerol in activation of CTP : phosphocholine cytidylyltransferase from rat lung. *J. Biol. Chem.*, **253**, 4980-6

25. Hallman, M., Saugstad, O. D., Porreco, R. P., Epstein, B. L. and Gluck, L. (1985). Role of myoinositol in regulation of surfactant phospholipids in the newborn. *Early Human Devel.*, **10**, 245-54

Discussion

Dr J. J. Batenburg	Phosphatidylinositol (PI) is lower in adult surfactant than in fetal surfactant. Did you compare the two type II cell preparations with regard to the rate of inositol synthesis and breakdown?
Dr M. Hallman	In the adult the serum inositol is low and the uptake is low. We have done limited numbers of experiments on the synthesis of *myo*-inositol in isolated type II cells. In the lung there is quite active endogenous inositol synthesis but in type II cells we find very little. We believe that the type II cells, at least in the adult, do not have inositol synthesis.
Dr B. Smith	Using your organ culture system I would be concerned about using protein as a 'denominator' because this kind of system generally shrinks with time. Therefore anything which makes the organ culture 'feel better' will increase the denominator making the numerator look smaller and thus risking exactly the opposite conclusion of what may be physiological. My second comment is perhaps more philosophical. If I heard correctly, you didn't see any difference in physical properties between PI surfactant and PG surfactant. You then told us you can change an adult rabbit surfactant to fetal type of PI surfactant by dietary means. What would be the ethics of undertaking any human trial?
Hallman	We have expressed the data also on the basis of DNA, and the results look very similar. Since both DNA and protein tended to be higher in cultures containing inositol, the effects that we observe cannot be due to 'shrinkage'. Our initial assumption was that PI or absence of PG made surfactant worse, but it didn't quite work out. The initial comparison was made between fetal and adult surfactant (Ref. 6 of Chapter 14). When a similar comparison was made in adults, using PG suppressed and normal surfactant, there was no difference in surfactant characteristics. Since we noticed a dip in serum inositol levels in very preterm babies, apparently as a result of lack of dietary inositol, we studied the association between the severity of RDS - especially the incidence of BPD - and serum inositol. We also studied the phospholipid composition in tracheal aspirates. In RDS patients of more than 32 weeks gestation, PG appears concomitantly with the recovery and the decrease in serum inositol. However, in very preterm infants the situation is quite different. Low serum inositol is associated with low PG and a high incidence of BPD. Since we knew that there were very high concentrations of inositol in the breast milk and especially in the colostrum of mothers of preterm babies, we felt that it is ethically sound to supplement the sick infants' artificial diet with inositol in similar quantity to that which would be present in their mother's breast milk, if these infants were on full breast feeding.
Dr L. M. G. van Golde	Did you look at the molecular composition of the PI which is disappearing and of the PG which is appearing?
Hallman	In a recent paper we reported (Ref. 17 of Chapter 14) the fatty acid structure of PG and PI in lungs from adults fed inositol. There were some differences in the fatty acid composition: PI contained more unsaturated fatty acid components than PG, but the difference was very small. We have obtained similar results in fetal rabbits.

207

Dr W. Seeger   With PI metabolism you touch a completely new field including the PI response (the breakdown of PI) which appears to be a receptor-operated mechanism affecting many cells with two consequences – release of unsaturated arachidonic acid and liberation of ITP3 (inositol-3-phosphate). As in granulocytes this could be an important mediator in type II cells.

Hallman   As you mentioned, PI is considered to be a second messenger of membrane-related functions, for instance action of many hormones, phagocytosis, and nerve transmission. In these cases we would expect rapid breakdown of PI and re-incorporation of diglyceride and inositol-P into PI by the inositol–PI cycle. We have detected a PI-specific phospholipase C activity in the lung (unpublished). However, the story of type II cells and surfactant PI seems quite different: I think there is no rapid degradation and resynthesis of surfactant PI which is more stable than surfactant PG. In addition the amount of inositol does not seem to be sufficient for the inositol–PI cycle. It is clear that the inositol–PI cycle operates in the lung, but the cell type(s) and the function(s) involved remain to be identified.

15
Absorption of Fetal Lung Liquid and Exogenous Surfactant in Premature Lambs

E. A. EGAN, M. S. KWONG AND
R. H. NOTTER

OVERVIEW

The studies discussed here concern general mechanisms of lung liquid and solute absorption in the immediate perinatal period, as well as specific characteristics of these phenomena in premature surfactant-deficient lambs. Descriptions of lung liquid and solute absorption are developed for such lambs, and correlated with experiments where the surfactant deficiency is ameliorated by instillation of an exogenous surfactant preparation prior to the start of ventilation. Of particular interest is the absorption of fetal lung liquid volume, surfactant phospholipid, and radiolabelled alveolar solutes of known radius (albumin, cytochrome C and cyanocobalamin), together with the transport of unlabelled proteins into alveoli during the first 90 min of ventilation.

INTRODUCTION

Premature lambs delivered at or prior to 135 days gestation (term = 150 days) are deficient in lung surfactant. If attempts are made to deliver such premature animals and sustain extrauterine life by mechanical ventilation, lambs less than 130 days typically die within the first hour, and those between 130 and 135 days have respiratory failure which is eventually fatal in many. Without pulmonary surfactant it is impossible to ventilate immature lambs effectively. Hypoxaemia and hypercapnoea progress, at a fast or slower rate depending on gestational age, regardless of efforts to mechanically ventilate the lung.

A remarkable prevention of this respiratory failure occurs with the instillation of natural lung surfactant (LS) or surfactant extract preparations (eg. calf lung surfactant extract, CLL) into the fetal lung liquid before the onset of breathing[1-3]. The lambs can then be ventilated with ease. Near-normal gas exchange is achieved and the mechanical properties of the lungs approach those expected for surfactant-sufficient animals. This effect is sustained for many hours, in contrast to the transient improvement in gas exchange observed if surfactant is administered after the onset of ventilation[4]. The success of CLL surfactant extract administration experiments in lambs *in vivo*[1,3] has recently been followed by two prospective clinical trials of this material in very premature infants, which demonstrated substantially less respiratory failure in treated infants compared to controls[5,6].

One interesting feature in the previous CLL surfactant replacement experiments carried out by Egan *et al.*[1] and Notter *et al.*[3] in premature lambs was the observation of a rapid decrease in the amount of alveolar phospholipid during the first hours of ventilation without any diminution in the efficiency of gas exchange[1,3]. In lambs less than 130 days gestation, only two-thirds of the instilled exogenous surfactant was still detectable in lung liquid after 30 min of breathing, less than half after 2 h, and only 10% after 8–14 h of breathing[3]. Similarly, Ikegami *et al.*[7] have reported that less than 25% of instilled natural surfactant could be recovered from the alveolar space of 122- and 130-day gestation lambs several hours after delivery.

The large loss of exogenous surfactants such as CLL from the alveolar space within the first hours of breathing poses the question of the route and destination of the lost phospholipid[1,3]. Uptake by the alveolar type II cell and reutilization as substrate for endogenous surfactant production is one possibility. Another possibility is that CLL is absorbed from the alveolar lumen with the fetal lung liquid and is cleared completely from the lung. If exogenous surfactant is being lost from the lung, the potential exists for a premature animal treated with exogenous surfactant to 'run out' before endogenous production and secretion are adequate to sustain normal lung function over the long term.

The first minutes of breathing for a newborn mammal are accompanied by many dramatic changes in the lung. The aeration of the alveoli and the initiation of oxygen and carbon dioxide exchange between pulmonary capillary blood and alveolar gas is the most apparent event. In addition, lung vascular resistance must decrease to allow the 10-fold increase in pulmonary blood flow needed for effective gas transport rates. The secretion of the liquid which distends the airspace of the fetus must also be reversed, and the liquid present at birth must be absorbed and cleared from the lung. Finally, a new alveolar hypophase liquid lining layer must be established as a site for surfactant action and the adult pattern of surfactant secretion, reabsorption, and synthesis established. In prematurely born animals, surfactant deficiency appears to be a major factor preventing these successful pulmonary adaptations. If the deficiency is reversed by instillation of exogenous surfactant, effective aeration occurs and the premature animal is able to achieve the other pulmonary adaptations needed for survival.

ABSORPTION OF FETAL LUNG LIQUID AND ITS MECHANISMS

As noted above, the fetal pulmonary airspace is filled with a specially secreted lung liquid prior to ventilation. Before the onset of labour, this liquid approximates the same volume as the functional residual capacity (FRC) after birth, i.e. 20–30 ml/kg body weight. In the first 1–2 h of life, if the lungs are degassed by absorption atelectasis, significant amounts of fetal lung liquid can be aspirated from the airspaces[8-10]. After 2 h it is usually impossible to aspirate liquid from the airspaces, indicating that liquid absorption from lumen to tissue has largely occurred by this time. However the weight of the lungs of newborn lambs continues to fall for 6 h or so after birth, indicating that complete clearance of liquid from the lung takes substantially more time than that involved in absorption from the alveolar lumen[11].

To date three mechanisms of liquid absorption have been determined to occur as fetal lung liquid leaves the alveolar space during labour and after birth.

1. *Absorption through inter-cellular pores*

   In 1975, Egan, Olver and Strang[8] reported on the absorption of fetal liquid from the airspaces in spontaneously breathing full-term lambs for the first hour of life. In addition, they measured the concentration of multiple tracer solutes placed into the fetal liquid before the onset of ventilation. The larger solutes, protein-sized, increased in concentration in the fetal liquid during absorption, while smaller ones decreased in concentration, and the rate of decrease was found to be proportional to molecular size. During the first hour of breathing the absorptive epithelium was described as one with pores averaging 4 nm in radius, 8 times larger than before breathing, and 4–5 times larger than the case for lambs 1–4 days of age[8].

   Absorption pathways 4 nm in radius are too large to represent cell membrane pathways, and must reflect an intercellular route for water and solute absorption. Since pores of this size are still virtually impermeable to protein, Egan, Olver and Strang[8] proposed that the conductivity of the epithelium for the absorption of fetal lung liquid was increased early in ventilation, but was small enough to preserve the large protein concentration gradient between fetal lung liquid and interstitial fluid, which provides a driving force for liquid absorption. Their study also stated that about 25% of the fetal lung liquid was absorbed in the first hour of breathing[8]. However, that estimate was based upon the concentration increase of large solutes in the fetal lung liquid, and did not allow for the possibility of some absorption by other mechanisms.

2. *Absorption by bulk flow through the epithelium*

   Another pathway for liquid and solute absorption is by bulk flow through the epithelium, without restriction of larger solutes. To help evaluate this mechanism, Egan *et al.*[10] performed intermittent measurements of alveolar liquid volume in breathing, exteriorized fetal lambs while the fetus remained attached to the umbilical circulation. The lung was degassed by absorption atelectasis, and a small amount of a radiolabelled solute added to the lung liquid, mixed, and the resulting dilution used to give an estimate of alveolar liquid volume. Egan et al.[10] used this method, together with measurements of changes in concentration of different-sized tracer solutes, to evaluate lung liquid absorption characteristics in premature lambs. It is in such premature animals, where the integrity of the epithelium may not be fully developed, that unrestricted solute transport by a bulk flow absorption mechanism might be expected.

In the experiments of Egan et al.[10], premature lambs with little surfactant in the fetal lung liquid were found to absorb over 50% of the volume within 20 min, but the concentration of radiolabelled albumin in the alveolar liquid remained unchanged. This implied that a large fraction of the radiolabelled protein was absorbed from the alveoli at the same rate as the lung liquid itself, i.e. a bulk flow solute absorption was present. Interestingly, lambs which released surfactant into the alveolar liquid during the first minutes of breathing showed only the intercellular pore pathway (described in item 1 above) after the first 20 min of breathing. Lambs that did not release significant amounts of surfactant continued to have bulk absorption for longer times, and did not demonstrate restriction of any solute to the alveolar space because of a pore size limit[10].

3. *Absorption through an intracellular pathway*

A third pathway of fetal lung liquid and solute absorption is one where transport occurs through the alveolar epithelial cells rather than between them. Although the actual contribution of such a pathway to liquid absorption in mammals is not well documented, its possibility does exist. For example, it has been found that secretion of lung liquid in fetal lambs can be reversed, and absorption initiated, by infusion of β-adrenergic agents[12]. Moreover, this absorption can be blocked by addition of the diuretic amiloride to the fetal lung liquid[13].

Amiloride is a sodium channel blocker, among other actions, so one interpretation of these results is that absorption due to β-adrenergic agents is associated with solute transfer through lung lining cells. However, this intracellular pathway for lung liquid absorption has only been studied in the fluid-filled fetal lung and not in the ventilated lung, and clearly requires further experiments to document its significance.

The possible presence, in principle, of three functionally different mechanisms for absorption of fetal lung liquid affects analyses and interpretations of data involving solutes in the airspaces. Retention in the alveoli of substances dissolved or suspended in alveolar liquid will depend upon the fraction of the liquid being absorbed by each pathway. For example, in terms of surfactant status and lung liquid absorption, the results of *Egan et al.*[10] showed that fetal lung liquid absorption changed from a bulk-flow predominance to a pore-limited predominance with rising alveolar surfactant content in some lambs. This suggests that preventilatory instillation of an exogenous surfactant such as CLL in premature lambs might similarly induce a pore-limited absorption mechanism. CLL phospholipid aggregates reaching the alveolar epithelial barrier during lung liquid absorption by this mechanism could be more available for surfactant recycling pathways, for example, compared to the case where CLL phospholipid is rapidly carried through the epithelium, without restriction, by a significant bulk flow. Consequently, it is appropriate to address questions about whether exogenous surfactant replacement affects the mechanisms or patterns of lung liquid absorption in premature lambs, and this is discussed in the experiments below.

CHARACTERIZATIONS OF LUNG LIQUID ABSORPTION RELATED TO EXOGENOUS SURFACTANT REPLACEMENT

Methods

The experimental protocols used for these experiments were similar to previous studies with premature lambs in our laboratory[1,3], and used lambs of 130 days gestation (term 150 days). The ewe was anaesthetized, maintained on halothane anaesthesia, and the fetus delivered by hysterotomy with the umbilical circulation kept intact. A tracheal cannula was then inserted, and lung liquid aspirated. To the lung liquid were added trace amounts of radiolabelled albumin, molecular radius 3.5 nm; cytochrome C, molecular radius 1.7 nm and cyanocobalamin, molecular radius 0.7 nm. From the dilution of these labelled solutes, all of which are restricted to the alveolar space in the fetal state prior to ventilation, the initial volume of the fetal lung liquid was calculated.

For surfactant-replacement studies, six lambs had 100 mg/kg body weight of calf lung surfactant lipid extract, CLL, added to the fetal lung liquid. Mechanical ventilation was then started using 100% oxygen with the umbilical circulation maintained. After 45 and 90 min of ventilation the ventilator was stopped, and the oxygen in the lung absorbed. A sample of lung liquid was aspirated via the trachea, and an aliquot taken for measurement of the concentrations of tracer solutes, phospholipids, and plasma proteins. An additional amount of labelled cyanocobalamin was added to the remaining lung liquid, which was then re-instilled and mixed for a few minutes in the lung and re-sampled in the absence of further ventilation. From the dilution of the added cyanocobalamin after re-instillation, the total volume of alveolar liquid was estimated[10]. The rate of liquid absorption was then calculated by subtracting the newly calculated volume from the initial lung liquid volume. In addition, the net flux of a substance into or out of the alveolar space was calculated as the difference between its amount at the sampling time and the previous amount found to be present, with amount determined as the product of concentration and volume.

Comparison of the concentrations of alveolar liquid solutes found by these techniques at different times permitted determination of their relative rates of loss, regardless of the absorptive pathways being utilized. Although the exogenous surfactant CLL exists largely as phospholipid

Table 15.1 Gas exchange and lung mechanics in control and surfactant extract (CLL)–treated premature lambs

	Control lambs	Surfactant-treated lambs
After 45 min of breathing:		
Pa_{O_2}	55 ± 10 torr	268 ± 51 torr
Pa_{CO_2}	50 ± 8 torr	42 ± 4 torr
TLC	18 ± 2 ml/kg	36 ± 4 ml/kg
FRC	7 ± 1 ml/kg	19 ± 2 ml/kg
After 90 min of breathing:		
Pa_{O_2}	73 ± 6 torr	363 ± 2 torr
Pa_{CO_2}	51 ± 5 torr	35 ± 4 torr
TLC	22 ± 2 ml/kg	44 ± 6 ml/kg
FRC	8 ± 1 ml/kg	20 ± 2 ml/kg

TLC is total lung capacity at 35 cmH_2O distending pressure and FRC is lung volume at 0 distending pressure (ml/kg)

vesicles in suspension, not solution, we also used comparisons, of phospholipid concentration changes to those of tracer solutes to define the fate of the instilled surfactant material.

Experimental results

The efficiency of oxygenation, and the mechanical properties of the lungs, of the six CLL pretreated and five control 130-day gestation lambs is presented in Table 15.1. As expected, the surfactant-pretreated lambs had excellent gas exchange and much higher total lung capacities and functional residual lung capacities than did the control animals, in agreement with our previous studies of lung surfactant replacement with CLL[1,3,5,6]. Most important for the present paper, the rate of lung liquid absorption from the alveolar space was significantly slower in CLL-treated animals compared to controls. A comparison of the change in alveolar liquid volume over the first 90 min of breathing for these animals is charted in Fig. 15.1. As shown there, surfactant-treated animals had larger volumes of alveolar liquid during the first 90 min of breathing, to go along with the better ventilation and higher lung gas capacities presented in Table 15.1.

Figure 15.2 shows the change over time of the alveolar concentration of labelled albumin, the largest tracer solute instilled into the fetal lung liquid before the onset of breathing. From 0 to 45 min labelled albumin left the alveolar space of CLL-treated lambs at the same rate as volume, indicating a bulk flow mechanistic process. However, from 45 to 90 min the albumin concentration rose in treated animals, reflecting a more rapid loss of volume than of labelled albumin. Control animals not treated with CLL

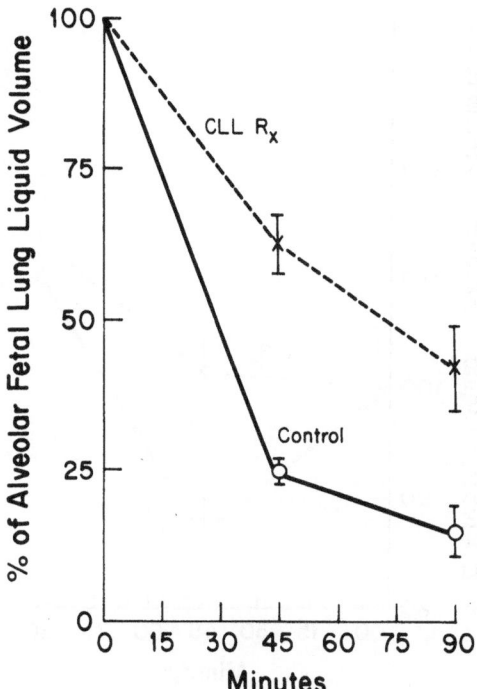

Figure 15.1 The volume of fetal alveolar liquid measured before breathing and at 45 and 90 min after the start of ventilation. CLL R_X denotes lambs treated with exogenous calf lung surfactant extract prior to ventilation (100 mg/kg)

showed a decline in labelled albumin concentration from 0 to 45 min, reflecting a more rapid loss of albumin than volume, despite the fact that these controls absorbed 75% of the total fetal lung liquid within the first 45 min (Figure 15.1). From 45 to 90 min there was a rise in labelled albumin concentration, just as was seen in CLL-treated animals.

The data in Figure 15.2 indicate that initially most of the liquid absorption was by bulk flow in both CLL-treated and control groups, although the CLL animals did lose albumin at a slower rate than controls. Moreover, the very rapid initial loss in labelled albumin by the control animals suggests that an additional transport mechanism may have been present for this group. Specifically, since the rate of labelled albumin loss by these animals in the first 45 min of ventilation was actually more rapid than volume loss, some transport passages must exist initially in the controls to allow diffusional or other loss of labelled albumin from the alveoli in addition to a strict bulk flow process. After 45 min of ventilation, bulk flow absorption continues in both groups, but a rising albumin concentration is exhibited for each in Fig. 15.2. Presumably this means that some liquid absorption is now through pathways which do not allow the passage of labell-

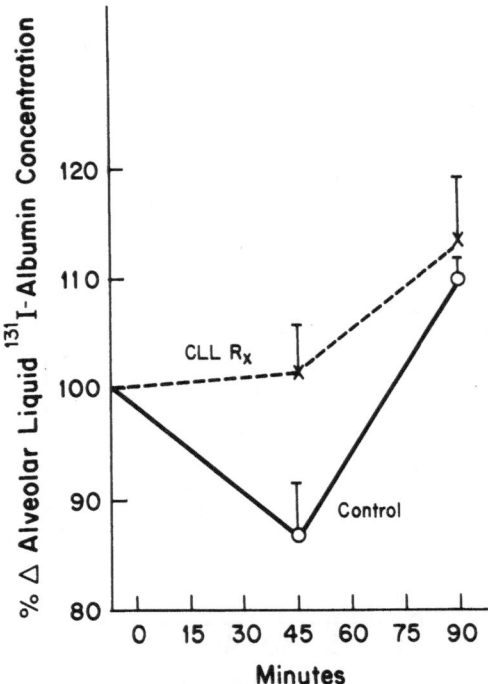

Figure 15.2 The change in concentration of labelled bovine albumin in fetal alveolar liquid as a function of time after ventilation. Protein is expressed as the percentage of its concentration present before the onset of breathing

ed albumin, thus retarding its absorption in comparison to water and resulting in a rise in its alveolar concentration. (Although it is likely that this rise in labelled albumin concentration from 45 to 90 min reflects a change in the mechanism of liquid absorption, part of the rise could also be due to re-entry of previously absorbed labelled albumin from the lung interstitial space, particularly for control animals.)

The absorption characteristics of labelled albumin instilled into lung liquid give one measure of the state and integrity of the alveolar epithelium. Another measure is provided by determination of the *total* protein concentration in the alveolar liquid, and this is shown in Fig. 15.3 for CLL-treated and control premature lambs. The measured rise in unlabelled protein found in Fig. 15.3 almost certainly represents plasma proteins crossing the epithelium into the alveolar lung liquid in a direction opposite to the absorption processes we have been discussing to this point. Both surfactant-treated and control animals show increasing total protein concentrations in alveolar liquid over the first 45 min after ventilation in Fig. 15.3, but the control group concentration is more than three times that of the surfactant-treated group. After 45 min there is a further rise in plasma protein content in the alveoli of both control and CLL-treated animals. Some of this

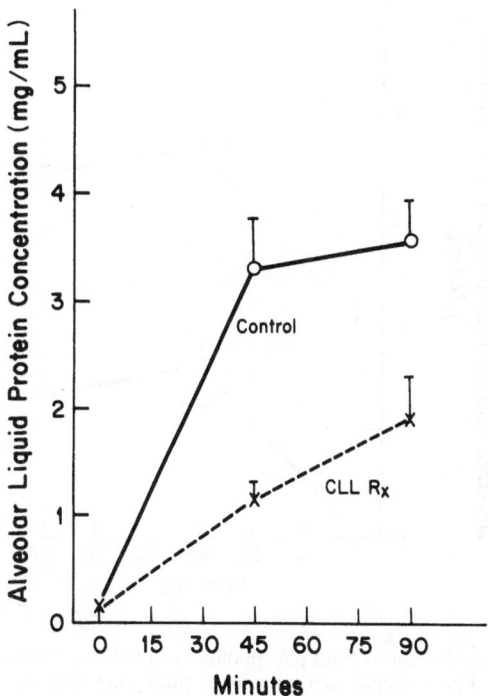

Figure 15.3 The total concentration of protein in fetal alveolar liquid during the first 90 min of ventilation. Total concentration is expressed as mg protein/ml liquid at any time

rise in total alveolar protein concentration from 45 to 90 min may be due to liquid absorption alone and not continuing influx of plasma proteins. However, the data in Fig. 15.3 demonstrate that significant plasma protein transfer occurs into the alveoli of these premature lambs early in ventilation, and that this transfer is greater in animals not receiving exogenous surfactant replacement.

The lower total alveolar protein concentrations in CLL-treated animals in Fig. 15.3 may have an additional functional significance in respiration aside from their indication of a more intact alveolar epithelium in terms of solute transport characteristics. This is because plasma proteins in sufficient quantitities have been shown to inhibit lung surfactant biophysical activity, leading to decreased dynamic surface tension lowering ability and decreased surfactant adsorption to the air–hypophase interface[14]. Moreover, the degree of such inhibition is now known to be dependent upon the amount of surfactant phospholipid present, with the most severe inhibition found at low phospholipid concentrations[14,15]. In premature animals (or infants) which are already marginal in terms of alveolar surfactant phospholipid, a large plasma protein influx to alveoli could lead to a vicious cycle of

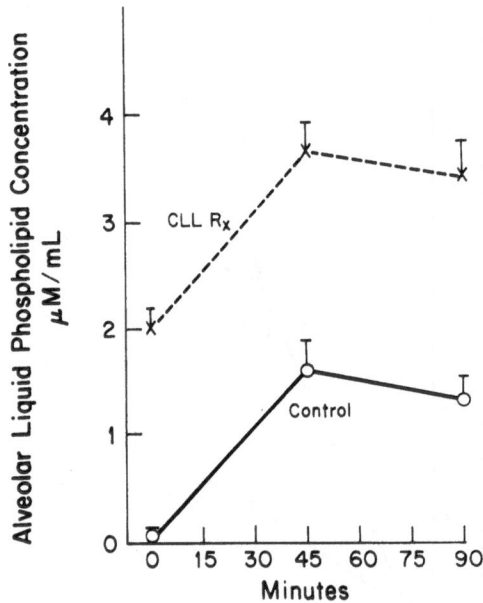

Figure 15.4 The concentration of total phospholipid in fetal alveolar liquid during the first 90 min of ventilation. Phospholipid concentration is total μmol lipid phosphorus/ml lung liquid

surfactant inactivation, followed by an increased driving force for pulmonary oedema[16], further protein influx and surfactant inactivation, and so on. Exogenous surfactant supplementation would appear to be protective against such a cycle, both by providing increased alveolar phospholipid and by decreasing the amount of alveolar protein present.

Changes in the phospholipid concentration in fetal lung liquid during the first 90 min of breathing are detailed for surfactant-supplemented and control lambs in Fig. 15.4. The CLL-pretreated group is seen to exhibit a rise in concentration during the first 45 min, which reflects the addition of significant amounts of exogenous phospholipid to the alveolar liquid at the start of the experiment and its subsequent concentration by alveolar liquid volume absorption. However, part of this initial rise in the CLL-treated group is probably due also to the release of endogenous surfactant into alveoli. Clearly, the rise in phospholipid concentration shown in control animals in the first 45 min in Fig. 15.4 can only reflect release of endogenous stores. After the initial rise in alveolar phospholipid concentration there is a slight decline in alveolar phospholipid concentration from 45 to 90 min found in both groups. Moreover, although not shown explicitly in Fig. 15.4, alveolar phospholipid levels (absolute amounts) are known to continue to decrease in CLL-treated animals as ventilation proceeds over 6–10 h[1,3].

Figure 15.5 expresses the changes in concentration for all three tracer

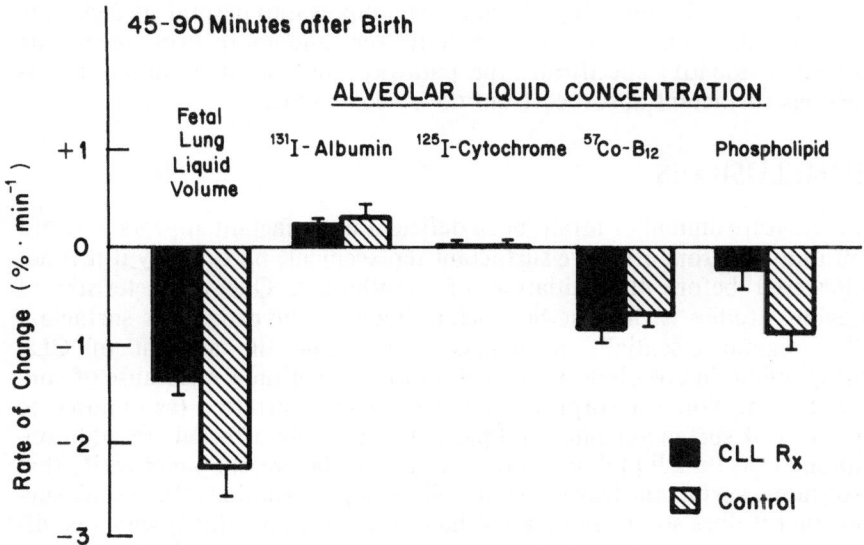

Figure 15.5 The rate of change of fetal alveolar liquid volume, labelled alveolar solute concentration, and alveolar phospholipid concentration between 45 and 90 minutes of ventilation. See text for details

solutes added to the alveolar liquid, the rate of alveolar liquid absorption, and the decline in phospholipid concentration in the alveolar liquid, for the period between 45 and 90 min after the start of ventilation. The rate of change, expressed as percentage per minute, is shown for each variable during this 45–90 min time period. For calculations, the total change in alveolar content for any substance was determined from the rate of volume change and the rate of its concentration change.

In interpreting the results in Fig. 15.5, the radiolabelled molecular tracers show a size-dependent pattern for both control and CLL-treated groups over the given time period: labelled albumin concentration increases with time, cytochrome C concentration is static, and cyanocobalamin concentration decreases with time. However, since the rate of labelled albumin increase is less than the rate of liquid absorption, some labelled albumin is still being removed from the alveolar space for both groups of animals over the 45–90 min time period of ventilation. In terms of phospholipid clearance, the alveolar phospholipid concentration is decreasing over this time period, despite the fact that CLL (and natural LS) phospholipid exists in liposomes and other microstructural aggregates in alveolar fluid, and these aggregates are much larger than albumin molecules[17]. The fact that the phospholipids in both CLL-treated and control groups do not increase in concentration over the 45–90 min period of ventilation, as would be predicted from their size, indicates that part of their loss must involve a mechanistic process of absorption different from typical solute molecules. One attractive hypothesis is that the loss of phospholipid in alveolar liquid over time, as shown in Fig. 15.5, reflects cellular uptake for recycling of the phospholipids into natural surfactant in type II cells[18]. This is speculative, however, and more experiments are needed to identify specifically the pathways and the destinations of exogenous surfactant absorbed from the alveolar space.

CONCLUSIONS

A premature animal or infant born deficient in surfactant appears to profit substantially from effective surfactant replacement, particularly if it is administered before the initiation of breathing[1-6]. One characteristic of previous studies is that the beneficial effects of the exogenous surfactant CLL remain essentially unchanged even while the amount of CLL phospholipid in alveoli decreases substantially over time[1,3]. Because of concurrent lung liquid absorption, the alveolar concentration (as opposed to amount) of surfactant phospholipid is less severely affected. In addition, although the lung liquid absorption studies of the present paper verify that exogenous surfactant leaves the alveoli during ventilation, the results suggest that it does so partly by a mechanism (as yet undefined) which is different from normal bulk flow or solute transport mechanisms. One possibility worthy of further study is that some of this material may enter a surfactant recycling pathway. Aside from considerations involving phospholipid uptake, the transport data here also show that the delivery of effective exogenous surfactant to premature lambs diminishes the influx of proteins into the alveolar space compared to controls. It also shows the overall rate of absorption of alveolar liquid compared to surfactant-deficient premature animals.

All of these observations are as yet not integrated into a coherent understanding of the actions of exogenous surfactant in affecting the many adaptations of the premature lung during the initiation of pulmonary ventilation and gas exchange. Indeed, there still exist substantial gaps in our knowledge of how perinatal pulmonary adaptations occur even in normal births of full-term gestation. However, the past few years have provided data from many sources to show that surfactant lack is important in the poor lung function found in premature animals and humans at birth, and that exogenous surfactant therapy can prevent respiratory failure. The experiments described here suggest that the physiological effects of surfactant interact with the mechanisms of lung liquid and solute absorption which occur at the start of ventilation.

Acknowledgement

This work was supported in part by NIH grants HL-25170, HL-22522, and HL-00945 (RCDA to R.H.N.).

References

1. Egan, E. A., Notter, R. H., Kwong, M. S. *et al.* (1983). Natural and artificial lung surfactant replacement in premature lambs. *J. Appl. Physiol.,* **55,** 875–83
2. Jobe, A., Ikegami, M., Jacobs, H. *et al.* (1984). Surfactant and pulmonary blood flow distributions following treatment of premature lambs with natural surfactant. *J. Clin. Invest.,* **73,** 848–56
3. Notter, R. H., Egan, E. A., Kwong, M. S. *et al.* (1985). Lung surfactant replacement in premature lambs with extracted lipids from bovine lung lavage: effects of dose, dispersion technique, and gestational age. *Pediatr. Res.,* **19,** 569–77
4. Jobe, A., Ikegami, M., Glatz, T. *et al.* (1981). Duration and characterization of treatment of premature lambs with natural surfactant. *J. Clin. Invest.,* **67,** 370–5
5. Enhorning, G., Shennan, A., Possmayer, F. *et al.* (1985). Prevention of neonatal respiratory distress syndrome by tracheal instillation of surfactant: a randomized trial. *Pediatrics,* **76,** 145–53
6. Kwong, M. S., Egan, E. A., Notter, R. H., *et al.* (1985). Double blind clinical trial of calf lung surfactant extract for the prevention of hyaline membrane disease in extremely premature infants. *Pediatrics,* **76,** 585–92
7. Ikegami, M., Jobe, A., Glatz, T. *et al.* (1981). Surface activity following natural surfactant treatment of premature lambs. *J. Appl. Physiol.,* **51,** 306–12
8. Egan, E. A., Olver, R. E., and Strang, L. B., (1975). Changes in the non-electrolyte permeability of alveoli and the absorption of lung liquid at the start of breathing in the lamb. *J. Physiol.,* **244,** 161–79
9. Egan, E. A., Nelson, R. M. and Beale, E. F. (1980). Lung solute permeability and lung liquid absorption in premature fetal goats. *Pediatr. Res.,* **14,** 314–18
10. Egan, E. A., Dillon, W. P. and Zorn, S. (1984). Fetal lung liquid absorption and alveolar epithelial solute permeability in surfactant deficient, breathing premature lambs. *Pediatr. Res.,* **18,** 566–70
11. Humphreys, P. W., Normand, I. C. S., Reynolds, E. O. R. and Strang, L. B. (1967). Pulmonary lymph and the uptake of liquid from the lungs of the lamb at the start of breathing. *J. Physiol.,* **193,** 1–29
12. Brown, M. J., Olver, R. E., Ramsden, C. A., Strang, L. B. and Walters, D. V. (1983). Effects of adrenaline and of spontaneous labour on the secretion and absorption of lung liquid in the fetal lamb. *J. Physiol.,* **344,** 137–52
13. Olver, R. E., Ramsden, C. A. and Strang, L. B. (1981). Adrenaline induced changes in net lung liquid volume flow across the pulmonary epithelium of the fetal lamb: evidence for active sodium transport. *J. Physiol.,* **319,** 38–39P
14. Holm, B. A., Notter, R. H. and Finkelstein, J. N. (1985). Surface property changes from interactions of albumin and natural lung surfactant and extracted lung lipids. *Chem. Physics Lipids.,* **38,** 287–98
15. Holm, B. A., Notter, R. H., Siegle, J. and Matalon, S. (1985). Pulmonary physiological and surfactant changes during injury and recovery from exposure to 100% oxygen. *J. Appl. Physiol.,* **59,** 1402–9
16. Notter, R. H. and Finkelstein, J. N. (1984). Pulmonary surfactant: an inter-disciplinary approach. *J. Appl. Physiol.,* **57,** 1613–24
17. Notter, R. H., Penney, D. D., Finkelstein, J. N. *et al.* (1986). Adsorption of natural lung surfactant and phospholipid extracts related to tubular myelin formation. *Pediatr. Res.,* **20,** 97–101
18. Jacobs, H., Jobe, A., Ikegami, M. *et al.* (1986). Accumulation of alveolar surfactant following delivery and ventilation of premature lambs. *Exptl. Lung Res.,* (In press)

Discussion

Dr D. V. Walters I'm a little worried about the way you measure lung liquid volume. Do you look in the plasma to see if your radiolabelled albumin is coming through, and if so to what extent; and have you thought of using an even bigger tracer than albumin since the channels in your experiments must be very big to allow unrestricted passage of albumin?

Dr E. A. Egan Yes. We've even gone to using something as big as blue dextran. But when you go through the calculations, our measurements of volume using albumin, while not totally accurate, are all within plus or minus 10% of the correct value. We have checked this by adding known volumes of saline to increase lung volume.

Walters Is there evidence from histological sections that bits of the epithelium are totally wrenched off in your experiments?

Dr L. B. Strang I don't know about Dr Egan's present experiments, but in earlier work on changes taking place at birth the normal mature animal was found to have a very moderate enlargement of the pathway for solute transport at the start of breathing. The channels remained sufficiently small to prevent almost all albumin transfer across the epithelium[1]. Surely these pathways you now describe are quite different and much larger. Should they be considered pathological?

Egan Yes, I think they should be considered pathological.

Strang Perhaps the best hope for exogenous surfactant treatment would be that it might prevent the epithelial damage characteristic of HMD.

Dr J. A. Clements Surfactant is sticky stuff and sticks to surfaces, including epithelia. It is difficult to distinguish between the sticking of the material on the surface of the epithelium, uptake into cells, and movement through passages into the interstitium. Your data show that the rate of removal from accessible lavagable spaces was 17 μmol/g of lung tissue per hour, which is 50 times the calculated normal surfactant secretion rate. If you postulate that the material is going to type II cells they would have to be awfully busy, and my interpretation would rather be that the material is not being lost from the alveolar spaces but getting stuck on top of cells where it might be potentially still available.

Egan From our experiments we have no way of distinguishing between these possibilities.

Dr B. Robertson One of the most striking effects of surfactant replacement is the prevention of epithelial lesions, not only in bronchioles where they are easily observed by light microscopy, but also at the alveolar level. I consider prevention of epithelial disruption to be one of the key effects of surfactant replacement.

Dr J. S. Wigglesworth I don't know if anyone has actually looked to see if surfactant particles ever do get into the pulmonary lymphatics which are most prominent in the first few hours after birth.

Dr J. P. Mortola A lamb at term has about 100 ml of fluid in its lungs. Thus, at the absorption rate shown, it would take about 2 hours to clear the lungs from the pulmonary fluid. How can the lamb breathe meanwhile?

222

Egan   At the time of taking the first breath, if there's been some prenatal absorption there should be less than 30 ml/kg body weight in the lung and the remainder should be absorbed through temporarily enlarged paracellular pathways as postulated by Egan et al.[1]. Nevertheless lung weight measurements show that liquid is removed from the lung as a whole rather slowly over a period of hours. During this period it is probably contained in the interstitial spaces and lymphatics of the lung as shown in histological studies by Aherne and Dawkins[2] and others[3].

References

1. Egan, E. A., Olver, R. E. and Strang, L. B. (1975). Changes in non-electrolyte permeability of alveoli and the absorption of lung liquid at the start of breathing in the lamb. *J. Physiol.*, **244**, 161–79
2. Aherne, W. and Dawkins, M. J. R. (1964). The removal of fluid from the pulmonary airways after birth and the effect on this of prematurity and prenatal hypoxia. *Biolog. Neonat.*, **7**, 214–29
3. Bland, R. D., Bressack, M. A. and McMillan, D. D. (1979). Labor decreases lung water content of newborn rabbits. *Am. J. Obstet. Gynecol.*, **135**, 364–67

REFERENCES

16
Surfactant Inhibitory Plasma-Derived Proteins

W. SEEGER, G. STÖHR AND H. NEUHOF

There are three potential mechanisms by which the alveolar surfactant system can be altered:

1. lack of surface-active material;
2. changes in the relative composition of its lipid or protein compounds;
3. inhibitory effect of a factor or factors leaked from the intravascular or interstitial space due to increased permeability of the capillary-endothelial and/or alveolo-epithelial barrier.

As the main line of pathogenesis of the respiratory distress syndrome of the adult includes alterations of the endothelial and/or epithelial barrier we have concentrated on the third point with three questions:

1. What are the consequences of a stimulation of the arachidonic acid cascade in the pulmonary vascular bed on lung mechanics?
2. What are the consequences of differently induced high permeability oedema on lung mechanics and surfactant function *in vitro?*
3. What is the influence of different proteins on the function of natural surfactant *in vitro?*

Most experiments were performed in the isolated rabbit lung[1,2]. Briefly, the lungs were excised from deeply anaesthetized adult animals without interruption of ventilation and perfusion, and were placed in a 38 °C warmed chamber, freely suspended from a force transducer. They were ventilated with 4% CO_2, 17% O_2, rest N_2. They were perfused with Krebs Henseleit albumin (bovine source, 92% purity, fatty acid free) buffer (KHAB) in a recirculating system. The alternate use of two different perfusion systems allowed different perfusion phases, each with fresh perfusion liquid with or without addition of a stimulus. Only those lungs which showed a homogeneous white appearance and revealed no change of perfusion pressure, ventilation pressure and organ weight during a steady-state period of least 30 min were used. Random light microscopical examination of these lungs revealed no oedema formation and no adhering leukocytes or platelets.

In this model a variety of stimuli activate the arachidonic acid cascade in the pulmonary vascular bed[2,3]. Experimentally this is mimicked by application of the calcium-ionophore A 23187, which is known to release free arachidonic acid from the membrane phospholipid pools. In isolated rabbit lungs A 23187 provokes an acute pulmonary artery pressor response, which appears to be mediated primarily by the arachidonic acid product thromboxane A2. It is accompanied by a release of this mediator, it is suppressed by inhibitors of cyclo-oxygenase and thromboxane synthetase and by a thromboxane receptor antagonist, and it can be mimicked by the stable thromboxane analogue U-46619[1-3]. Additionally, increased availability of free arachidonic acid is accompanied by a gain in lung weight, which is not suppressed by inhibition of cyclo-oxygenase. It is caused by an increased permeability of the pulmonary vascular bed[1,4], which must be ascribed to non-cyclo-oxygenase pathways of arachidonic acid action.

The consequences of calcium ionophore-induced oedema on lung mechanics were investigated with the following protocol[5]:

On the one hand oedema formation in the isolated lungs was induced by mechanically increasing the capillary filtration pressure. This was performed by repeated obstruction of the pulmonary venous outflow by means of a Swan–Ganz balloon catheter. The total amount of oedema was standardized at 7 g/kg bodyweight of the animal from which the lung originated. The time of oedema development ranged between 30 and 60 min. On the other hand the same amount of oedema was induced by stimulation of the arachidonic acid cascade with the calcium ionophore A 23187 in the following ways:

1. Repeated application of A 23187 (2–3 μmol/l), allowing pulmonary artery pressure peaks between 25 and 40 mmHg (time of oedema formation 3–4.5 h).

2. Repeated application of A 23187 (2 μmol/l) in the presence of indomethacin (60 μmol/l), thus suppressing any increase in pulmonary artery pressure (time of oedema formation 3–4.5 h).

3. Repeated application of A 23187 (2 μmol/l) in presence of indomethacin (60 μmol/l) and reduced glutathione (13 μmol/l), thus reinforcing the increase in vascular permeability (time of oedema formation 30–60 min).

4. Application of a high dose of A 23187 (4 μmol/l), allowing pulmonary artery pressure peaks of 50 $\pm$ 5 mmHg, with rapid formation of the standardized amount of oedema within 3–10 min.

After the period of oedema formation, classical pressure volume diagrams and pneumoloop diagrams of the isolated lungs were performed (Fig. 16.1). In comparison to control lungs all lungs with oedema formation showed alterations of lung mechanics, namely decrease of total compliance and decrease of the compliance quotients of the classical pressure–volume diagrams and of the pneumoloop diagrams[5]. The alterations were,

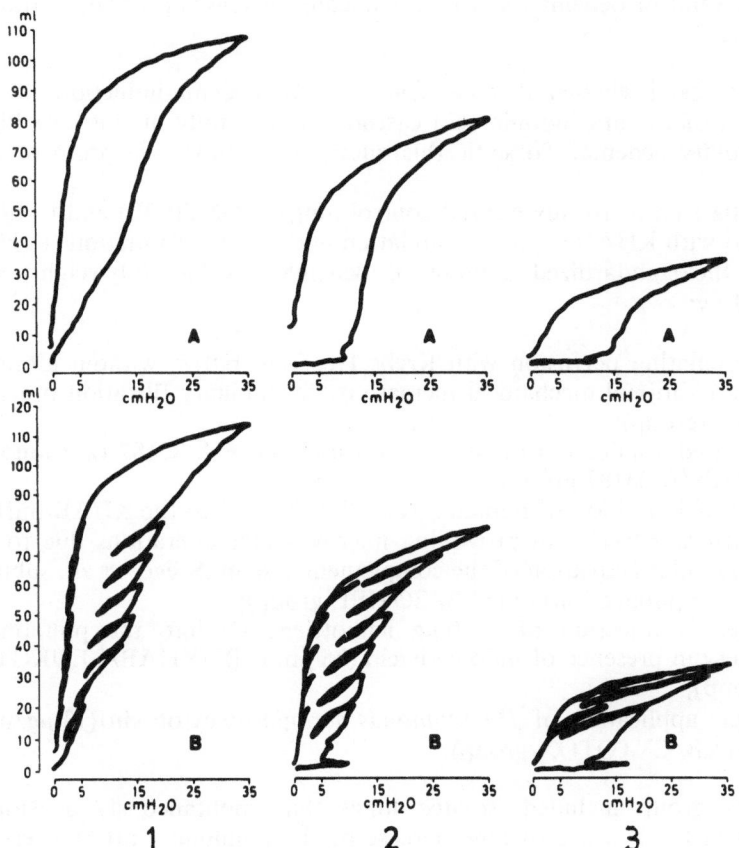

Figure 16.1   Classical pressure–volume diagrams (A) and pneumoloop diagrams (B) of a control lung (1), a lung that developed 7 g oedema/kg bodyweight due to mechanical increase in the capillary filtration pressure (2) and a lung that developed the same amount of oedema following stimulation of the pulmonary vascular arachidonic acid cascade (A 23187 + indomethacin + GSH) (3). The marked differences in pressure–volume characteristics are evident. (Classical PV diagrams: continuous inflation and deflation with room air up to a maximum inflation pressure of 35 cmH₂O. Pneumoloop diagrams: inflation and deflation in form of loops at changing functional residual capacity)[5].

however, significantly more severe in all oedematous lungs after application of the calcium ionophore than they were in the lungs with oedema formation due to repeated obstruction of the pulmonary venous outflow. In separate experiments this was also the case for oedema-induction due to direct application of free arachidonic acid in comparison to lungs with mechanically induced oedema. Within the groups of lungs with repeated application of A 23187 the degree of alteration in lung mechanics correlated with the speed with which the oedema had developed.

We concluded that *high permeability oedema* due to stimulation of the pulmonary vascular *arachidonic acid cascade* in rabbit lungs causes alterations of *lung mechanics* markedly more severe than those induced by the same amount of oedema due to mechanically *increased capillary filtration pressure.*

Next we asked whether this was true only for oedema-induction via stimulation of the arachidonic acid cascade, or generally in states of high-permeability oedema. To settle this question the following protocol was chosen[6]:

In comparison to freshly excised control lungs (CONTROL) and to lungs perfused with KHAB without stimulation and oedema formation (KHAB-group) the standardized amount of oedema (7 g/kg bodyweight) was induced by:

1. recirculating perfusion with Krebs Henseleit buffer without albumin and additional mechanical increase in the capillary filtration pressure (KHB-group);
2. repeated application of the calcium ionophore A 23187 (2–3 μmol/l) KHAB/A 23187-group);
3. repeated addition of human serum (8–16% v/v) to the KHAB-buffer, which is effective in provoking microvascular alterations due to intravascular activation of the complement system (Seeger *et al.,* submitted for publication) (KHAB/COMPL-group);
4. repeated injection of 5–10 μg leukotriene C4 into the pulmonary artery in presence of indomethacin (35 μmol/l)[7] (KHAB/LEUKOTR-group);
5. single application of *Pseudomonas aeruginosa* cytotoxin (13 μg/ml)[8] (KHAB/CYTOTOX-group).

The last group included isolated lungs that spontaneously developed oedema in the absence of any increase of the pulmonary artery pressure for unknown reasons (KHAB/sp.OEDEMA-group).

After the lungs had developed the standardized amount of oedema (7 g/kg bodyweight) classical pressure–volume diagrams and pneumoloop diagrams were recorded and extensive bronchoalveolar lavage of the whole lungs with saline was performed. The lavage phospholipid (organic phosphorous) and protein content was determined, and the surface activity of the lavage fluid was measured at a standardized phospholipid concentration of 50 μg/ml in a modified Langmuir–Wilhelmy Teflon surface balance according to Clements *et al.*[9] and Hildebran *et al.*[10] (Fig. 16.2).

There was no difference in the total lavage phospholipid content between the different groups of lungs (Fig. 16.3). There was, however, a marked difference in the lavage protein content: low protein in the control lungs, in the perfused non-oedematous lungs and in the lungs that developed oedema in the absence of circulating protein; and markedly increased (up to 25 times) lavage protein in all lungs with high permeability oedema (Fig. 16.3). SDS polacrylamide gel electrophoresis of the lavage proteins revealed that the proteins had leaked from the intravascular space. As expected from the previous experiments all lungs with protein-

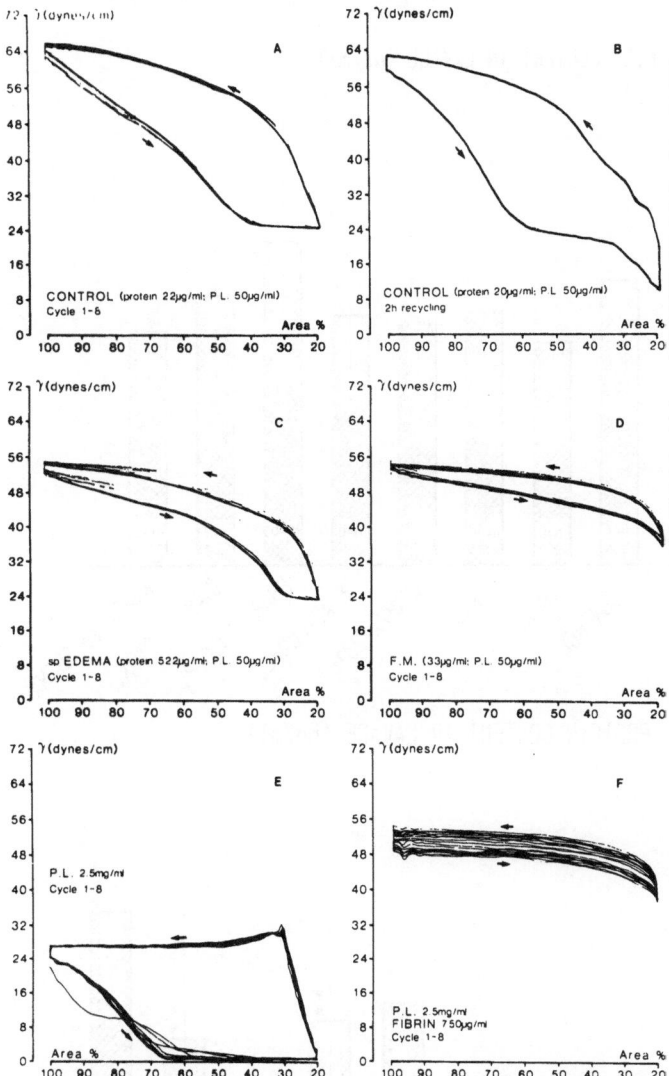

Figure 16.2 Original records of the surface tension characteristics of control lavage fluid (A), control lavage fluid recycled for 2 h (B), protein-rich lavage fluid from a spontaneously oedematous lung (C) and control lavage fluid in presence of 33 µg/ml bovine fibrin monomer (F.M.) (D). The experiments were performed with a phospholipid concentration of 50 µg/ml, at 38 °C, with cyclic area variation between 100% and 20% within 2.5 min. The first eight cycles after sonication are shown (except for B), the 8th cycle being plotted as a thicker line. The alterations of surface tension in presence of protein-rich oedema and fibrin monomer are evident. Panels E and F show the surface tension–area diagrams of lavage surfactant pooled from eight rabbits and concentrated to a phospholipid concentration of 2.5 mg/ml. After addition of 6 mg/ml bovine fibrinogen and 0.1 NIH/ml thrombin the bulk of the fibrin(ogen) was removed as a fibrin clot. The remaining 'soluble' fibrin was measured as 750 µg/ml. After this procedure the surface activity is markedly altered (F compared to E)[6]

229

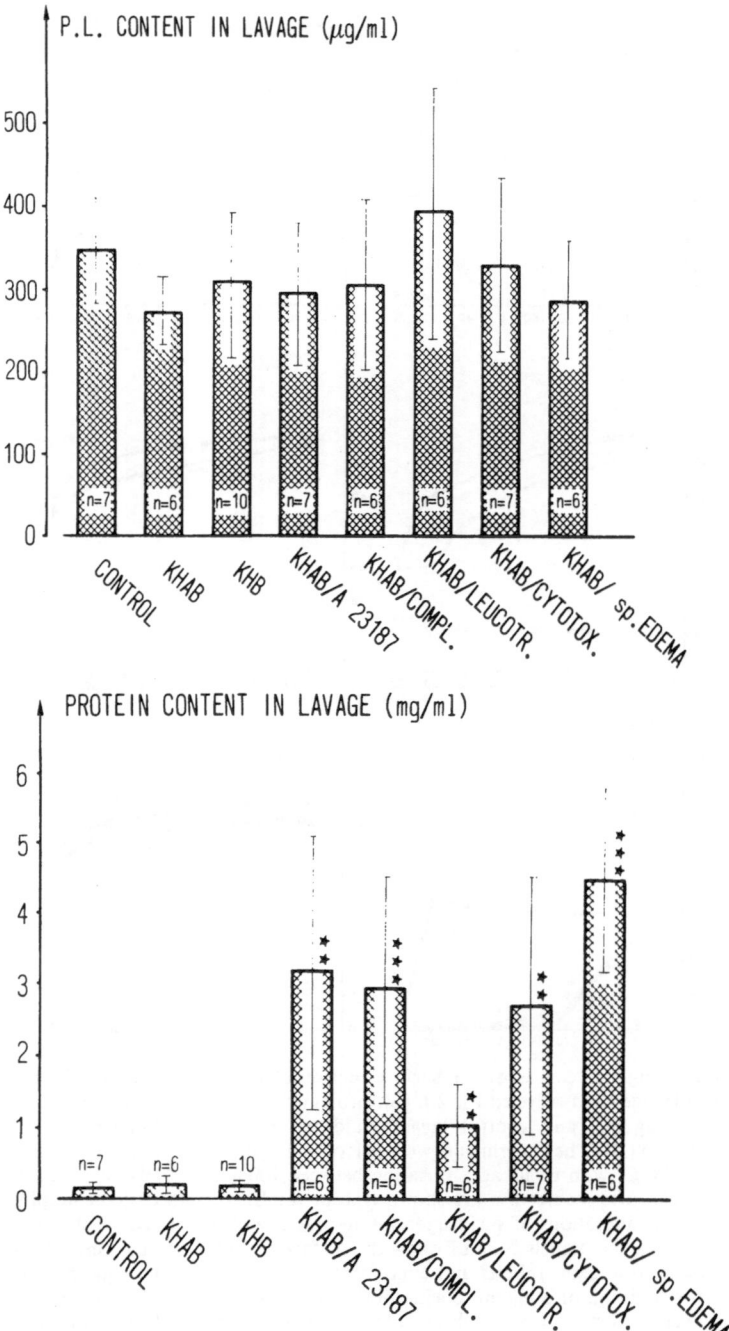

Figure 16.3 Phospholipid and protein concentration in the bronchoalveolar lavage fluid of non-oedematous lungs (CONTROL, KHAB) and of lungs with differently induced oedema. The manoeuvres of oedema induction are explained in the text. The columns show mean ± SD[6]

rich oedema showed markedly altered pressure–volume characteristics (decrease of the total compliance and of the compliance quotients of the classical PV – and the pneumoloop diagrams). There was a significant correlation between the lavage protein content and the alteration of lung mechanics, as shown for the compliance quotient of the pneumoloop diagrams in Fig. 16.5. Furthermore the lavage fluids of all lungs with protein-rich oedema showed marked alterations of surface activity, despite the standardization of the phospholipid concentration: decreased hysteresis area, increased minimal surface tension and increased minimal compressibility. The difference between the lungs with protein-rich oedema and the lungs without protein leakage into the alveolar space is best demonstrated

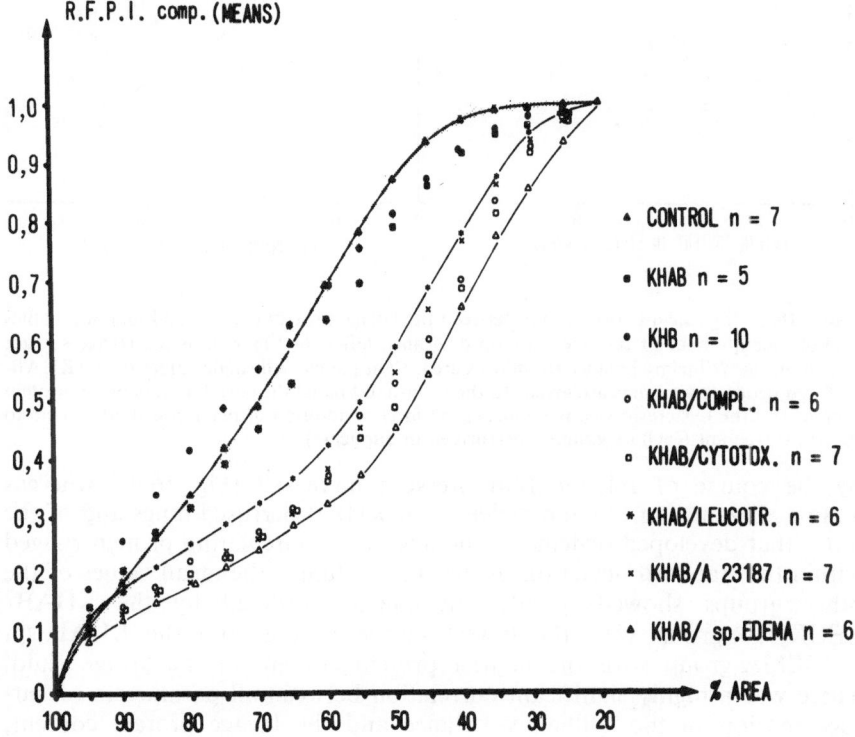

Figure 16.4 Course of relative film pressure increase during compression (R.F.P.I. comp.). Each point represents the mean of one group at the given percentage area. The shaded area gives the standard deviation of the control group. All groups of lungs with protein-rich oedema show a completely different course of film pressure increase, bordered by the KHAB/LEUKOTR. group and the KHAB/sp.OEDEMA group. The different groups are explained in the text[6]

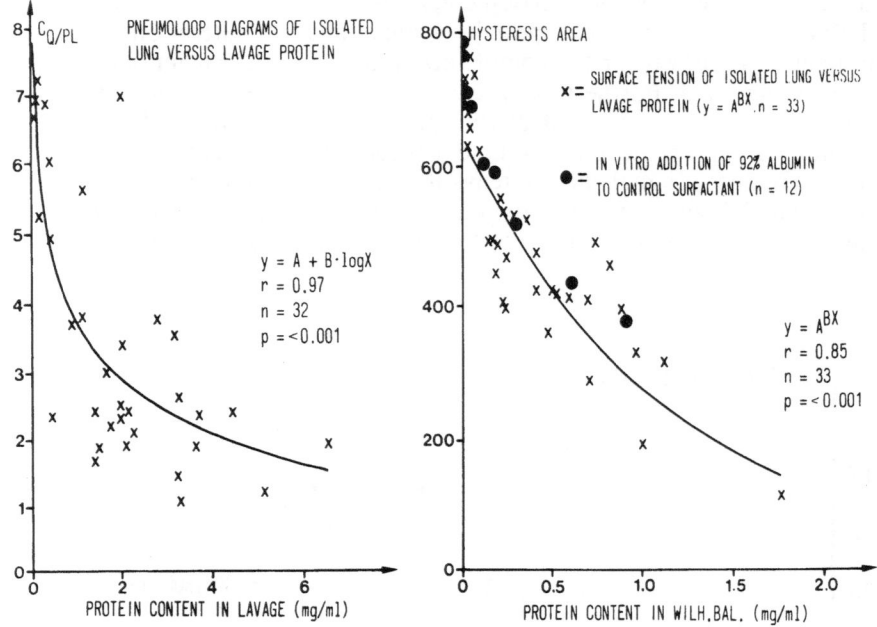

Figure 16.5 Significant correlations between the lavage protein content and lung mechanics (compliance quotient of the pneumoloop diagrams, left panel) as well as the lavage surface activity in the Wilhelmy balance (hysteresis area, right panel). All single values of the KHAB-perfused oedematous lungs are given. In the right-hand panel the correlation between protein content and the hysteresis area is mimicked by *in vitro* addition of perfusion fluid protein to control surfactant (each experiment performed in duplicate)[6]

by the course of relative film pressure increase[11] (Fig. 16.4): whereas almost all values of the non-oedematous KHAB-perfused lungs and of the lungs that developed oedema in the absence of circulating protein ranged within the standard deviation of the control lungs, the mean values of the other groups showed a different course bordered by the KHAB/LEUKOTR-group with the lowest lavage protein and the KHAB/sp. OEDEMA-group with the highest protein content in the lavage fluid. There was a highly significant correlation between all parameters of surface tension in the Wilhelmy balance and the lavage protein content, demonstrated for the hysteresis area in Fig. 16.5. Addition of perfusion fluid protein to control surfactant in the Wilhelmy balance mimicked the surface tension alterations qualitatively and quantitatively.

Our conclusion was that *protein leakage* into the alveolar space appears to be the common cause of *altered lung mechanics* and *altered surfactant function in vitro* after different manoeuvres which induced *high permeability oedema*.

Next the effect of different purified proteins on natural surfactant func-

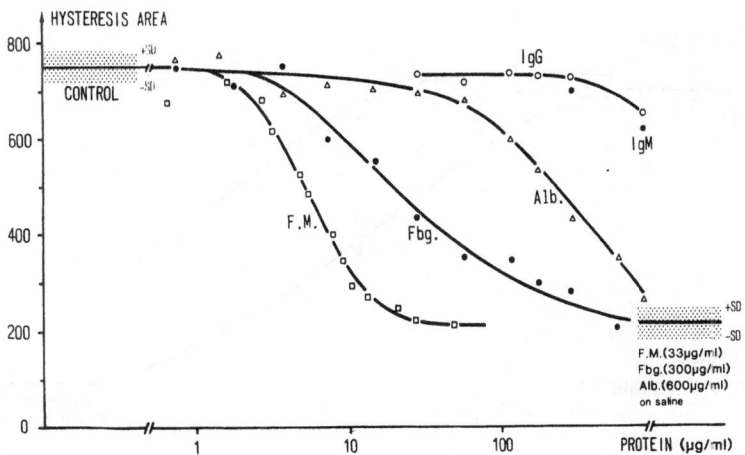

Figure 16.6 Dose–effect curves of IgG (human), IgM (human), albumin (bovine; Alb.), fibrinogen (bovine; Fbg.) and fibrin monomer (bovine; F.M.) on surface tension characteristics (hysteresis area) of control surfactant (each experiment was performed in duplicate). The shaded areas give the standard deviation of the control surfactant without protein addition and the standard deviation of the protein effects on pure saline, respectively. The true fibrin monomer concentration is corrected for polymerization according to Fig. 16.8. The marked rank order of potency in interfering with surfactant function is evident[6]

tion *in vitro* was investigated. The proteins were admixed to surfactant at a standardized phospholipid concentration of 50 μg/ml and surface activity was measured as in Fig. 16.2. All proteins provoked the same pattern of surface tension alterations: decrease of hysteresis area, increase in minimal surface tension and minimal compressibility and altered course of relative film pressure increase, similar to that shown in Fig. 16.4. The dose–effect curves of the different proteins, however, revealed a marked rank order of potency in interfering with surfactant function: IgG, IgM and elastin < albumin < fibrinogen < fibrin monomer (Fig. 16.6). The latter is effective down to concentrations of nearly 1 μg/ml. Species differences appear to be of minor importance: there was no significant difference between fibrinogen or fibrin monomer from bovine, human or rabbit source. The greater effectiveness of fibrinogen over albumin and globulin in raising the minimal compressibility of a lipoprotein from lung homogenate has been described by Abrams and Taylor[12,13]. The greater effectiveness of fibrin monomer compared with fibrinogen was confirmed in a second experimental set. Incubation of a surfactant–fibrinogen mixture with thrombin caused a further deterioration of surface activity despite the removal of the majority of protein material as a fibrin clot, mimicking the shift between the fibrinogen curve and the fibrin monomer curve. Thrombin itself, and the resulting fibrinopeptides A and B, were shown to be ineffective. This experiment is in agreement with those of Balis *et al.*[14], who found an increase in minimal surface tension of natural surfactant after

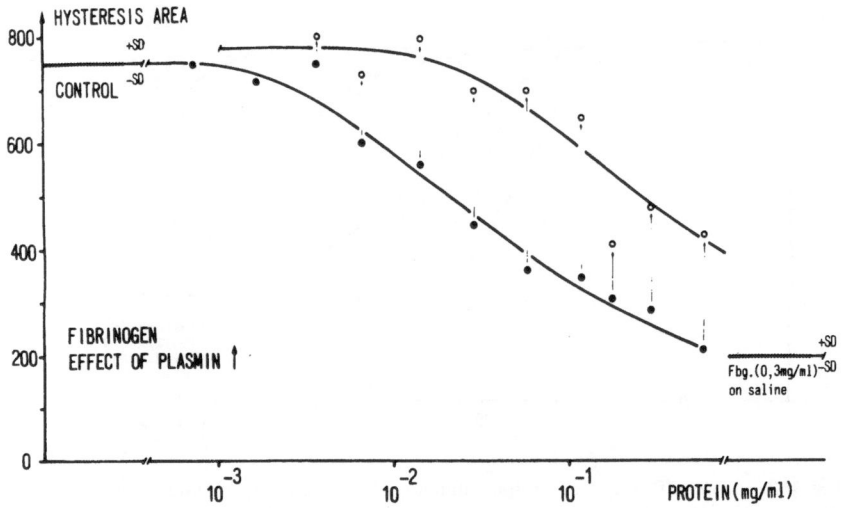

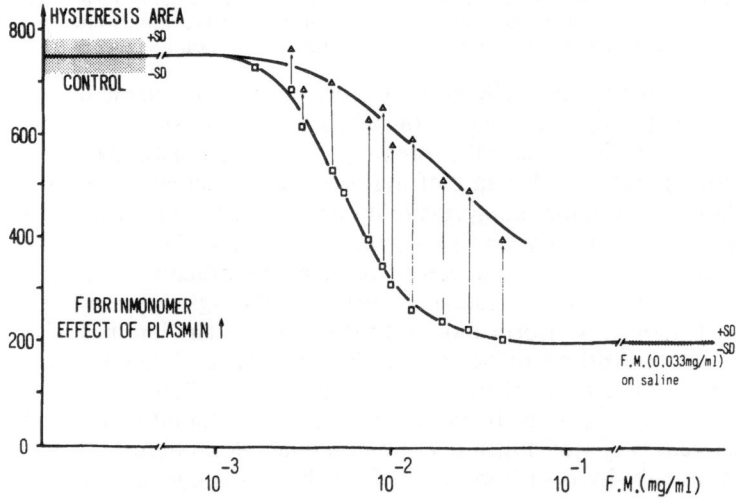

Figure 16.7 Reversibility of the fibrinogen (bovine; Fbg.) and fibrin monomer (bovine, F.M.) effects on surface tension behaviour of natural surfactant by subsequent application of plasmin underneath the film. After recycling the surfactant protein mixture eight times, plasmin (0.15 CU/ml) was injected into the hypophase without disturbance of the film, cycling was continued for 30 min and surface tension characteristics were evaluated again. Each experiment was performed in duplicate. In the concentration used plasmin is without any effect on the surface tension behaviour of control surfactant. The shaded areas give the standard deviation of the control surfactant without protein addition and the standard deviation of the effect of fibrinogen or fibrin monomer on pure saline. The dose–effect curves of both fibrinogen and fibrin monomer are shifted by almost one order of magnitude.

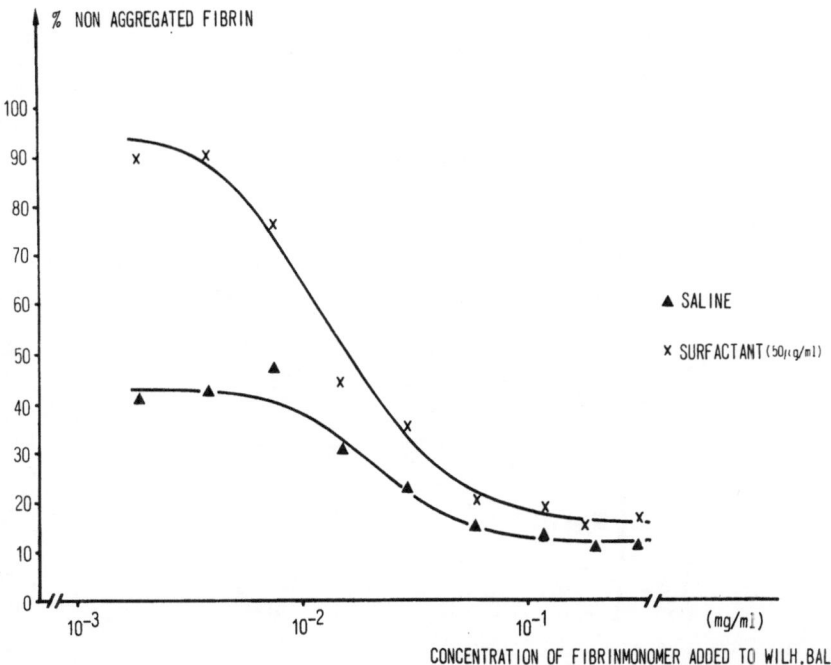

Figure 16.8 Curve of fibrin monomer polymerization (bovine fibrin monomer mixed with 3% ^{125}I-labelled human fibrin monomer) after injection of the monomer, dissolved in urea (3M)–tris (50 mmol/l) buffer, into saline or natural surfactant in the Wilhelmy balance (Wilh.Bal.). The percentage of dissolved (non-aggregated) fibrin monomer was calculated from the ^{125}I found in the aqueous phase versus the ^{125}I detected in the pellet after spinning and in the filter cloth after passage of the fluid. Experiments were performed in duplicate. In presence of natural surfactant the polymerization of fibrin monomers is markedly reduced[6].

addition of recalcified plasma to the hypophase, which was even reinforced after coagulation and clot removal. As the clot removal was accompanied by a 50% loss of phospholipids from the hypophase, they blamed this effect on a coagulative type of surfactant depletion. In the present experiments, however, there was no significant phospholipid loss accompanying clot removal (<10%), thus the generated fibrin monomer was most probably responsible for these observations. The effects of fibrin monomer were also visible at lower and at higher phospholipid concentrations (example given in Fig. 16.2). The dose–effect curves of fibrinogen and of fibrin monomer could be shifted by almost one order of magnitude by subsequent application of plasmin underneath the film without removal of the (split) protein material (Fig. 16.7). The specificity of the fibrin molecule in interacting with one or more functionally important surfactant compounds is suggested not only by the over 50 times greater effectiveness compared with albumin (or IgG and IgM) and by the reversibility of its effect on surfactant activity upon splitting with plasmin, but also by the marked inhibition of fibrin monomer polymerization in the presence of

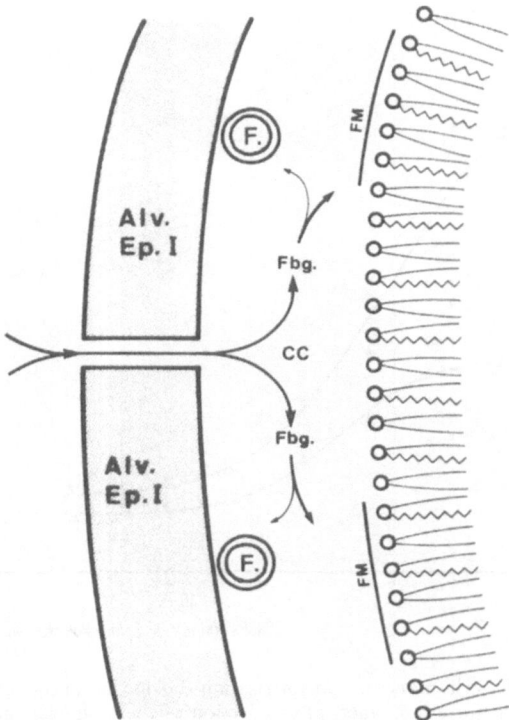

Fig. 16.9 Schematic arrangement of plasmaprotein-leakage interfering with surfactant function. Fbg = fibrinogen; CC = proteins of the coagulation cascade; FM = fibrin monomer; F = polymerized fibrin; Alv.Ep. I = alveolar epithelial cells type I. For explanation see text

natural surfactant, shown in Fig. 16.8. When applied on pure saline in absence of surfactant, there is no difference in the surface tension effects between the different proteins, including fibrin monomer.

CONCLUSIONS

An overall conclusion from the summarized experiments is depicted in Fig. 16.9. The *primum movens* of the manoeuvres undertaken to provoke surfactant alterations is an increase in the capillary–endothelial and alveolo – epithelial barrier, followed by leakage of plasma proteins, including fibrinogen and proteins of the coagulation cascade, into the alveolar space. High albumin concentrations, fibrinogen and possibly further distinct proteins, as suggested by Jobe, Ikegami and co-workers for premature lambs[15,17], may directly interfere with surfactant function. On the other hand it is known that natural surfactant has procoagulant activity, first described by Abrams and Taylor[12,13]. It is probably a combination of a thromboplastin-like activity, which is possibly released from the alveolar macrophages[18] and is effective on the extrinsic coagulation pathway, and a cephalin-like activity, effective on the intrinsic coagulation pathway. Arising thrombin generates fibrin monomer from leaked fibrinogen. Instead of aggregating to a fibrin clot low monomer concentrations appear to interact with one or more surfactant compounds, with severe impairment of surfactant function. This may be an important intermediate step between increased alveolar-epithelial permeability and massive fibrin aggregation in form of the well-known hyaline membranes. In the respiratory distress syndrome of the newborn this pathogenetic sequence may be of importance when the primary lack of surface-active material is accompanied, or followed, by an increase in alveolar-epithelial permeability, as described in premature ventilated goats and lambs[17,20], which results in a marked increase in the protein content of the alveolar wash of these animals.

References

1. Seeger, W., Wolf, H., Stähler, G., Neuhof, H. and Roka, L. (1982). Increased pulmonary vascular resistance and permeability due to arachidonate metabolism in isolated rabbit lungs. *Prostaglandins,* **23,** 157–73
2. Seeger, W., Bauer, M. and Bhakdi, S. (1984). Staphylococcal alpha-toxin elicits hypertension in isolated rabbit lungs. Evidence for thromboxane formation and the role of extracellular calcium. *J. Clin. Invest.,* **74,** 849–58
3. Seeger, W., Wolf, H. R. D., Neuhof, H. and Roka, L. (1982). Release and oxygenation of arachidonic acid: nonspecific triggering and pathophysiological consequences in isolated rabbit lungs. In Samuelsson, B. *et al.* (eds.) *Advances in Prostaglandin, Thromboxane and Leukotriene Research.* Vol 12, pp.99–105. (New York: Raven Press)
4. Seeger, W., Radinger, H. and Neuhof, H. (1984). Increase in the capillary filtration coefficient of isolated rabbit lungs due to non-cyclooxygenase pathway of arachidonic acid (Abstract). *Int. J. Microcirc. Clin. Exp.,* **3,** 351
5. Seeger, W., Wolf, H. R. D., Stähler, G. and Neuhof, H. (1983). Alteration of pressure–volume characteristics due to different types of edema induction in isolated rabbit lungs. *Respiration,* **44,** 273–81
6. Seeger, W., Stöhr, G., Wolf, H.R.D. and Neuhof, H. (1985). Alteration of surfactant function due to protein leakage: special interaction with fibrin monomer. *J. Appl. Physiol.,* **58,** 326–38
7. Seeger, W., Wolf, H., Bauer, M., Neuhof, H. and Roka, L. (1982). Comparative influence of LTC4, LTD4 and LTE4 on the pulmonary vaculature in isolated rabbit lungs. (Abstract). *V. Int. Conf. Prostaglandins,* Florence, May 1982, Abstract Book, p.350
9. Lutz, F., Seeger, W., Schischke, B., Weiner, R. and Schramm, W. (1983). Effects of a cytotoxic protein from pseudomonas aeruginosa on phagocytic and pinocytic cells: in vitro and in vivo studies. *Toxicon Suppl.,* **3,** 257–60
10. Clements, J. A., Hustead, R. F., Johnson, R. P. and Gribetz, I. (1961). Pulmonary surface tension and alveolar stability. *J. Appl. Physiol.,* **16,** 444–50
11. Hildebran, J. N., Goerke, J. and Clements, J. A. Pulmonary surface film stability and composition. *J. Appl. Physiol.,* **47,** 604–11
12. Reifenrath, R. and Zimmerman, I. (1973). Surface tension properties of lung alveolar surfactant obtained by alveolar micropuncture. *Respir. Physiol.,* **19,** 369–93
13. Abrams, M. E. (1966). Isolation and quantitative estimation of pulmonary surface-active protein. *J. Appl. Physiol.,* **21,** 718–20
14. Taylor, F. B. and Abrams, M. E. (1966). Effect of surface active lipoprotein on clotting and fibrinolysis, and of fibrinogen on surface tension of surface active lipoprotein. *Am. J. Med.,* **40,** 346–50

15. Balis, J. U., Shelley, S. A., McCue, M. J. and Rappaport, E. S. (1971). Mechanisms of damage to the lung surfactant system. *Exp. Mol. Pathol.,* **14,** 243–62
16. Ikegami, M., Jobe, A. and Glatz, T. (1981). Surface activity following natural surfactant treatment in premature lambs. *J. Appl. Physiol.,* **51,** 306–12
17. Jobe, A., Ikegami, M., Jacobs, H., Jones, S. and Conaway, D. (1983). Permeability of premature lambs to protein and the effect of surfactant on that permeability. *J. Appl. Physiol.,* **55,** 169–76
18. Ikegami, M., Jobe, A., Jacobs, H. and Lam, R. (1984). A protein from airways of premature lambs that inhibits surfactant function. *J. Appl. Physiol.,* **57,** 1134–42
19. Wasi, S., Burrowes, C. E., Hay, J. B. and Movat, H. Z. (1983). Plasminogen activator and plasminogen activity from sheep alveolar macrophages. *Thrombos. Res.,* **30,** 27–45
20. Egan, E. A., Nelson, R. M. and Beale, E. F. (1980). Lung solute permeability and lung liquid absorption in premature ventilated fetal goats. *Pediatr. Res.,* **14,** 314–18

Discussion

Dr. B. Robertson	Why did you choose hysteresis as the main parameter of surface activity?
Dr. W. Seeger	Everything was also true for all the other parameters – compressibility, minimum surface tension, etc.
Dr. C. A. R. Boyd	Do your experiments allow you to decide whether the inhibition is a stoichiometric or a catalytic effect of the protein?
Seeger	I can't decide that from these data.
Dr. J. A. Clements	Would you recommend treating patients with respiratory distress syndrome with plasmin or steptokinase? Ambrus *et al.*[1] thought they had quite good success with that some years ago but it seems to have fallen out of favour.
Seeger	One would have to do a lot of experiments to see whether topical application in the animal model had a reproducibly good effect without damage to the alveolar epithelial barrier. With regard to the endothelial barrier, for example, there are suggestions that a fibrinogen lining layer may be a necessary barrier and that splitting of fibrinogen might have an effect on the endothelium.
Dr. L. B. Strang	Could one go so far as to suggest that the critical step in RDS and related disorders is a disturbance in epithelial solute permeability? These large proteins such as fibrinogen normally pass from the capillaries into the interstitial space and can be found in lung lymph, but none normally cross the epithelial barrier either in the fetus or during the period of lung expansion at birth[2]. If we are to be reductionists (something that Dr Bryan doesn't like), perhaps we could say that anything – be it over-distension of the lung or some more specific epithelial toxin – which damages the pulmonary epithelium, will allow these large proteins to get into the lumen of the lung which should normally be reserved for only a thin film of fluid surfactant and alveolar gas.
Seeger	It is clear that all the procedures I used to increase capillary filtration also damaged the alveolar epithelial barrier.
Strang	I wonder if I could use this occasion to clear up some points of ignorance from which I still suffer. Is it quite clear how much difference the polar head of the phospholipid makes to the physical properties of a surface film? We understand the importance of whether the fatty acids are saturated or unsaturated but does it matter whether the molecule is phosphatidylcholine, phosphatidylinositol, phosphatidylglycerol or phosphatidylethanolamine.
Clements	In truth it is an enormously complicated question and the literature does not contain enough data on which to base a comprehensive answer. The problem should be divided into at least two parts, one of which has to do with the velocity of film formation for which a certain complex of properties may be required; the second part has to do with the maintenance of film stability once the monomolecular film has been formed. We could state some requirements for an adequate rate of film formation. For this the system needs fluidity but that's not to say that surfactant may not be in a mosaic and contain solid parts. It is a complication that experiments to test adsorption rate involve an enormous excess of material, the surface film being formed from 1% or 0.1% of the material

present in the subphase. This material is heterogenous and we do not know which of the structures in the mix actually take part in film formation. All the kinds of phospholipids we are interested in *can* form a film quite rapidly, giving an equilibrium film pressure corresponding to a surface tension of 24 to 28 mN/m, but then the second part of the problem arises: the film must remain stable when compressed, allowing surface tension to go down close to zero. While this property, like film fluidity, depends on the melting temperature of the hydrocarbon chains, it is also affected by the structure of the polar head. Thus phosphatidylethanolamine absorbs very rapidly to a surface and generates an equilibrium film, but this film collapses readily when compressed even at a temperature below its phase transition temperature. The complexity gets even greater when we consider mixtures of lipids rather than individual substances and allow that the phospholipids may undergo lateral phase separation in a film. In these circumstances the film may contain domains with a composition different from the average. It is even more complicated when we have structures as different as those seen by electron microscopy. So are the polar heads important? I think in a word, yes; because we know that when the acyl chains are kept constant and the polar heads changed, some of the resulting species have appropriate physical properties and others do not.

Dr C. J. Morley Some of the phospholipids bear acidic charges which may be very important to the way in which the surfactant reacts with ions. Calcium is important and it seems likely that this ion may react not only with the apoprotein but also with the acidic phospholipids.

Clements I think it's useful to distinguish between natural surfactant and the artificial mixes invented to imitate its activity. There are anionic phospholipids which are significant components of the natural material and, as Dr Morley said, their interaction with calcium may be important. Nevertheless, studies with recombinant mixtures show an order of magnitude difference in the *effective* ionic concentration of Ca when the lipids are alone and when the apoprotein is present. You need ten times less calcium to promote adsorption when the apoprotein is present than when it is absent[3]. Magnesium does not substitute for calcium in this effect[3].

References

1. Ambrus, C. M., Choi, T. S., Cunnanan. E., Eisenberg, B., Staub, H. P., Weintraub, S. H., Couvey, N. G., Patterson, R. J., Jockin, H., Pickren, J. W., Bross, I. D., Jung, O. S. and Ambrus, J. L. (1977). Prevention of hyaline membrane disease with plasminogen. *J. Am. Med. Assoc.*, **237**, 1837–41
2. Strang, L. B. (1976). The permeability of lung capillary and alveolar walls as determinants of liquid movements in the lung. In Porter, B. and O'Connor, M. (eds.) Ciba Foundation Symposium, *Lung Liquids.* pp. 49–58. (Amsterdam and New York: Elsevier)
3. Hawgood, S., Benson, B. J. and Hamilton, R. L. (1985). Effects of a surfactant-associated protein and calcium ions on the structure and surface activity of lung surfactant lipids. *Biochemistry,* **24**, 184–90.

17
Surfactant Replacement: Theory and Practice

B. ROBERTSON

INTRODUCTION

Treatment of the neonatal respiratory distress syndrome (RDS) with exogenous surfactant is a logical step, as the disease is caused by a deficiency
of surface-active phospholipids in the alveolar spaces. The efficacy of this
therapeutic approach has been demonstrated in animal models as well as in
clinical trials, as reported elsewhere in this book (Chapters 18 and 19) and
earlier by other investigators[1-6]. Encouraging preliminary data from several
current clinical trials were also presented at the recent Special Ross Conference on 'Clinical trials of the use of surfactant in the neonatal respiratory distress syndrome'[7]. The impression from these reports is that
surfactant replacement effectively improves lung expansion and gas exchange in patients with severe RDS, and that prophylactic treatment with
synthetic[8,9] or natural[10] surfactant soon after birth reduces the incidence
of severe RDS in immature babies.

In spite of these promising results, some important problems remain to
be solved. This chapter will discuss the timing of surfactant replacement
therapy in relation to the pathology and pathophysiology of neonatal RDS,
the dosage and optimal composition of exogenous surfactant, and the
possible synergistic effect of surfactant replacement and ventilation by
high frequency oscillation (HFO).

TIMING OF SURFACTANT REPLACEMENT THERAPY;
EPITHELIAL LESIONS AND SURFACTANT INHIBITORS

In the surfactant-deficient lung the ventilatory movements do not result in
uniform alveolar expansion. Furthermore, the alveoli tend to collapse (or
become refilled with unresorbed fetal lung liquid) at end-expiration. These
well-known pathophysiological features of neonatal RDS trigger shear
forces in the bronchiolar and alveolar walls, with disruption of the epithelial lining. Electron microscopic studies of lungs from experimental

animals and babies with neonatal surfactant deficiency have documented necrosis of bronchiolar and alveolar epithelium within a few minutes after birth[11-13]. These lesions become aggravated by artificial ventilation, and eventually develop into the typical hyaline membranes, containing cell debris and protein leaking from denuded epithelial surfaces (for review, see Ref. 14). In a baby with severe RDS, terminal bronchioles may become literally plugged by necrotic epithelial cells. To ensure efficacy of replacement therapy, surfactant should be given before such obstructive features have become unduly prominent.

The proteins leaking into the airspaces of the immature lung include at least one potent inhibitor of pulmonary surfactant. This particular protein, recently isolated and characterized by Ikegami et al.[15], has a molecular weight of 110 000 daltons, and its ability to inhibit surfactant function is significantly higher than that of other serum proteins.. It has been demonstrated in the airways of immature lambs[15] as well as in tracheal effluents from babies with RDS[16].

The inhibitory activity of the leaking proteins can be quantified with, for example, pulsating bubble[16], by determining the amount of protein required to raise the minimum surface tension of a standard suspension of natural surfactant above zero. Data from such experiments indicate that the 'specific' surfactant inhibitor interferes with surfactant function at a concentration of about 0.2 mg protein per μmol surfactant phosphatidylcholine; the corresponding figure for serum albumin is about 2 mg/μmol phosphatidylcholine[15].

Treatment of immature newborn experimental animals with natural surfactant prevents the development of epithelial lesions during artificial ventilation and reduces the leakage of protein into the airspaces[17,18]. Recent experiments on rabbit neonates, delivered on day 27 of gestation, have revealed that about 3% of the pool of serum albumin enters the airspaces during a 1 h period of artificial ventilation; this leakage was only half as large in animals treated with natural surfactant before the onset of ventilation[18]. The proteins accumulating in the alveoli of control animals also had a relatively higher inhibitory activity than had the proteins entering the airspaces of surfactant-treated littermates.

These experimental and clinical observations indicate that surfactant inhibitors are involved in the pathogenesis of neonatal RDS[19]. Such inhibitors might also compromise the effect of surfactant replacement, accounting for the transient effect of replacement therapy in some babies treated with surfactant after several hours of artificial ventilation. The same mechanism could explain why, in immature lambs, the improvement of lung function is more long-standing in animals receiving surfactant at birth than in those treated after the onset of respiratory failure. Alternatively, the less striking effect in the latter group might reflect a non-homogeneous distribution of the exogenous surfactant, associated with a ventilation–perfusion imbalance[20]. The most uniform distribution of surfactant is obtained when the exogenous material is added to the fetal pulmonary fluid before the first breath (Fig. 17.1).

All the above-mentioned factors argue for early treatment with surfac-

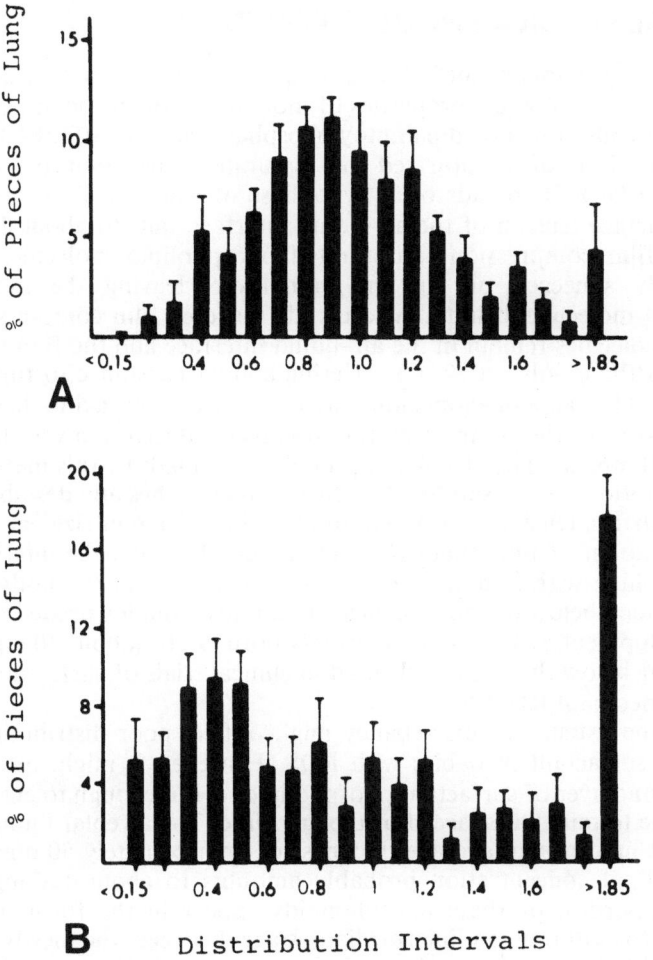

Figure 17.1 Normalized distributions of labelled surfactant instilled into the lungs of immature newborn lambs (gestational age 120 days). The diagrams illustrate mean ± SEM percentage of label in pieces of lung tissue vs. the 10% distribution intervals. The 1.0 bars indicate the average content of label per piece of lung tissue in each experiment. **A**: Data from six animals treated with surfactant at birth, showing fairly regular distribution, with most values clustered in the middle of the diagram. **B**: Irregular surfactant distribution in six lambs treated with surfactant at about 23 min of age. A significant number of lung pieces contain either very much or very little label. From Jobe et al.[20]. (Reproduced by copyright permission of the American Society for Clinical Investigation)

tant in neonatal RDS, or prophylactic replacement therapy at birth in babies at risk, as originally suggested by Enhörning and Robertson[21]. In patients receiving exogenous surfactant at a later stage the inhibitory activity of proteins in tracheal effluents should be determined, to clarify whether a variability in the clinical response is correlated to the magnitude of the protein leakage and to the amount of surfactant inhibitors in the airspaces.

DOSAGE OF EXOGENOUS SURFACTANT

The role of pulmonary surfactant in lung mechanics is usually explained by referring to the physical properties of monolayers of surfactant phospholipids, especially films of dipalmitoylphosphatidylcholine (DPPC). When a composite film of unsaturated and saturated surfactant phospholipids (including DPPC) spreads on a hypophase of water at 37 °C, the equilibrium surface tension of the air–liquid interface falls to about 25 mN/m. During film compression, unsaturated phospholipid molecules are preferentially squeezed out of the monolayer, leaving the more rigid, saturated molecules behind. At a certain stage of film compression, only DPPC molecules remain in the air–liquid interface and the film then turns solid (DPPC is solid at 37 °C), offering a great resistance to further compression. The same phenomenon may be described by saying that the contractile force of the compressed film becomes reduced to a very low value, close to 0 mN/m. The alveoli are probably 'splinted' by this mechanism at end-expiration, as the solidified surface film abolishes any destabilizing effect of surface tension in a system of alveoli of different size[22,23].

The amount of phosphatidylcholine required to coat the interior of the neonatal lung with a monolayer is approximately 5 mg/kg body weight[24]. This is much below the dose of surfactant phospholipids needed to prevent the development of RDS in prematurely born lambs (about 50 mg/kg)[25]. It is also far below the dose levels used in clinical trials of surfactant replacement in neonatal RDS[1-6].

To some extent this discrepancy might reflect poor distribution of exogenous surfactant in babies with RDS. However, it might also indicate that a monolayer of surfactant phospholipids is not enough to ensure stability of the terminal airspaces for a longer time. The alveolar lining layer of the adult lung has an average thickness of approximately 50 nm[26], and its phospholipid concentration probably amounts to about 120 mg/ml[27]. A large proportion of these phospholipids appear in the form of tubular myelin, constituting an intermediate stage between the newly excreted lamellar bodies and the surface film; other phospholipid complexes may represent material desorbed from the air–liquid interface to be taken up by the alveolar epithelium in a process of very effective reutilization. Jacobs et al.[28] have calculated that more than 90% of the alveolar surfactant phosphatidylcholine is reutilized in the full-term neonatal lung. Pathways for surfactant recycling are probably disturbed in RDS patients with widespread epithelial lung lesions, further explaining the need for a large reservoir of exogenous surfactant in the airspaces. An excess of surfactant might be required in these patients also to balance the noxious effect of surfactant inhibitors.

Some synthetic surfactants, showing only limited physiological activity in artificially ventilated immature newborn animals, may still have a beneficial effect when administered to newborn babies prophylactically, before the development of epithelial lesions in the lungs. Such preparations could increase the pool size of intra-alveolar DPPC available for recycling, without providing material immediately available for spreading in the air–liquid interface. For example, treatment with synthetic DPPC and un-saturated phosphatidylglycerol soon after birth reduces the incidence of severe RDS in immature babies, but the improvement of lung function is not apparent until after several hours[8,9].

NON-ENRICHED VS. ENRICHED NATURAL SURFACTANT

The 'natural' surfactant that can be isolated from minced lung tissue con-tains a mixture of unsaturated and saturated phospholipids. Such prepara-tions exhibit rapid film adsorption at 37 °C, but the content of DPPC is usually so low that a large degree of surface compression (> 50%) is re-quired to solidify the film. With these observations in mind, Fujiwara *et al.*[29] and Tanaka *et al.*[30] tried to improve the physical properties of natural bovine surfactant by adding certain synthetic lipids, until a minimal surface tension of nearly zero (implying film solidification) could be obtained with only moderate surface compression. This is the rationale of the enrichment procedure applied in the making of 'Surfactant TA', a mixture of bovine surfactant, DPPC, tripalmitin, and palmitic acid[31].

Unfortunately, there is no conclusive evidence from animal experiments or clinical trials that the unique surface properties of Surfactant TA are, in-deed, essential for the therapeutic effect. Studies in our laboratory have confirmed that the *in vitro* surface properties of natural surfactant, isolated from minced lungs, can be 'improved' by enrichment with various synthetic phospholipids including DPPC; however, variations in spreading rate and film compressibility within a fairly wide range did not seem to in-fluence the physiological activity of the surfactant preparations in static pressure–volume recordings or in *in vivo* experiments on immature newborn rabbits[32].

In a recent non-randomized clinical trial of replacement therapy in neonatal RDS we have used a non-enriched preparation of natural surfac-tant phospholipids. This material, isolated from bovine or porcine lungs by chloroform : methanol extraction and liquid-gel chromatography, differs from other natural surfactant preparations[1-4] by being devoid of cholesterol, triglycerides, cholesteryl esters, and the major (35 000-dalton) apoprotein. However, it contains about 1% of small apoproteins (< 15 000 daltons) which have an unusually high proportion of hydrophobic amino acids (explaining why the molecules move with the phospholipids in chro-matography systems).

We have now treated a total of 13 'emergency cases' of neonatal RDS with this new type of surfactant. All these babies were severely ill, requir-ing artificial ventilation with an average FiO$_2$ of 0.88 before replacement therapy. Each patient received about 200 mg of phospholipids per kg body weight, instilled via the tracheal cannula. As reported in detail else-where[33], there was a striking improvement of gas exchange, with an aver-age increase of the PaO$_2$/FiO$_2$ quotient by approximately 200% within 2 h after surfactant replacement (Fig. 17.2). In most patients there was also a rapid improvement of the radiological findings in chest films (Fig. 17.3). Five of the eight surviving patients had an uneventful recovery, and three

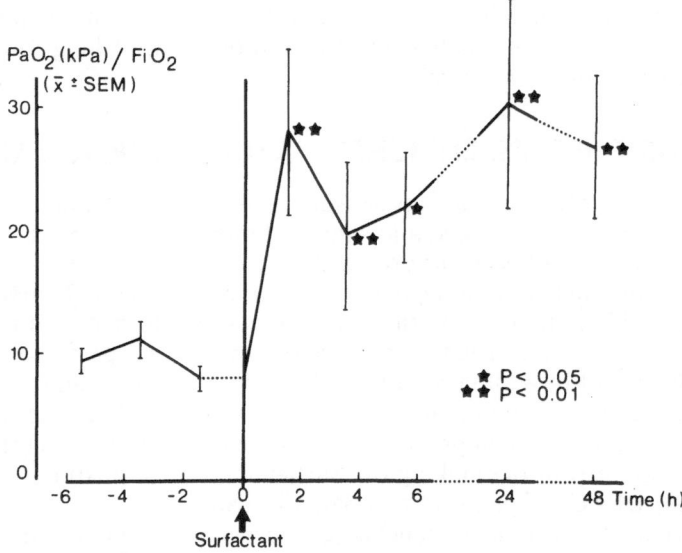

Figure 17.2 PaO_2/FiO_2 in a first series of eight RDS patients, before and after surfactant replacement. The babies were treated at a mean age of 12 h. Statistical evaluation with the Wilcoxon signed-ranks test for pair samples (two-tailed): *p vs. last observation before surfactant replacement <0.05; **p <0.01. From Noack *et al.*[6]. (Copyright Munksgaard International Publishers Ltd, Copenhagen, Denmark)

other babies survived with clinical and radiological evidence of bronchopulmonary dysplasia. Five babies showed a transient therapeutic response and died from various complications including cerebral haemorrhage, patent ductus arteriosus, pulmonary interstitial emphysema, and pneumothorax.

The comparatively high mortality in this trial (38%) almost certainly reflects a 'negative bias' in the selection of cases: the series included only critically ill patients, in whom surfactant replacement was applied as a last resort. The data from this pilot study have encouraged us to use the same surfactant preparation in a current randomized multicentre trial of replacement therapy in neonatal RDS.

APOPROTEIN-BASED ARTIFICIAL SURFACTANT

All surfactant preparations used for replacement therapy contain a small amount of proteins, even if the material has been isolated by repeated chloroform : methanol extraction. The physiological properties of natural surfactant probably depend on these specific apoproteins, which seem to enhance the adsorption of phospholipids to an air–liquid interface, perhaps by promoting the formation of tubular myelin in the hypophase[34]. The amino-acid sequence of the major human surfactant apoprotein (35 000 daltons) has recently been clarified[35] and the gene encoding this molecule has been cloned, facilitating the large-scale, commercial produc-

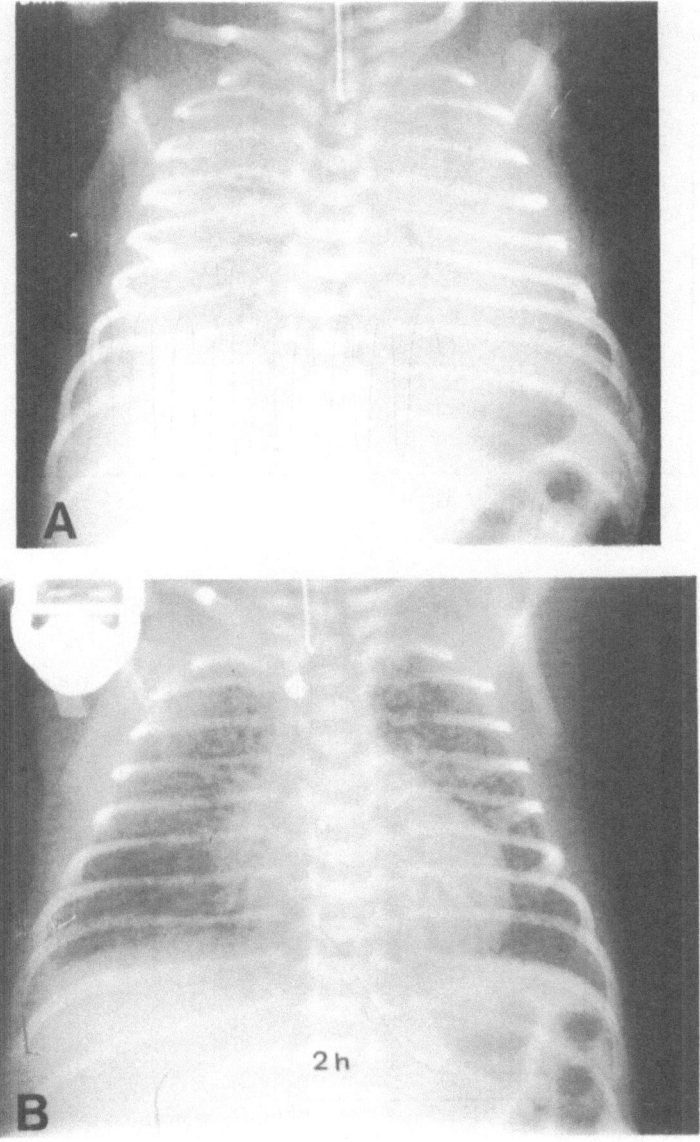

Figure 17.3 Radiograms demonstrating the striking effect of surfactant replacement in neonatal RDS. This male infant (1035 g) developed severe RDS shortly after birth, required artificial ventilation from the age of 4 h, and was treated with surfactant 5 h later. Chest films before surfactant replacement **(A)** show reduced lung volume, marked exudative abnormalities, and air bronchogram. Two hours after surfactant replacement **(B)** there is a dramatic improvement of lung aeration, but a moderate amount of fluid is still present in the interstitial spaces and in the right pleura. The bronchioles remain slightly dilated in the lower part of the lungs. Courtesy Dr Wigher Mortensson, Stockholm

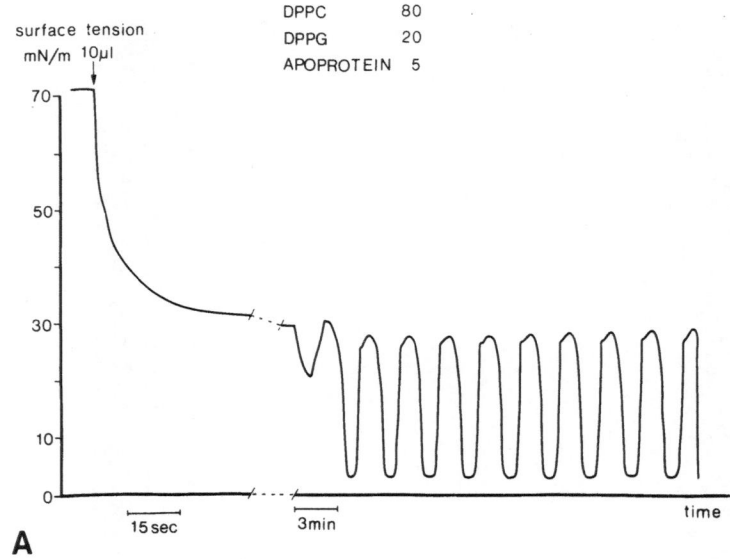

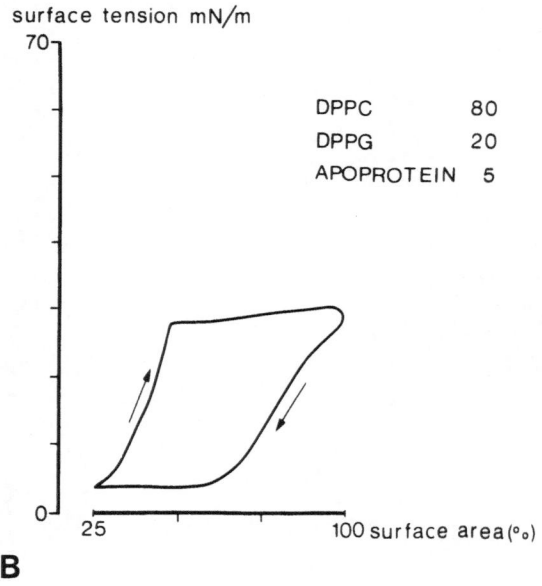

Figure 17.4 Surface properties of artificial surfactant made from DPPC, dipalmitoylphosphatidylglycerol, and the 15 000-dalton apoprotein (phospholipid concentration 3.5 mg/ml), evaluated with Wilhelmy balance at 37°C; 10 μl of the sample are applied (**A**, arrow) onto a hypophase of saline (surface area 60 cm²). From the second cycle, surface tension is reduced to about 4 mN/m during surface compression. Variations in surface tension are reproducible in subsequent cycles. **A**: 'Longitudinal' recording, **B**: XY-recording from the 10th cycle. From Suzuki *et al.*[38]. (Copyright Munksgaard International Publishers Ltd., Copenhagen, Denmark)

tion of the protein in cell culture systems[36]. Most likely, several attempts will soon be made to develop new artificial surfactant preparations, based on this particular apoprotein and selected synthetic phospholipids.

The smaller surfactant apoproteins ($\leqslant$ 15 000 daltons) also enhance the spreading of DPPC and other saturated phospholipids in an air–liquid interface[37]. Suzuki *et al.*[38] recently studied the physical and physiological properties of a surfactant prepared from DPPC, dipalmitoylphosphatidylglycerol, and small apoproteins isolated from porcine lungs. The three components were combined in proportions 80 : 20 : 5 (w : w : w). This artificial surfactant exhibited a comparatively slow spreading (about 30 s) but it reduced surface tension close to zero (indicating film solidification) during cyclic film compression in a Wilhelmy balance system (Fig. 17.4). It improved lung compliance in artificially ventilated immature newborn rabbits, although it was difficult to administer this comparatively viscous surfactant in a concentration higher than 5 mg/ml. However, the *in vivo* effect was similar to that of natural surfactant administered in the same low concentration[39]. Further studies are required to clarify whether a more 'fluid', yet physiologically active, artificial surfactant can be prepared from other combinations of synthetic phospholipids and the small apoproteins.

SURFACTANT REPLACEMENT AND HIGH FREQUENCY OSCILLATORY VENTILATION (HFO)

Several experimental observations indicate that the effects of surfactant replacement might be modified by the ventilatory pattern. For example, the clearance of surfactant from the alveolar spaces depends on the minute ventilation[40]. It has also recently been suggested that the intracellular pathways for degradation and recycling of surfactant are modified by various ventilatory patterns[41,42]. Furthermore, the spreading of exogenous surfactant within the lungs might be enhanced by periods of pro-longed inspiration, similar to those normally observed during the first few breaths.

We have recently tested the combination of surfactant replacement and HFO in experiments on immature newborn rabbits, delivered on day 27 of gestation. The animals were treated at birth with the isolated phospholipid fraction of natural bovine surfactant, i.e. with the same type of surfactant as used in our current clinical trial. They were then ventilated with HFO (8 Hz), 100% oxygen, and a mean airway pressure of 6–8 cmH$_2$O. Animals receiving surfactant could be kept alive for 1 h under these experimental conditions, whereas nearly all control animals died. Surfactant-treated animals had very well-expanded lungs, without evidence of epithelial lesions in the finer airways (Fig. 17.5A). The lungs of control animals, on the other hand, were characterized by poorly expanded alveoli and widespread necrosis of bronchiolar epithelium[43] (Fig. 17.5B). These experimental findings suggest that the combination of HFO and surfactant replacement might be useful in the clinical management of neonatal RDS, especially as this combination allows ventilation of the lungs with a comparatively low mean airway pressure.

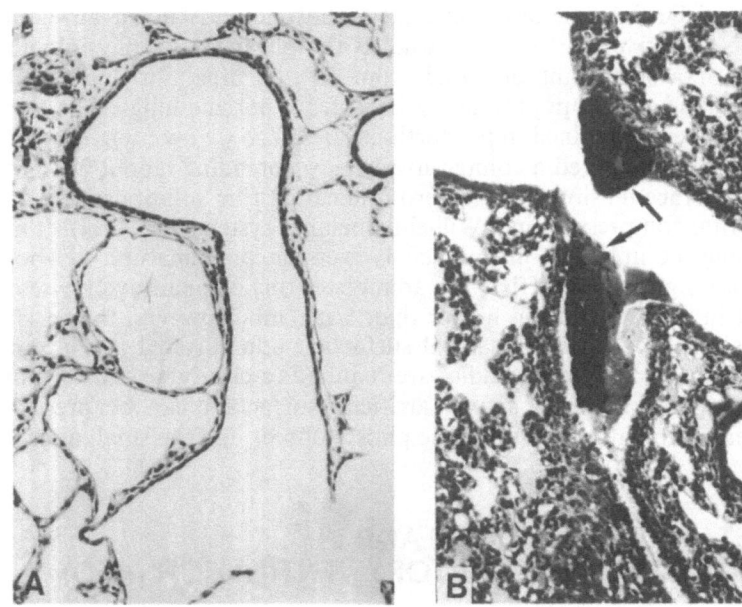

Figure 17.5 Light microscopic fields of bronchioles and surrounding alveoli, documenting the combined effects of surfactant replacement and HFO. Both animals were ventilated for 60 min with 100% oxygen, a frequency of 8 Hz, and a mean airway pressure of 6–8 cmH$_2$O. In the surfactant-treated animal (**A**), the alveoli are well aerated and the bronchiole is coated with intact, but flattened epithelium. In the non-treated control animal (**B**), there is poor alveolar air expansion and very prominent necrosis and desquamation of bronchiolar epithelium (arrows). Haematoxylin and eosin, × 195 (**A**), × 180 (**B**). From Nilsson *et al.*[43]

POSSIBLE ADVERSE EFFECTS OF SURFACTANT REPLACEMENT

Treatment of neonatal RDS with exogenous surfactant leads to a rapid improvement of alveolar aeration in most patients, with a consequent fall in pulmonary vascular resistance. As these babies usually have a patent ductus arteriosus, they tend to develop a significant left-to-right shunt following surfactant replacement. This phenomenon has also been documented in immature lambs treated with surfactant[44]. The shunt through the ductus may lead to overloading of the pulmonary circulation, with recurrent respiratory failure. Furthermore, some babies receiving surfactant exhibit large swings in arterial oxygenation, from 'flip-flop' changes in the direction of the ductal shunt. It cannot be excluded that these swings may be associated with corresponding variations in cerebral blood flow, perhaps increasing the risk of intraventricular haemorrhage. If so, treatment with indomethacin or mefenamic acid[31] is urgently indicated, or the ductus has to be closed surgically.

The risk of sensitization has been a matter of concern ever since the first RDS patients were treated with heterologous surfactant[1]. However, no allergic complications have been reported so far; perhaps because immature newborn infants have a limited immunological response capacity. Nevertheless, the protocol of forthcoming clinical trials should include a careful follow-up, with particular attention to the possible development of serum antibodies against foreign proteins in the exogenous surfactant.

Acknowledgements

This study was supported by The Swedish Medical Research Council (Project No. 3351), The Swedish National Association against Heart and Chest Diseases, The Swedish Society of Medical Sciences, The 'Expressen' Prenatal Research Foundation, The Research Funds of the Karolinska Institute, Allmänna Barnbördshusets Minnesfond, and Stiftelsen Samariten.

References

1. Fujiwara, T., Maeta, H., Chida, S., Morita, T., Watabe, Y. and Abe, T. (1980). Artificial surfactant therapy in hyaline-membrane disease. *Lancet,* **1,** 55–9
2. Hallman, M., Merritt, T. A., Schneider, H., Epstein, B. L., Mannino, F., Edwards, D. K. and Gluck, L. (1983). Isolation of human surfactant from amniotic fluid and a pilot study of its efficacy in respiratory distress syndrome. *Pediatrics,* **71,** 473–82
3. Smyth, J. A., Metcalfe, I. L., Duffty, P., Possmayer, F., Bryan, M. H. and Enhorning, G. (1983). Hyaline membrane disease treated with bovine surfactant. *Pediatrics,* **71,** 913–7
4. Nohara, K., Muramatsu, K. and Oda, T. (1983). Six cases of RDS treated with Surfactant CK. *J. Jpn. Med. Soc. Biol. Interface,* **14,** 173–8
5. Berggren, P., Curstedt, T., Grossmann, G., Herin, P., Mortensson, W., Nilsson, R., Noack, G. and Robertson, B. (1984). Gynnsam effekt av surfaktantbehandling vid IRDS. *Läkartidningen,* **81,** 4180–2
6. Noack, G., Berggren, P., Curstedt, T., Grossmann, G. and Robertson, B. (1986). Treatment of the neonatal respiratory distress syndrome with isolated surfactant phospholipids. *Eur. J. Respir. Dis.* (In press)
7. Lucey, J. F. (ed.) (1984). *Clinical Trials of the Use of Surfactant in the Neonatal Respiratory Distress Syndrome.* (Columbus, Ohio: Ross Laboratories)
8. Morley, C. J., Bangham, A. D., Miller, N. and Davis, J. A. (1981). Dry artificial lung surfactant and its effect on very premature babies. *Lancet,* **1,** 64–8
9. Morley, C., Greenough, A., Miller, M., Bangham, A., Wood, S., Hill, C. and Gore, S. (1984). In von Wichert, P. (ed.) *Current Concepts in Surfactant Research. Prog. Respir. Res.* Vol. 18, pp. 274–8 (Basel: Karger)
10. Enhorning, G., Shennan, A., Possmayer, F., Dunn, M., Chen, C. P. and Milligan, J. (1985). Prevention of the neonatal respiratory distress syndrome by tracheal instillation of surfactant: A randomized clinical trial. *Pediatrics,* **76,** 145–53
11. McAdams, A. J., Coen, R., Kleinman, L. I., Tsang, R. and Sutherland, J. (1973). The experimental production of hyaline membranes in premature rhesus monkeys. *Am. J. Pathol.,* **70,** 277–90
12. Finlay-Jones, J. M., Papadimitriou, J. M. and Barter, R. A. (1974). Pulmonary hyaline membrane: Light and electron microscopic study of the early stage. *J. Pathol.,* **112,** 117–24

13. Nilsson, R., Grossmann, G. and Robertson, B. (1980). Bronchiolar epithelial lesions induced in the premature rabbit neonate by short periods of artificial ventilation. *Acta Pathol. Microbiol. Scand. [A]*, **88**, 359–67

14. Robertson, B. (1983). Pathology and pathophysiology of neonatal surfactant deficiency ('respiratory distress syndrome', 'hyaline membrane disease'). In Robertson, B., Van Golde, L. M. G. and Batenburg, J. J. (eds.) *Pulmonary Surfactant*. pp. 383–418. (Amsterdam: Elsevier)

15. Ikegami, M., Jobe, A., Jacobs, H. and Lam, R. (1984). A protein from the airways of premature lambs that inhibits surfactant function. *J. Appl. Physiol.*, **57**, 1134–42

16. Ikegami, M., Jacobs, H. and Jobe, A. (1983). Surfactant function in the respiratory distress syndrome. *J. Pediatr.*, **102**, 443–7

17. Jobe, A., Ikegami, M., Jacobs, H., Jones, S. and Conaway, D. (1983). Permeability of premature lamb lungs to protein and the effect of surfactant on that permeability. *J. Appl. Physiol.*, **55**, 169–76

18. Robertson, B., Berry, D., Curstedt, T., Grossmann, G., Ikegami, M., Jacobs, H., Jobe, A. and Jones, S. (1985). Leakage of protein in the immature rabbit lung; effect of surfactant replacement. *Respir. Physiol.*, **61**, 265–76

19. Jobe, A. (1984). Respiratory distress syndrome – new therapeutic approaches to a complex pathophysiology. *Adv. Pediatr.*, **30**, 93–130

20. Jobe, A., Ikegami, M., Jacobs, H. and Jones, S. (1984). Surfactant and pulmonary blood flow distributions following treatment of premature lambs with natural surfactant. *J. Clin. Invest.*, **73**, 848–56

21. Enhörning, G. and Robertson, B. (1972). Lung expansion in the premature rabbit fetus after tracheal deposition of surfactant. *Pediatrics*, **50**, 58–66

22. Clements, J. A. (1977). Functions of the alveolar lining. *Am. Rev. Respir. Dis.*, **115**, 67–71

23. Bangham, A. D., Morley, C. J. and Phillips, M. C. (1979). The physical properties of an effective lung surfactant. *Biochim. Biophys. Acta*, **573**, 552–6

24. Enhörning, G., Grossmann, G. and Robertson, B. (1972). Morphometric analysis of lung expansion in the premature rabbit foetus after pharyngeal deposition of surfactant. *Acta Pathol. Microbiol. Scand. [A]*, **80**, 694

25. Ikegami, M., Adams, F. H., Towers, B. and Osher, A. B. (1980). The quantity of natural surfactant necessary to prevent the respiratory distress syndrome in premature lambs. *Pediatr. Res.*, **14**, 1082–5

26. Gil, J. and Weibel, E. R. (1969). Improvements in demonstration of lining layer of lung alveoli by electron microscopy. *Respir. Physiol.*, **8**, 13–36

27. Kobayashi, T. and Robertson, B. (1983). Surface adsorption of pulmonary surfactant in relation to bulk-phase concentration and presence of $CaCl_2$. *Respiration*, **44**, 63–70

28. Jacobs, H., Jobe, A., Ikegami, M. and Conaway, D. (1983). The significance of reutilization of surfactant phosphatidylcholine. *J. Biol. Chem.*, **258**, 4156–65

29. Fujiwara, T., Tanaka, Y. and Takei, T. (1979). Surface properties of artificial surfactant in comparison with natural and synthetic surfactant lipids. *IRCS Med. Sci.*, **7**, 311

30. Tanaka, Y., Takei, T., Kanazawa, Y., Kiuchi, A. and Fujiwara, T. (1982). Reconstitution of lung surfactant by adjusting chemical composition. *J. Jpn. Med. Soc. Biol. Interface*, **13**, 43–50

31. Fujiwara, T. (1984). Surfactant replacement in neonatal RDS. In Robertson, B., Van Golde, L. M. G. and Batenburg, J. J. (eds.) *Pulmonary Surfactant*. pp. 479–503 (Amsterdam: Elsevier)

32. Nohara, K., Berggren, P., Curstedt, T., Grossmann, G., Nilsson, R., Robertson, B. (1986). Correlations between physical and physiological properties of various preparations of lung surfactant. *Eur. J. Respir. Dis.* (In press)

33. Robertson, B., Noack, G., Bevilacqua, G., Berggren, P., Cosmi, E. V., Curstedt, T. and Grossmann, G. (1986). Surfactant replacement in severe neonatal respiratory distress syndrome. In Vignali, M., Cosmi, E. V. and Luerti, M. (eds.) *Diagnosis and Treatment of Fetal Lung Immaturity* pp. 193–197, (Milano: Masson)

34. Benson, B. J., Williams, M. C., Hawgood, S. and Sargeant, T. (1984). Role of lung surfactant-specific proteins in surfactant structure and function. In von Wichert, P. (ed.) *Current Concepts in Surfactant Research. Prog. Respir. Res.* Vol. 18, pp. 83–92. (Basel: Karger)

35. Benson, B., Hawgood, S., Schilling, J., Clements, J., Damm, D., Cordell, B. and Tyler White, R. (1985). Structure of canine pulmonary surfactant apoprotein; cDNA and complete amino acid sequence. *Proc. Natl. Acad. Sci. USA,* **82,** 6379–83

36. Tyler White, R., Damm, D., Miller, J., Spratt, K., Schilling, J., Hawgood, S., Benson, B. and Cordell, B. (1985). Isolation and characterisation of the human pulmonary surfactant apoprotein gene. *Nature,* **317,** 361–3

37. Suzuki, Y. (1982). Effect of protein, cholesterol, and phosphatidylglycerol on the surface activity of the lipid–protein complex reconstituted from pig pulmonary surfactant. *J. Lipid Res.,* **23,** 62–9

38. Suzuki, Y., Curstedt, T., Grossmann, G., Kobayashi, T., Nilsson, R., Nohara, K. and Robertson, B. (1986). Experimental studies on the role of the low-molecular weight ($\leqslant$ 15 000-dalton) apoproteins of pulmonary surfactant. *Eur. J. Respir. Dis.* (In press)

39. Suzuki, Y. (1986). The role of apoprotein and phosphatidylglycerol in artificial surfactant. In Cosmi, E. V. and Di Renzo, G. C. (eds.) *Selected Topics in Perinatal Medicine* pp. 211–217, (Rome: CIC Edizioni Internazionali)

40. Oyarzun, M. J., Clements, J. A. and Baritussio, A. (1980). Ventilation enhances pulmonary alveolar clearance of radioactive dipalmitoyl phosphatidylcholine in liposomes. *Am. Rev. Respir. Dis.,* **121,** 709–21

41. Ennema, J. J. T., Reijngoud, D. J., Wildevuur, C. R. H. and Egberts, J. (1984). Effects of artificial ventilation on surfactant phospholipid metabolism in rabbits. *Respir. Physiol.,* **58,** 15–28

42. Ennema, J. J., Reijngoud, D. J., Egberts, J., Mook, P. H. and Wildevuur, C. R. H. (1984). High-frequency oscillation affects surfactant phospholipid metabolism in rabbits. *Respir. Physiol.,* **58,** 29–39

43. Nilsson, R., Berggren, P., Curstedt, T., Grossmann, G., Renheim, G. and Robertson, B. (1985). Surfactant treatment and ventilation by high frequency oscillation in premature newborn rabbits; effect on survival, lung aeration and bronchiolar epithelial lesions. *Pediatr. Res.,* **19,** 143–7

44. Clyman, R. I., Jobe, A., Heymann, M., Ikegami, M., Roman, C., Payne, B. and Mauray, F. (1982). Increased shunt through the patent ductus arteriosus after surfactant replacement therapy. *J. Pediatr.,* **100,** 101–7

Discussion

Dr van Hellen   You showed that animals treated with high-frequency oscillation without surfactant replacement develop striking epithelial lesions. Do you have any information about animals treated with surfactant and conventional ventilation?

Dr B. Robertson   Without surfactant we see the same type of lesions after 1 h of conventional ventilation, although perhaps they are less severe than with high-frequency oscillation. You can reduce these lesions during conventional ventilation by adding an end-expiratory pressure. Although the movements of the lungs during oscillation are very small, they are apparently enough to produce lesions at least as severe as those seen following conventional ventilation.

Dr A. C. Bryan   Robertson is absolutely right. If you cannot get the lung inflated but insist on 'rattling' it some 900 times a minute, the possibility of causing damage is very high.

Robertson   Because the lung may have the capability to refine a film of surfactant from whatever mixture is provided, the surface balance may show one thing but *in vivo* measurements another. Indeed there seems to be little correlation between minimum surface tension on the balance and the *in vivo* effect.

18
The Cambridge Experience
Of Artificial Surfactant

C. J. MORLEY

We have been treating very premature babies with artificial surfactant in Cambridge (UK) since 1979. In this paper I would like to share our experience and ideas about its prophylactic use.

Surfactant treatment is used by ourselves and others on the assumption that a deficiency of surfactant is the major cause of respiratory distress syndrome (RDS). Although this seems an attractive hypothesis for which there is considerable evidence, two things must be remembered. Firstly, surfactant deficiency and RDS are closely associated with prematurity, and it is difficult to disentangle this association from the specific role surfactant deficiency might play in causing RDS. Secondly, premature babies have immaturity of all systems concerned with respiration. This leads to a number of problems which in most cases contribute substantially to the baby's respiratory failure. Some of them are:

1. difficulty clearing the lung fluid after birth;
2. very immature structure of the airspaces and capillaries;
3. immature pulmonary circulation with relative pulmonary hypertension and shunting of blood through and past the lungs;
4. patent ductus arteriosus;
5. soft, easily deformed ribs and weak respiratory muscles;
6. respiratory control and rhythms which are erratic;
7. proteinaceous exudation onto the alveolar surface which interferes with effective surfactant function;
8. surfactant with an immature composition which will mix with exogenously applied surfactant and may alter its function.

RDS is therefore a complex condition, the severity of which is compounded by many interrelating factors. Before clinical trials are designed or the results of exogenous surfactant therapy discussed it is important to consider what effects can realistically be expected in this complicated condition and how they can be assessed. An increased level of inspired oxygen is a major part of the treatment of RDS and reflects the severity of the disease. What effect could surfactant therapy be expected to have on the oxygen requirements of a baby with RDS? Would it be reasonable in a very premature baby to expect a reduction in inspired oxygen by 10%, 25% or 80%? If so, over what time period: 1 hour, 5 hours or 1 day? As we don't expect all babies to respond in the same way how much variation can we expect to find? Would 50% of treated babies not responding be acceptable? If a reduction in inspired oxygen is a good outcome, how should we take into account changes in other aspects of respiratory support such as continuous positive airway pressure (CPAP) and mechanical ventilation?

Which are the most important effects, short-term improvements or long-term benefits? Would any effect still be worthwhile if it was lost within the next day or two? Which are the long-term factors which are likely to be influenced by surfactant treatment at birth? Time in oxygen, time being ventilated, complications such as pneumothoraces, or should we just try to define the outcome in terms of the severity of RDS?

All outcome effects are compounded by babies dying. The loss of these babies censors any possibility of accurately calculating the time each group spends in oxygen or being ventilated, and if they have died early it reduces the number with complications. If more babies die in one group than another this makes the analysis complicated. The length of time babies are receiving oxygen or ventilation might be good measurements of the effect of surfactant but these are also affected by other factors unrelated to RDS, such as infections, surgery and apnoea.

If surfactant therapy improves RDS it should reduce the serious complications, but it is possible that with improved lung expansion there might be an increase in pneumothoraces and patent ductus arteriosus. These complications might reduce any benefit gained from the treatment.

Another problem is the large number of factors which cannot be anticipated but affect the outcome. Such factors are antenatal problems and drugs, type of delivery, labour, complications, effectiveness of resuscitation, intrauterine or neonatal infection, and the variations in quality of staff. There are many neonatal problems and various neonatal therapies which may be important in the outcome. For example some babies may 'fight the ventilator'; they are then treated with pancuronium. If this is effective it may reduce the number of pneumothoraces and severity of the respiratory problem and completely alter the course of the disease. If this is only given to the worst babies it may be used much more in one group than the other.

Lastly, the outcome will be different when surfactant is given prophylactically at birth to all babies at risk of RDS, than when it is given to selected babies with established RDS several hours after birth.

The statistical analysis of this type of trial is difficult because even when the treatment has been carefully randomized there are many factors which influence the outcome. This can be overcome by using multiple regression analysis for ordered categorical data. In this the outcomes are divided into several groups equivalent to good, moderate and bad. For example hours of ventilation could be divided up to be less than 1 day, 2 to 10 days, more than 10 days, and dead. This technique can then take into account the effect of other factors such as sex, gestational age and delivery.

Following the work of Enhorning, Robertson and others[1-4] we became convinced that therapy with extracts of natural surfactant should benefit babies with RDS. However, we decided against using natural animal surfactant because of the difficulties of extracting and purifying enough material, the potential variation between batches in the composition and physical properties, and the difficulty of convincing our collegues that it was sterile and not contaminated with proteins which might sensitize the babies.

We developed a synthetic mixture of naturally occurring phospholipids which could mimic the important properties of natural surfactant[5]. This consists of dipalmitoylphosphatidylcholine and phosphatidylglycerol in a ratio of 7 : 3 mol/mol. The phospholipids are pure and protein-free. The mixture is made into a powder, packed into capped vials under nitrogen and stored at 4 ^{0}C. Batches have been cultured but no organisms have been grown. I named this surfactant ALEC, which stands for artificial lung-expanding compound, as a tribute to my collegue Dr Alec Bangham[6]. The main physical properties of this surfactant are:-

1. On an aqueous surface, in a crystalline state, at 37 ^{0}C it spreads rapidly to a monolayer with an equilibrium surface pressure above 43 mN m^{-1}.
2. With 50% compression of an equilibrium monolayer the surface pressure rises to 72 mN m^{-1}.
3. On expansion the surface pressure does not fall below 25 mN m^{-1} while there is a reservoir of surfactant on the surface.
4. In a fully hydrated state it only replenishes the monolayer slowly.

We have now conducted two large clinical trials of this surfactant and are over halfway through a multicentre study.

The first clinical trial was planned without statistical advice. It was a pilot study of ALEC powder given prophylactically to very premature babies intubated at birth for resuscitation. We decided to use ALEC at birth because we wanted to answer the question, 'Will ALEC reduce the severity of RDS?' There was good evidence that it was likely to be most effective before protein exudation and cell damage had occurred. Asphyxiated babies were chosen because they have a high risk of developing RDS, are intubated at birth, and therefore easy to treat with an endotracheal dose of ALEC.

The ALEC was blown down the endotracheal tube as a powder on the premise that at 37 ^{0}C it would melt and spread over the available surface. It was not expected that the particles of powder would reach the alveoli. A dose of 25-50 mg was used for three reasons: (1) it is 10 times more than enough to form a monolayer on the surface of a premature baby's lungs; (2) the excess is needed because not all the ALEC delivered in this way reaches the lungs; (3) larger amounts might block the endotracheal tube.

The first part of this trial of 78 babies was published in 1981[7]. Having started in September 1979 it was extended to 130 babies and finished in

January 1982. The trial had the following protocol:

1. all babies were born in Cambridge;
2. they were less than 34 weeks 6 days gestation;
3. they were intubated for resuscitation at birth;
4. ALEC was only given when Dr Greenough or I attended the delivery;
5. if we were unable to attend, the babies became controls;
6. the ALEC was given as one dose of powder blown down the endotracheal tube from a modified Laerdal resuscitation bag;
7. the clinical decisions were determined by the duty paediatric team.

Table 18.1 Treatment score

Oxygen		CPAP (not PEEP) (cmH_2O)	IPPV	Pressure (cmH_2O)	Peak rate (Breaths/min)
Air	+ 0	+ 5	+ 12	<15 + 0	<15 + 0
21–30%	+ 1			15–19 + 1	15–30 + 1
31–49%	+ 2			20–25 + 2	31–40 + 2
50–75%	+ 3			26–30 + 3	>40 + 3
>75%	+ 4			>31 + 4	

The score is recorded every hour for the first 48 hours. It is obtained by adding the component scores. For example a baby in 40% head box oxygen scores 2 per hour, i.e. 48 in 24 hours. A baby ventilated scores 12, in 75% oxygen scores 3, at a peak pressure of 30 cmH_2O scores 3, and at a rate of 90/min scores 3; therefore the score is 21 per hour or 504 in 24 hours. A score of less than 360 in a day means that the baby is either off IPPV or on minimal settings

To overcome some of the problems of the babies' respiratory therapy changing we devised a scoring system which enabled us to quantify the treatment given, even though the baby's respiratory therapy was being altered. A score was assigned every hour. As shown in Table 18.1 it is based on the inspired oxygen concentration, ventilation pressures and rates. In retrospect, we realized this score is biased heavily in the direction of ventilation with comparatively little weight given to inspired oxygen.

Table 18.2 shows the predisposing factors for RDS. There were 130 babies in the trial. One with Potter's syndrome was excluded from analysis, leaving 129 eligible babies. There was no statistical difference, between the groups, in any of the factors. I will show some of the results for the whole trial although the more significant results were to be found in the subgroup in the babies less than 30 weeks gestation who are at highest risk of RDS and its complications.

Figure 18.1 shows the treatment score for the two groups averaged for each of the 12 h during the first 48 h. The maximum score for a living baby is 24. There is no easy way to analyse the data including the worst babies who have died. In this analysis dead babies are scored at 25. All babies are

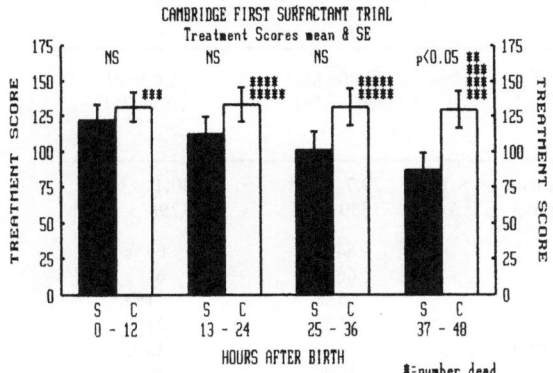

Figure 18.1 Cambridge first surfactant trial. Surfactant treatment is represented by filled blocks and controls by open ones. They are shown as the mean and standard error. The asterisks show the number of babies dead in each group at each time. There were 54 babies treated with ALEC and 75 controls. The differences between these groups were not significantly different except for 37–48 h at $p<0.05$

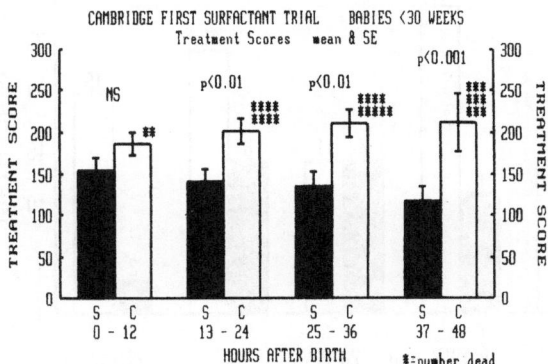

Figure 18.2 Cambridge first surfactant trial: babies <30 weeks. Surfactant treatment is represented by filled blocks and controls by open ones. They are shown as the mean and standard error. The asterisks show the number of babies dead in each group at each time. There were 28 babies treated with ALEC and 34 controls. The significance of the differences were as follows: 0–12 h NS; 13–24 h $p<0.01$; 25–36 h $p<0.01$; 37–48 h $p<0.001$

included even though 40% of the ALEC group and 38% of the controls did not need ventilation, and 5% of the ALEC and 12% of the controls needed no oxygen. By the end of the first 48 h the ALEC-treated group had significantly lower scores. Interestingly, this effect was barely apparent in the first few hours after birth. Figure 18.2 shows the scores for the babies for less than 30 weeks gestation during the first 48 h. The ALEC-treated babies needed progressively less treatment than the controls, and this trend continued.

It is not satisfactory to show the average time each group spent in oxygen

Table 18.2 First surfactant trial (predisposing factors for RDS)

	Surfactant (n = 54)	Control (n = 75)
Gestational age (mean ± S.E.)	29.7 ±0.3	30.1 ±0.3
Birth weight (mean ± S.E.)	1359 ±55	1398 ±54
Males	54%	68%
Caesarian section	66%	61%
Steroids	5%	1%
Beta-stimulants	26%	23%
Toxaemia or hypertension	26%	16%
Prom	19%	16%
Gestation <30 weeks	52%	45%

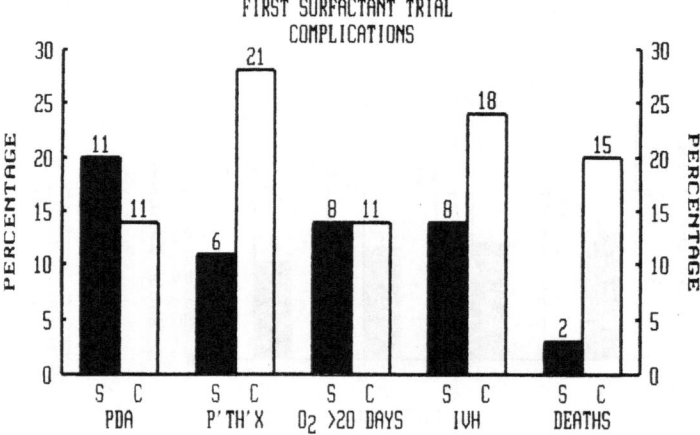

Figure 18.3 Complications. The numbers are the actual numbers of babies with the complication in each group. There were 54 ALEC-treated babies and 75 controls. The ALEC babies are represented by the filled blocks and the controls by open blocks. The only differences which were significant are pneumothoraces (p=0.011) and deaths (p=0.002)

or being ventilated, because it is meaningless when more than twice as many babies died in the control group.

Figure 18.3 shows the complications in the two groups as percentages. The complications shown are patent ductus arteriosus (PDA), pneumothorax (PTX), number of surviving babies who were in oxygen for more than 20 days, periventricular haemorrhages (IVH) and deaths. The incidence of PDA was similar in the two groups, but there were reductions in pneumothoraces, periventricular haemorrhages and deaths.

Figure 18.4 shows the same groups of complications in the babies of less

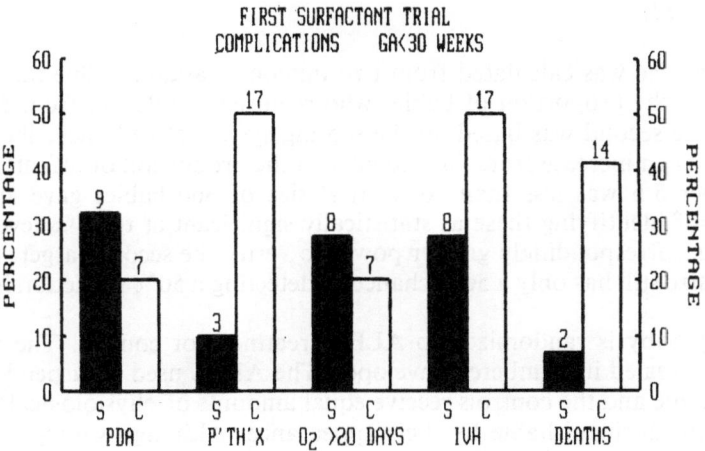

Figure 18.4 Complications. The numbers are the actual numbers of babies with the complication in each group. There were 28 ALEC-treated babies and 34 controls. The ALEC babies are represented by the filled blocks, and the controls by open ones. If there was any significant difference it is shown above each pair. The only differences which were significant are pneumothoraces ($p=0.0002$) and deaths ($p=0.0005$)

than 30 weeks who have most of the complications. One of the main effects of ALEC is a reduction in the incidence of periventricular haemorrhage and death. It is therefore possible that the increased number of survivors in the ALEC group might have had a more prolonged illness than the controls. In consequence it was interesting to note that the proportion in oxygen for more than 20 days was not increased. The mean age at death for the treated babies was 80.5 h and the controls 21.0 h. Although the effect on IVH was not statistically significant it might have biological significance.

These results were encouraging, but it is not possible to determine from this study whether one small dose of ALEC powder blown into the trachea at resuscitation really does have a beneficial effect because of the non-randomized nature of the study and the different doctors at the delivery. However, these results encouraged us to start a randomized controlled trial.

The second trial was a collaborative study between Cambridge and Nottingham. It was designed with the help of Sheila Gore, the MRC trial statistician. It started in January 1982 and finished on 31 May 1985[8]. There were several differences from the first trial:

1. The ALEC used was suspended in 1 ml cold saline. In this state it remains as a crystalline suspension below 37 °C and therefore maintains the properties of the powder.
2. The first dose was placed into the pharynx at birth, so that some was inhaled with the first breaths.

3. Further doses were given at 10 min, 1 h and 24 h if the baby was intubated.

The trial size was calculated from two outcome variables. One target was to reduce the proportion of babies who required ventilation from 50% to 35%. The second was based on the scoring system already described, and was set as an increase from 40% to 60% in the proportion of infants whose score per 6 h was less than 90. A trial size of 360 babies gave an 80% chance of identifying these as statistically significant at the 5% level. The trial has correspondingly greater power to verify the second target. A trial of this size still has only a 50% chance of detecting a 50% reduction in mortality.

Every baby is randomized to ALEC treatment or control. The allocations are sealed in numbered envelopes. The ALEC used is suspended in 1 ml of saline and the controls receive equal amounts of physiological saline. These are distinguishable by their appearance. Although we try to mask the given substance from the clinicians and nurses the trial is not assuredly single-blind.

The protocol for this trial was:

1. Babies entered the trial if one of the research teams attended the delivery.
2. Babies were less than 33 weeks gestation.
3. Babies were randomized, from data in sealed envelopes, before delivery.
4. ALEC suspension was made up at 4 °C just before delivery with 1 ml saline.
5. The control substance was 1 ml cold saline.
6. Amniotic fluid, gastric aspirate or pharyngeal aspirate were collected at delivery for subsequent L : S ratio and phosphatidylglycerol analysis.
7. At delivery, and as near to the first breath as possible, the baby received either ALEC or saline delivered deep into the pharynx so that it might be inhaled. If the baby was intubated for resuscitation a second dose of ALEC or saline was instilled through the endotracheal tube. If an endotracheal tube was present at 1 h and 24 h, third and fourth doses were given. A quantity of 1 ml of saline was chosen because this is the volume used during routine endotracheal lavage and suction of intubated babies.
8. The treatment given was not disclosed to the nurses or doctors caring for the baby. When the designated substance was given, they were asked to look away.
9. All clinical decisions were taken by the duty paediatric teams.
10. Respiratory compliance was measured at 1 h, 24 h, 48 h and at 7 days.
11. Babies having been entered into the trial were only excluded from the final analysis if they were stillborn or had gross congenital malformations.

This trial assesses the prophylactic effect of ALEC on all eligible babies with no exclusions and no prior screening for complicating factors. In consequence, babies are included in the trial with a variety of conditions that might adversely influence their outcome.

The trial is analysed according to treatment as randomized, rather than treatment as given. This pragmatic approach to clinical trials compares treatment policies and subsumes individual deviations from intended treatment for whatever the reason – innocent or idiosyncratic. If the analysis is not done this way it does not take account of the fact that the groups may have been biased by switching the randomized treatment; e.g. the smallest, sickest babies could have been given ALEC because someone was emotionally involved and thought that it might help a baby who had little chance of survival or, conversely, because such babies have little chance of survival the allocated treatment with ALEC might have been withheld. Eight babies did not receive the treatment registered for them on the randomization master list.

The trial lasted 40 months. During this time there were time trends which influenced the outcome. Forty-five per cent of babies were entered in 1982, 18% in 1983, 25% in 1984 and 11% in 1985. With each year the babies were smaller and sicker, so that 38% were less than 30 weeks in 1982, 42% in 1983, 49% in 1984 and 54% in 1985 with 33% ventilated in 1982, 62% in 1983, 63% in 1984 and 76% in 1985.

Three hundred and forty-one babies entered the trial. This was less than the target of 360 because after the first interim analysis we reduced the gestational age to less than 33 weeks and therefore needed less babies. Of the 14 ineligible babies, seven were fresh stillbirths and seven had malformations. Lung hypoplasia from prolonged rupture of the membranes was a problem. There have been eight clinical cases. Because of the difficulty diagnosing this from severe RDS we deferred to Jonathan Wigglesworth. Four were definite cases and are included in the ineligible babies. The other four are included in the trial analyses. Three babies could not be resuscitated, but as they were randomized and treated they are included in the analysis. The trial eventually contained 327 eligible babies, 163 ALEC-treated and 164 controls.

Table 18.3 shows the basic data for the trial, and the distribution of factors which might influence subsequent lung disease. Although the trial was planned to include only babies of less than 34 weeks, one baby of 34 weeks was randomized and is included, as are all babies down to 23 weeks. There are some differences between the groups which do not reach statistical significance but may have biological significance.

There are several problems in analysing this trial. The analysis of all aspects of treatment is complicated because the worst babies die. Distribution of the treatment score is skewed because 50% of babies breathed without assistance. Both of these difficulties are resolved by categorizing the factors into ordered categories. The first category is no assistance and the final category is death. Tables 18.4–18.8 show regression analyses for some of the major outcome factors. They compare the influences of ALEC on several categorized outcome parameters with the following other prognostic factors: being female instead of male, 1 extra week of gestational age and the year of randomization. The variables sex and gestational age are chosen for comparison because they are well known to effect RDS, and the year of randomization is included to monitor general time trends. An additional effect for babies randomized in 1984/85 who received ALEC is included because at final analysis, compared with interim analyses, the beneficial effect of ALEC on second day treatment score, hours of ventilation and pneumothoraces had diminished, although the reduction in periventricular haemorrhage and mortality persisted. This prompted the question: had there been some change in delivery of the surfactant or

Table 18.3 Basic data and factors which might influence outcome, shown as percentages or mean and standard deviation

	Surfactant		Controls	
Number	170	(71)	171	(70)
Ineligible	7	(2)	7	(3)
Eligible	163	(69)	164	(67)
Randomized in Cambridge	138	(61)	138	(61)
For eligible babies				
Birthweight	1426.0 ± 434		1423.0 ± 448	
Birthweight <30 weeks	1092.0 ± 229		1047.0 ± 270	
Gestational age	29.9 ± 2.6		29.8 ± 2.6	
Gestational age <30 weeks	27.4 ± 1.7		27.4 ± 1.6	
L : S ratio*	1.7 ± 0.58		1.7 ± 0.58	
L : S ratio** <30 weeks	1.7 ± 0.60		1.7 ± 0.59	
Males	50%	(57%)	54%	(61%)
Membrane rupture >2 days	19%	(23%)	19%	(22%)
Pre-eclampsia	17%	(14%)	22%	(22%)
Caesarian section	54%	(51%)	57%	(61%)
Labour	68%	(72%)	60%	(61%)
Mothers age <20 years	14%	(14%)	14%	(6%)
Steroids	8%	(10%)	6%	(9%)
Beta stimulants	25%	(32%)	23%	(34%)
Second twin	9%	(7%)	17%	(21%)

Data for babies of <30 weeks gestation are given in parentheses or separately.
The data are numbers of babies, mean and one standard deviation, or percentages. The L : S ratios were analysed from amniotic or gastric aspirate collected at delivery.
* L : S ratios were analysable only in 136 surfactant babies and 134 controls
** L : S ratios were analysable only in 59 surfactant babies and 54 controls

neonatal care which partially compromised the ALEC versus control differential towards the end of the trial?

Investigation of the dose increase and change from capsules to vials did not explain the phenomenon. However, as the trial progressed there was a change in the population of babies. Recall that two-thirds of the trial babies were born in 1982/3 and one-third in 1984/5. One-third of the babies born in 1982/3 were less than 30 weeks compared with half the babies born in 1984/5. There were also changes in neonatal management. One-third of the babies who were treated with pancuronium were born in 1982/3 and two-thirds in 1984/5. Control babies were treated with pancuronium nearly twice as often as ALEC-treated babies. This is circumstantial evidence for associating the use of pancuronium with a differential effect of ALEC prophylaxis according to year of randomization. As the trial progressed there was an increase in the use of higher ventilator rates, which may also have reduced the incidence of pneumothoraces.

Table 18.4 First day treatment score

Prognostic factors	Coefficient (SE)		p-value
ALEC	0.21	(0.37)	0.6
Female	0.50	(0.29)	0.08
One week gestation	0.64	(0.07)	0.0001
1983	-1.25	(0.38)	0.001
1984/85	-0.84	(0.43)	0.05
1984/85 and ALEC	-0.11	(0.58)	0.85

Regression analysis giving the coefficients with the standard error of the mean and the significance value. The baseline values scoring zero are control, male sex and 1982. One week of gestation means an effect equivalent to being 1 week older at birth. The coefficients give the comparative effect of each factor on the first day score (e.g. a control male baby born in 1982 has a coefficient of zero, whereas a surfactant-treated female baby born 1 week later in 1984 has a weighting of $0.21 + 0.50 + 0.64 - 0.84 - 0.11 = 0.40$)

Table 18.5 Second day treatment score

Prognostic factors	Coefficient (SE)		p-value
ALEC	0.84	(0.37)	0.03
Female	0.57	(0.28)	0.04
One week gestation	0.53	(0.07)	0.0001
1983	-0.86	(0.37)	0.02
1984/85	-0.19	(0.40)	0.63
1984/85 and ALEC	-1.09	(0.56)	0.05

Regression analysis giving the coefficients with the standard error of the mean and the significance value. The baseline values scoring zero are control, male sex and 1982. One week of gestation means an effect equivalent to being 1 week older at birth. The coefficients give the comparative effect of each factor on the second day score (e.g. a control male baby born in 1982 has a coefficient of zero, whereas a surfactant-treated female baby born 1 week later in 1983 has a coefficient of $0.84 + 0.57 + 0.53 - 0.86 = 1.08$)

Table 18.6 Hours on ventilation

Prognostic factors	Coefficient (SE)		p-value
ALEC	0.72	(0.32)	0.02
Female	0.59	(0.24)	0.02
One week gestation	0.78	(0.07)	0.0001
1983	− 1.15	(0.32)	0.02
1984/85	− 0.64	(0.16)	0.07
1984/85 and ALEC	− 0.94	(0.48)	0.05

Regression analysis giving the coefficients with the standard error of the mean and the significance value. The baseline values scoring zero are control, male sex and 1982. One week of gestation means an effect equivalent to being one week older at birth. The coefficients give the comparative effect of each factor on hours of ventilation (e.g. a control male baby born in 1982 has a coefficient of zero whereas a surfactant treated male baby born one week later in 1983 has a weighting of $0.72 + 0.78 - 1.15 = 0.35$)

Table 18.7 Hours of oxygen therapy

Prognostic factors	Coefficient (SE)		p-value
ALEC	0.27	(0.26)	0.3
Female	0.84	(0.21)	0.0001
One week gestation	0.68	(0.06)	0.0001
1983	− 0.99	(0.28)	0.0005
1984/85	− 0.33	(0.32)	0.3
1984/85 and ALEC	− 0.57	(0.43)	0.02

Regression analysis giving the coefficients with the standard error of the mean and the significance value. The baseline values scoring zero are control, male sex and 1982. One week of gestation means an effect equivalent to being 1 week older at birth. The coefficients give the comparative effect of each factor on hours of oxygen therapy (e.g. a control male baby born in 1982 has a coefficient of zero, whereas a surfactant-treated female baby born 2 weeks later in 1982 has a coefficient of $0.27 + 0.84 + 1.36 = 2.47$)

Regression coefficients are estimated by regressing the logit (or log odds) of the cumulative proportion of babies who score below successive category boundaries in each outcome on the foregoing prognostic factors. Prognostic factors whose regression coefficient is positive benefit the baby, and those factors whose regression coefficient is negative are associated with a relative impairment of outcome. Control, male sex and randomized in 1982 are the baseline. For any outcome the coefficients can be added to give a cumulative risk score. Comparing the magnitude of regression coefficients between prognostic factors gives an idea of their relative contribution to the baby's risk score in respect of a particular outcome, the

Table 18.8 Mortality

Prognostic factors	Coefficient	SE	p-value
ALEC	1.54	(0.65)	0.02
Female	0.95	(0.50)	0.06
One week gestation	0.91	(0.13)	0.0001
1983	−0.29	(0.63)	0.7
1984/85	−0.79	(0.66)	0.2
1984/85 and ALEC	−1.21	(0.95)	0.2

Regression analysis giving the coefficients with the standard error of the mean and the significance value. The baseline values scoring zero are control, male sex and 1982. One week of gestation means an effect equivalent to being 1 week older at birth. The coefficients give the comparative effect of each factor on the mortality (e.g. a control male baby born in 1982 has a coefficient of zero, whereas a surfactant-treated male baby born 3 weeks later in 1983 has a weighting of 1.54 + 0.95 + 2.73 = 5.22)

statistical significance of the contribution is given by the associated p-value.

The interaction with ALEC and 1984/5 is significant only at the 5% level, and only for the second day score and hours of ventilation; moreover, consideration of it is a consequence of data monitoring.

All outcomes were best for babies born in 1982 (the year with the biggest babies), particularly so for the first day score and hours of oxygen. The regression analyses show that ALEC has a small beneficial effect on first day treatment score which is neither statistically significant nor large in relation to the effect of being female (Table 18.4). The effect on mortality was little influenced by year of treatment.

Interpretation of the effect of ALEC on different outcomes, as shown by regression analysis on the above prognostic factors, depends upon how strongly one believes that some change of practice occurred during the trial which could have influenced second day treatment score, hours of ventilation and the incidence of pneumothorax more than the first day score, periventricular haemorrhage and mortality. If one dismisses such a change, the effect of ALEC on second day treatment score and hours of ventilation is modest, approximating to half a week of gestational age, and fails to achieve statistical significance. Alternatively, if a differential effect of ALEC according to period of randomization is believed; prior to 1984 the surfactant effect was equivalent to being born female rather than male or to an additional week of gestation, but in the later part of the trial the surfactant effect on second day score and hours of ventilation was negated.

In this analysis the net effect of surfactant prophylaxis, in respect of hours in oxygen, is inconclusive.

The incidences of the main complications of RDS are shown in Fig. 18.5, with 95% confidence intervals and p-values for the difference in incidence. In respect of each complication, the majority of cases are accounted for by babies less than 30 weeks gestation (see Fig. 18.6). The wide confidence intervals for the differences in incidence show the trial's relatively low power for detecting even dramatic changes in complication rates.

ALEC treatment did not appear to have any adverse effects, particularly with respect to postnatal infection or any other major neonatal complication. However, very large numbers would be needed for complete assurance.

Babies were included in the deaths if they died while receiving 'neonatal' intensive care, even though some died when they were many weeks old. There was a reduced mortality of 9% in the ALEC-treated group compared with 14% in the controls for the whole trial, and 19% compared with 34% in the babies less than 30 weeks. Of the 24 control deaths, 21 had obvious RDS and its complications (88%), 1 had possible lung hypoplasia (4%), 1 was not resuscitable (4%) and one was septicaemic at birth (4%). Of the 14 ALEC deaths, 7 died from complications of RDS (50%), 2 had possible lung hypoplasia (14%), 1 was non-viable at 23 weeks gestation (7%), 1 was not resuscitable (7%) and 4 had infections (29%).

In the regression analysis of mortality (Table 18.8) ALEC is associated with a one-third reduction in mortality, significant at the 10% level without covariate adjustment (see Fig. 18.5), at the 5% level for the subset of babies less than 30 weeks (see Fig. 18.6) or at the 2% level if the factors in the regression analysis are taken into account. The unadjusted 95% confidence interval for the surfactant versus control difference in mortality is from -11 to $+1$ for the trial as a whole; wide but nonetheless any possible detriment from surfactant is slight and the benefit could be considerable. In the babies of less than 30 weeks the surfactant versus control difference in mortality is from -31 to -1, showing that there is a beneficial effect on mortality in this subset of the trial but, as the confidence intervals are wide, how beneficial an effect still remains to be ascertained from a larger multicentre trial.

The incidence of periventricular haemorrhages (PVH) was reduced in the ALEC-treated babies to 8% compared with 18% in the controls for the whole trial (Fig. 18.5) and 19% in the ALEC babies of less than 30 weeks compared with 40% of the controls (Fig. 18.6). The PVH were diagnosed in Nottingham only at postmortem. In Cambridge they were diagnosed by ultrasound scan performed weekly by a group unaware of the babies' trial status. PVH were categorized by the Papile method[9]. The Cambridge ultrasound data are shown in Fig. 18.7. Each group is subdivided by the grade of PVH. ALEC treatment is associated with a significant reduction in the total number of haemorrhages and particularly grade 4 bleeds. PVH was associated with approximately two-thirds of the deaths in both groups.

Whereas the incidence of pneumothoraces at the second interim analysis had been 21% in control and 14% in ALEC-treated babies, the final difference in overall incidence of pneumothorax in Cambridge babies is more modest with 18% of the ALEC-treated babies and 20% of the controls developing a pneumothorax. In the babies of less than 30 weeks gestation 28% of the ALEC-treated and 36% of the controls developed a pneumothorax.

Pancuronium was only prescribed in Cambridge. Its usage is considered

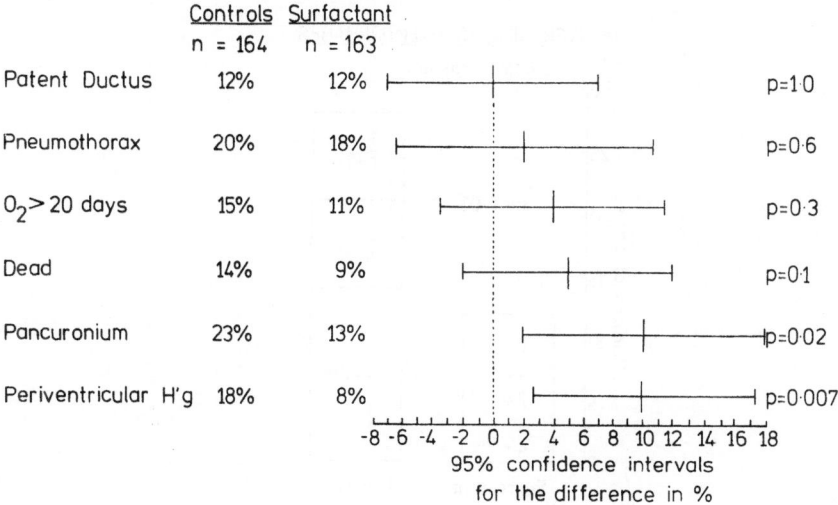

Figure 18.5 Effect of surfactant on complications. This shows the major complications in the whole trial. Pancuronium incidence is shown as a proportion of all babies. The deaths include deaths from all causes. Patent ductus was diagnosed from clinical criteria. Periventricular haemorrhages were mainly diagnosed by ultrasound scan, but in babies who died early they were found at postmortem

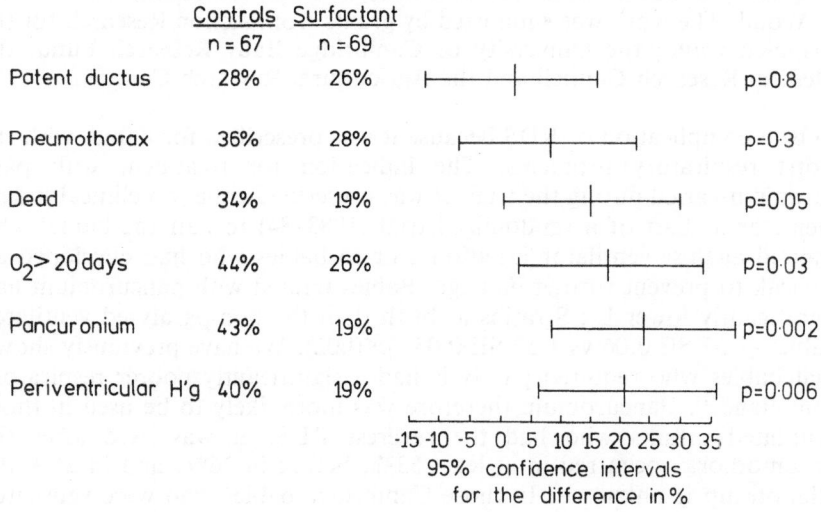

Figure 18.6 Effect of surfactant on complications – babies <30 weeks. Pancuronium is shown for the whole trial although it was only used in Cambridge where the incidence was 45% for controls and 21% for ALEC babies. The deaths include deaths from all causes. Patent ductus was diagnosed from clinical criteria. Periventricular haemorrhages were mainly diagnosed by ultrasound scan, but in babies who died early they were found at postmortem

269

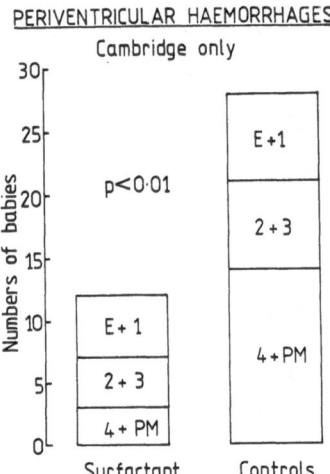

Figure 18.7 Periventricular haemorrhages diagnosed in the Cambridge subgroup. They are grouped according to the Papile classification: E = equivocal, 1 = grade 1, 2 = grade 2, 3 = grade 3, 4 = grade 4 and PM = haemorrhage diagnosed at postmortem. The p-value is for the comparison of the numbers in the two groups. The statistical significance for the comparison of the numbers with grade 4 or PM is $\chi^2 = 6.268$ ($p<0.05$)

Hopkins, N. G. A. Miller, A. D. Milner, J. Pool, M. South, H. Vyas and S. Wood. The work was supported by grants from Action Research for the Crippled Child; the University of Cambridge Baby Research Fund; the Medical Research Council and the Agricultural Research Council.

to be a complication of RDS because it was prescribed for babies with the worst respiratory problems. The indication for treatment with pancuronium varied during the trial. It was prescribed either on clinical judgement, or as part of a randomized trial (1983–84) to half the babies who expired against ventilator inflation[10], or to babies who had developed an air leak to prevent further damage. Babies treated with pancuronium had significantly lower L : S ratios at birth than the non-paralysed ventilated babies (1.37 SE 0.06 vs 1.57 SE 0.05; $p<0.02$). We have previously shown that babies who required paralysis had a significantly poorer respiratory compliance[11]. Pancuronium therefore was more likely to be used in those ventilated infants who had the severest RDS. It was used after the pneumothorax occurred in at least 53%, before in 26%, and in 21% the relationship is unknown. In those Cambridge babies who were ventilated 28% of the ALEC-treated babies were paralysed compared with 49% of the controls. These data are slightly different from those shown in Figs. 18.5 and 18.6, which include the use of pancuronium for both the ventilated and non-ventilated babies in the whole trial.

Table 18.9 Deaths

Gest.	Weight (g)	Sex	Age (h)	Trial Number	Cause of death
Control					
Cambridge					
24	738	F	936	C180	IVH-hydrocephalus, BPD
25	604	F	3	C264	HMD
25	625	M	51	C235	HMD, IVH, pulm. haemorrhage, liver haemorrhage
25	700	M	1	C133	Unsuccessful resuscitation
25	700	F	570	C187	HMD, IVH, PIE, pulm. haemorrhage, perforation
25	829	M	654	C267	Haemophilus septicaemia, HMD, IVH
26	517	F	2	C102	HMD, IPPV discontinued
26	688	M	2016	C104	BPD, renal failure, abdo. haemorrhage, peritonitis
26	697	M	362	C292	HMD, IVH, perforation, renal failure
26	904	M	16	C33	Possible lung hypoplasia
27	985	M	12	C3	HMD, IVH, pneumothorax
27	1048	M	46	C289	Group B strep. septicaemia
27	1081	M	122	C128	HMD, IVH, renal failure
27	1133	M	229	C174	HMD, IVH, pneumothorax
27	1138	M	40	C60	HMD, IVH, pneumonia
27	1224	M	648	C59	HMD, IVH, intestinal obstruction
27	1259	M	773	C87	HMD, IVH-hydrocephalus
27	1387	M	232	C109	HMD, IVH, renal failure
28	1238	M	56	C159	HMD, IVH
29	1098	M	201	C221	HMD, IVH, pneumothorax
Nottingham					
25	780	M	27	N2	HMD, IVH, pneumothorax, PIE
25	840	M	20	N34	HMD, IVH, pneumothorax
29	1100	F	48	N43	HMD, IVH, leucomalacia
29	1600	M	82	N8	HMD, pneumothorax, leucomalacia
ALEC					
Cambridge					
23	530	M	12	C35	Extreme prematurity
24	796	M	1	C146	Unsuccessful resuscitation
25	804	M	336	C81	Cord prolapse, HMD, IVH
25	867	M	3597	C68	Congenital CMV pneumonia
26	542	M	29	C178	HMD, pulm. haemorrhage, renal failure
26	873	M	113	C210	HMD, IVH, pulm. haemorrhage, pneumothorax
26	957	M	851	C134	Serratia septicaemia
27	1004	M	9	C51	Possible lung hypoplasia, Klebsiella septicaemia
27	1190	M	105	C23	HMD, IVH, renal failure, GC infection
27	1253	M	6	C275	Haemophilus septicaemia
31	1562	M	9	C195	Possible lung hypoplasia, HMD
31	1983	F	257	C208	Echo 7 infection
Nottingham					
25	780	M	14	N33	HMD, IVH, pneumothorax
26	650	M	296	N50	HMD, PIE, ventilation stopped

All deaths are shown for the eligible babies according to randomized groups (IVH = intraventricular haemorrhage; BPD = bronchopulmonary dysplasia; PIE = pulmonary interstitial emphysema; HMD = hyaline membrane disease; Group B Strep = Group B Streptococcus; CMV = Cytomegalovirus; GC = Gonococcus)

There was a slight reduction, compared with the controls, in the proportion of surviving babies treated with ALEC who were in prolonged oxygen. This was significant only in the babies of less than 30 weeks gestation. This effect is important because the reduced mortality in the ALEC group might have been expected to result in more surviving very premature babies requiring prolonged oxygen therapy.

The identical overall 12% incidence of patent ductus arteriosus (diagnosed clinically) in both treatment groups raises no concern about PDA being an adverse effect from ALEC prophylaxis. The wide confidence interval, however, cautions that the difference in incidences is not precisely estimated in this trial.

Over the past 6 years we have collected data on the use of this ALEC as a prophylaxis for RDS. These have included a non-randomized trial of the powder, and a randomized trial of a suspension of the ALEC. Both have shown similar trends in outcome. Table 18.8 summarizes the effect on mortality for 218 babies treated with ALEC compared with 236 randomized and non-randomized controls.

I would like to conclude that powdered artificial surfactant made from a mixture of dipalmitoylphosphatidylcholine and unsaturated phosphatidylglycerol in a ratio of 7 : 3, when given at birth into the pharynx of babies with gestations ranging from 23 to 34 weeks, is effective. The improvements can be summarized as follows.

The respiratory treatment required is reduced equivalent to 1 week of gestation or the effect of being female rather than male. In the babies less than 30 weeks gestation who have the worst RDS it has approximately halved the mortality, the incidence of periventricular haemorrhages and the number of babies in oxygen for more than 20 days.

Acknowledgements

This work was undertaken with considerable help from: A. D. Bangham,

References

1. Enhörning, G. and Robertson, B. (1973). Lung expansion in the premature rabbit fetus after tracheal deposition of surfactant. *Pediatrics,* **50,** 58–66
2. Adams, F. H., Tower, B., Osher, A., Ikegami, M., Fujiwara, T. and Nozaki, M. (1978). Effects of tracheal instillation of natural surfactant in premature lambs. *Pediatr. Res.,* **12,** 841–8
3. Enhörning, G., Hill, D., Sherwood, G., Cutz, E., Robertson, B. and Bryan, C. (1978). Improved ventilation of prematurely delivered primates following tracheal deposition of surfactant. *Am. J. Obstet. Gynecol.,* **132,** 529–36
4. Cutz, E., Enhörning, G., Robertson, B., Sherwood, W. G. and Hill, D. E. (1978). Hyaline membrane disease. Effect of surfactant prophylaxis on lung morphology in premature primates. *Am. J. Pathol.,* **92,** 581–94
5. Bangham, A. D., Morley, C. J. and Phillips, M. C. (1979). The physical properties of an effective lung surfactant. *Biochim. Biophys. Acta,* **573,** 552–6
6. Bangham, A. D., Miller, N. G. A., Davies, R. J., Greenough, A. and Morley, C. J. (1984). Introductory remarks about artificial lung expanding compounds (ALEC). *Colloid and Surfaces,* **10,** 337–47

7. Morley, C. J., Bangham, A. D., Miller, N. and Davis, J. A. (1981). Dry artificial surfactant and its effect on very premature babies. *Lancet*, 1, 64–8

8. Morley, C. J., Gore, S. M., Greenough, A., Miller, N. G. A., Hill, C. M., Brown, B. D., Pool, J. and Bangham, A. D. (1986). Randomized trial of artificial surfactant at birth. 1. Pragmatic analysis. (In press)

9. Papile, L. A., Burstein, J., Burstein, R. and Koffler, H. (1978). Incidence and evolution of subependymal and intraventricular haemorrhage. A study of infants with birthweight less than 1500 gm. *J. Pediatr.*, 92, 529–34

10. Greenough, A., Morley, C. J., Wood, S. and Davis, J. A. (1984). Pancuronium prevents pneumothoraces in ventilated babies who actively expire against positive pressure inflation. *Lancet*, 1, 1–3

11. Greenough, A., Morley, C. J. and Johnson, P. (1985). An active expiratory reflex in preterm ventilated infants. In *The Physiological Development of the Fetus and Newborn*. (New York: Academic Press)

Discussion

Dr B. Smith	In the large mass of data which you have shown I think I saw a trend that, in 1984, the babies did worse if given surfactant than if not given surfactant. Can you tell us about your compliance data?
Dr C. J. Morley	There have certainly been differences over the years. There is a statistical interaction between '1984' and 'surfactant' which we don't understand, except that in 1984 we were dealing with very much sicker and smaller babies. The compliance data are still to be analysed, but we have lost about a third of the measurements because the equipment broke on two occasions.
Dr F. Geubelle	Why should we expect saline put into the pharynx to be inhaled?
Morley	We were trying to get the surfactant and saline inhaled with the first breath, but we may have been naive to expect this. In our first trial a large number of the babies whose birth we attended were not intubated but later developed RDS, so in our second trial we felt that we would try to get surfactant in by putting it in the pharynx. If the infant was intubated, we put the surfactant down the endotracheal tube. About half the babies were given surfactant into the pharynx only.
Dr C. L. Gaultier	To measure compliance – did you use a balloon or a water-filled catheter?
Morley	We used an oesophageal balloon.
Gaultier	That must have meant the introduction of an oesophageal balloon many times during 2 days.
Morley	We tried to measure compliance at 1 hour of age after the neonatal team had put in the catheters. We measured it again at 6 hours in the early cases but later found that was too much to cope with, and restricted our measurements to 25 hours, 48 hours and 7 days. We did not leave the balloon *in situ*.
Dr C. A. Ramsden	Could you give us some assurance that the difference that you observed in ventilator score between groups was not due to a different incidence of pancuronium treatment. It has been our experience, and that of many others, that more ventilator support is needed following pancuronium treatment.
Morley	I cannot give a complete assurance because I haven't looked at that bit of our data yet, but I doubt whether the influence is large since only 50% of the babies in our trial needed ventilator treatment and only a few of these were paralysed with pancuronium.

19
Surfactant Supplementation: Toronto Trial

G. ENHÖRNING

INTRODUCTION

Some 25 years ago, when I first became interested in problems associated with the neonatal respiratory distress syndrome (RDS), a paper had just been published offering evidence that the condition was caused by, or at least connected with, a surfactant deficiency[1]. This pointed out the need for methods to evaluate the surface properties of fetal pulmonary fluid. The Wilhelmy balance, the only instrument used at that time, made possible the important observation that pulmonary surfactant has an equivalent surface tension of approximately 25 mN m^{-1}, and it is around this value that surface tension oscillates when a surfactant film, formed at the surface of the balance trough, is compressed to a smaller, or expanded to a larger, surface area[2]. From the observation that surface tension would approach zero during surface compression, Clements[3,4] concluded that the tendency for an alveolus to collapse because of surface tension would be inhibited during expiration. Usually the material to be examined with the modified Wilhelmy balance is applied to the surface when dissolved in chloroform, hexane, or other solvents. This allows an exact quantitation of the material and a calculation of the surface area available for each molecule.

When the main single component of pulmonary surfactant, dipalmitoylphosphatidylcholine (DPPC), was examined with this method, it was found to have surface properties quite similar to those of natural surfactant, an equivalent surface tension of about 27 mN m^{-1} and a surface tension clearly approaching zero during surface compression. It has been speculated, therefore, that in the final film of an alveolus, at least during surface compression, the molecule at the surface might be DPPC almost exclusively[5]. DPPC clearly was the most important component of pulmonary surfactant[6], in quantity and in quality, and I suspect it was partly because of the similarity between the final surface properties of DPPC, as observed with the Wilhelmy balance, and those of pulmonary surfactant, that the decision was made to treat severe RDS with DPPC. This was done in two clinical trials, one in Montreal, Canada[7], and the other in Singapore[8]. The results of these trials were not encouraging and did not offer support for the concept of surfactant supplementation. Yet the animal data we collected in the 10 years following these first clinical trials offered strong support, and encouraged us to embark on still another clinical trial.

When the newborn infant takes its first breath, the air–liquid interfaces formed in the cylindrical airways move in the direction of the alveolar sacs, a movement that will be resisted by surface tension in the hemispherical interfaces. According to the law of Laplace, $\triangle P = 2 \eth / R$, the resistance or pressure difference, $\triangle P$, that has to be overcome will be directly proportional to the surface tension, $\eth$, of pulmonary fluid and inversely related to the airway radius, R. Hence the resistance will increase as the menisci enter narrower airways and, with a high surface tension, the resistance in the smallest airways may be impossible for the infant to overcome. As a result large sections of the lung parenchyma may remain non-aerated, but with strong inspiratory efforts by the neonate, often aided by the resuscitator/ neonatalogist, the respiratory bronchioli and alveoli, expanded with air, tend to become overexpanded. The outlining pulmonary epithelium, normally with pores no larger than 0.6 nm in radius[9], may then lose its barrier function, and proteins, finding their way into the airways, will perhaps make the surfactant even more inadequate by exerting an inhibiting effect[10]. With this scenario the surfactant available most likely will be unable to exert a stabilizing effect. It is obvious, however, that problems were already encountered with the first breath before there were any alveolar air–liquid interfaces requiring stability.

The perception that RDS developed as outlined above called for a method that would make it possible to assess the resistance surface tension offers to the first breath, when hemispherical air–liquid interfaces are forced to move in the direction of the liquid. The maximal bubble pressure method seemed to be ideal. Modifications of this method were used to study surface tension of amniotic fluid[11] and of the pulmonary fluid from guinea pig fetuses at varying degrees of maturity[12]. Not surprisingly, we found that surface tension of the pulmonary fluid decreases with increasing fetal weight, and hence maturity, but we were unable to ascertain whether the surface activity detected with this dynamic method was due to the same agent as the one, so important for alveolar stability, forming a monomolecular film in the trough of the Wilhelmy balance. We are presently exploring the possibility that there are different components of fetal pulmonary fluid responsible for two types of surface activity: one that will counteract surface tension expressed at hemispherical air-liquid interfaces moving at high speed through a narrow tube in the direction of the liquid, and the one that will lower surface tension to an equilibrium value of 25 mN m $^{-1}$ and to a minimum value of close to zero with surface compression. The two types are of importance for the reduction of resistance to the first breath and for the stabilization of aerated alveoli. The maximal bubble pressure method yielded results that were interesting, but incomplete because no information was obtained regarding the ability of pulmonary fluid to stabilize aerated alveoli. One way of carrying out the method was to force air to move down a vertical glass capillary into a chamber filled with the sample. Air moved down the capillary until bubbles formed at its lower tip because the sample was being continuously withdrawn from the chamber. The principle of the pulsating bubble technique was a simple further development. The withdrawal was limited so that only *one* bubble formed at the capillary tip, and this bubble was made to oscillate by alternating infusion and withdrawal. This development of the maximal bubble pressure method, the pulsating bubble technique[13,14], made it possible to study the rate of adsorption, i.e. the speed with which a surfactant film forms at the air–liquid interface. It could also be seen whether the film was able to exert a high surface pressure, bringing surface tension close to zero at minimal bubble size. The method had the advantage of requiring a sample volume of only 20 μl, permitting an assessment of the small amount of fluid obtainable from the airways of rabbit fetuses. It was found that at a gestational age of 29 days the airway fluid usually had properties indicating maturity and adequate surface activity but, only 2 days earlier, surfactant seemed to be totally inadequate. With the pulsating bubble technique it was also found that natural surfactant, obtained by lavaging the airways of adult rabbits, had surface properties similar to the pulmonary fluid of a rabbit fetus at term and they did not change noticeably when, with centrifugation, the surfactant from the lavage fluid was given a concentration some ten times higher than that in pulmonary fluid at term. This observation suggested the possibility of instantaneously upgrading the lung maturity of a neonate by depositing a surfactant concentrate into its upper airways. The surfactant would then lower surface tension at the air–liquid interfaces of the airways, be evenly distributed, and finally reach the respiratory broncheoli and alveoli and offer them stability (Fig. 19.1).

That the concept of surfactant supplementation had a foundation in reality, and was not just a product of armchair thinking, was demonstrated by a series of animal experiments carried out in the seventies. Natural surfactant, instilled into the pharynx or trachea of rabbit neonates delivered on the 27th day of gestation, resulted in improved aeration[15,16], lung stability[17], gas exchange[18], and survival[19]. The importance of early installation, soon after birth, was demonstrated by Jobe *et al.*[20]; if the treatment was withheld until respiratory problems became manifest, the response was less conspicuous and of shorter duration. A delay of only a few minutes could result in damage to the airway epithelium, as reported by Nilsson *et al.*[21]. The favourable results of instillation could be ascribed to the use of natural surfactant rather than a synthetic preparation consisting of some of the natural product's main components[22].

THE CLINICAL TRIAL

A clinical trial clearly was called for, but natural surfactant, which at that time seemed to be the only preparation that worked, could not be used; it had a high protein content and could not be sterilized without losing activity. Most of the protein could be removed, however, by repeated extraction of the surface-active phospholipids, and when these lipids were

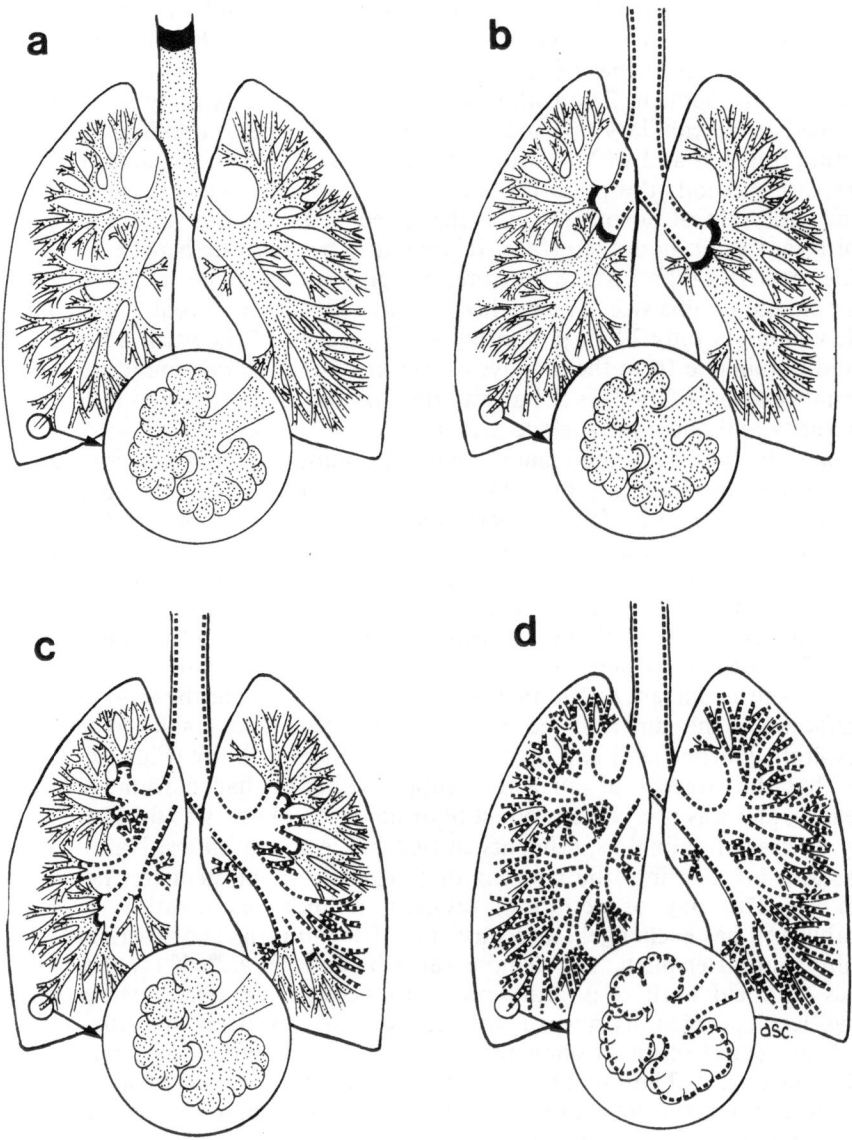

Fig. 19.1 The principle of supplementing pulmonary surfactant prior to the first breath of a newborn infant. The concentrated surfactant (black) is instilled into the upper airways (**a**). It will remain at air–liquid interfaces as they move down towards the alveoli (**b–d**). Resistance to the first breath is reduced and the surfactant, outlining airways and alveoli, offers stability. (Reprinted from Nelson G. H. (ed.) *Pulmonary Development*, vol. 27, p. 287; New York: Marcel Dekker, 1985, with permission)

resuspended in an electrolyte solution they yielded a product with high surface activity, even following sterilization by autoclaving. The preparation thus obtained seemed to satisfy all requirements[23,24]. It had the necessary surface properties, a high adsorption rate, an equivalent surface tension of around 25 mN m^{-1} and, within a few pulsation cycles, the ability to lower surface tension to zero at minimal bubble size. The protein content was less than 1% and the surfactant tolerated sterilization by autoclaving without a significant loss of surface activity. The raw material was the lung lavage fluid from calves, obtained within minutes after the animal had been killed. For the clinical trial the surfactant was prepared by Dr Fred Possmayer, University of Western Ontario, in 90 doses, all from a single batch. Each dose, in a sealed vial, consisted of a 4 ml suspension, with 25 mg phospholipids per ml. These vials were kept frozen until needed.

With an acceptable and effective surfactant preparation at hand, we started planning a clinical trial, and most of our efforts went into this stage. The trial was carried out at Women's College Hospital in Toronto under the direction of Dr Andrew Shennan. The study is in press[25], and I will limit myself to a short review of our project design and the most important observations.

The Department of Obstetrics and Gynaecology at Women's College Hospital is the tertiary care centre for several departments of obstetrics in Ontario, and there are some 120 to 180 deliveries per year at a gestational age of less than 30 weeks, the age group to which we limited our study. We did not expect that we would be able to obtain informed consent from more than half of the women delivering so much prior to term; but we felt the number available for a 1 year trial, 60–90 infants, would be adequate for a demonstration of improved gas exchange following the prophylactic surfactant treatment. We planned a stratification based on gestational age. The infants born at 27–29 weeks would receive 4 ml of the surfactant, approximately 100 mg/kg, whereas those born at less than 27 weeks would receive only 3 ml. Further stratification was based on betamethasone treatment given to the mother, according to Liggins and Howie[26], being (1) completed, (2) started but not completed, or (3) not given at all. Thus we had six strata, each randomized in subgroup blocks of 10 (Fig. 19.2). When a patient had been entered into the study and was close to delivery, the next numbered envelope was opened and the instructions on the enclosed card carried out by an individual who administered the surfactant, or air to the controls, but from then on had nothing to do with the neonatal care of the infant. Efforts were made to carry out the instillation prior to the first breath. Immediately after birth, inspiration was inhibited by gentle compression of the thorax while a neonatologist intubated the infant. As soon as the tracheal tube was in place, the instillation was carried out with a concealed syringe. The baby was bagged and connected to a respirator, the setting of which made it possible to control the $PaCO_2$ to within the range of 30–45 mmHg, and the PaO_2 was maintained at 50–70 mmHg by adjustments of the FiO_2.

There were 72 infants enrolled in the trial – 39 in the treatment and 33 in the control group. The randomization process functioned well, in that

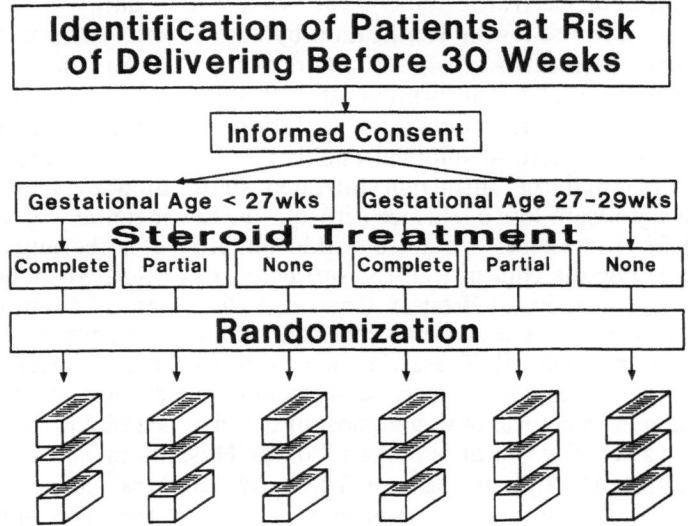

Figure 19.2 Stratification and randomization of surfactant trial (from reference 25; reproduced with permission of *Paediatrics*)

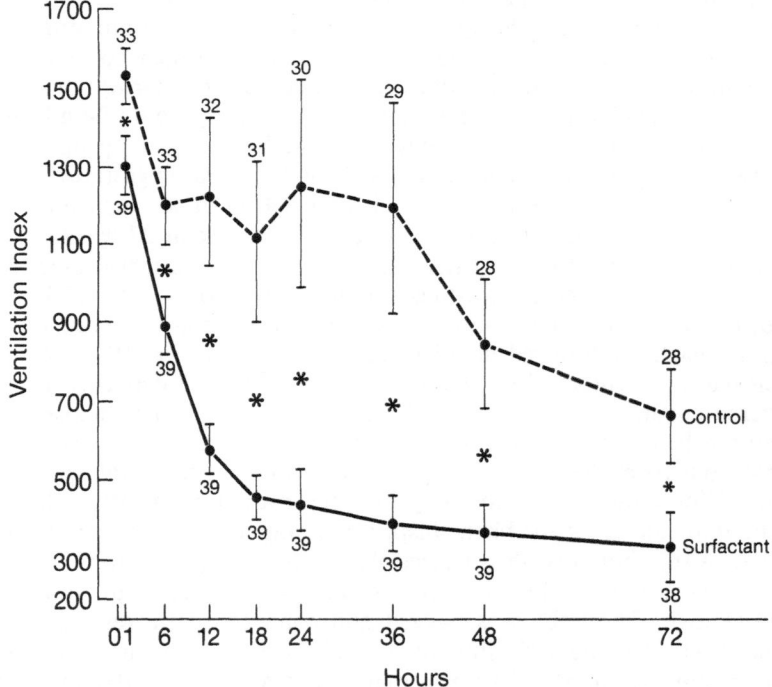

Figure 19.3 Ventilation index (peak inspiratory pressure × frequency) was significantly lower for treated infants. Values are mean ± SE and the number of infants alive and contributing to value of specific hour. Large asterisk indicates $p < 0.005$, small asterisk $p < 0.05$. (From reference 25; reproduced with permission of *Paediatrics*)

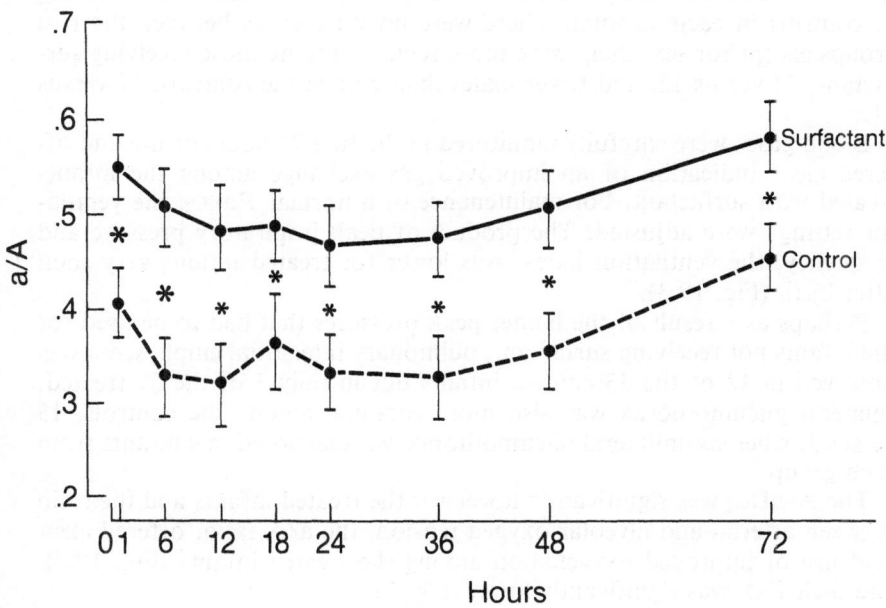

Figure 19.4 Ratio between arterial (a) and alveolar (A) oxygen tension was significantly higher for surfactant-treated infants. Asterisks as defined in Fig. 19.3. (From reference 25; reproduced with permission of *Paediatrics*)

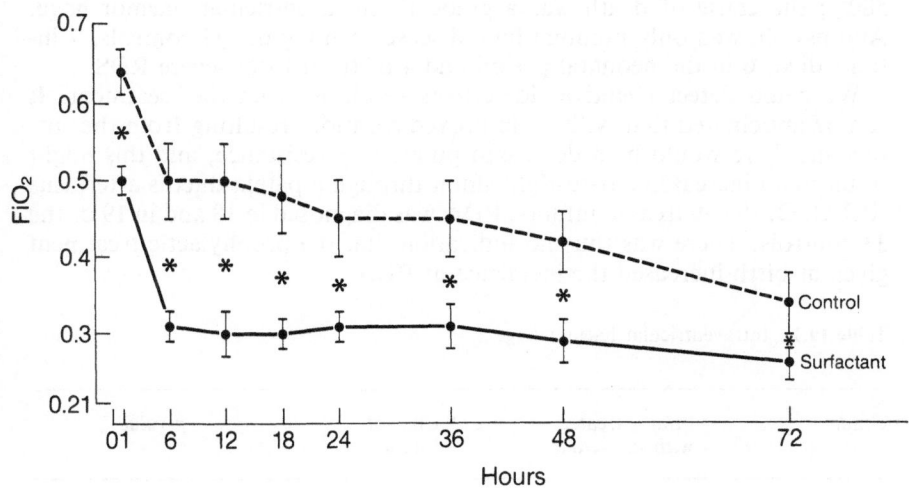

Figure 19.5 Oxygen fraction of inspired air (FiO_2) could be kept lower for treated infants. Asterisks as defined in Fig. 19.3. (From reference 25; reproduced with permission of *Paediatrics*)

there were approximately the same number of infants treated and serving as controls in each stratum. There were no differences between the two groups except for sex; there were more females among those receiving surfactant, 22 versus 12, and fewer males than among the controls, 17 versus 21.

Blood gases were carefully monitored in the first 72 hours of life and offered clear indication of an improved gas exchange among the infants treated with surfactant. For maintenance of a normal $PaCO_2$, the ventilator settings were adjusted. The product of peak inspiratory pressure and frequency, the ventilation index, was lower for treated infants very soon after birth (Fig. 19.3).

Perhaps as a result of the higher peak pressures that had to be used for the infants not receiving surfactant, pulmonary interstitial emphysema was observed in 13 of the 33 control infants but in only 3 of the 39 treated. Bilateral pneumothorax was also more common among the controls, 13 versus 3, whereas unilateral pneumothorax was diagnosed in 4 infants from each group.

The $A-aDO_2$ was significantly lower for the treated infants and the ratio between arterial and alveolar oxygen tension, the a/A ratio, offered clear evidence of improved oxygenation among the treated infants (Fig. 19.4). and their FiO_2 was significantly lower (Fig. 19.5).

We did not expect the surfactant treatment to result in a lower mortality, but in the neonatal period we found that it did. Of the 39 infants treated with surfactant, 2 died, but 1 not until after 14 months, and initially this baby had only mild respiratory distress. The only treated infant dying in the neonatal period was born at a gestational age of 25 weeks and weighed 580 g; the cause of death was a grade IV intraventricular haemorrhage. Autopsy showed only minimal lung disease. Among the 33 controls, 7 infants died, 6 in the neonatal period and 4 of them from severe RDS.

We could detect negative side-effects resulting from the treatment. It can be anticipated that with an improved aeration, resulting from the surfactant, there would be a decreased pulmonary resistance, and this might result in an increased left-to-right shunt through a patent ductus arteriosus (PDA). Of the 39 treated infants, PDA was diagnosed in 18 and in 19 of the 33 controls. There was thus no indication that the prophylactic treatment given at birth increased the incidence of PDA.

Table 19.1 Intraventricular haemorrhage

Grade	Infants treated with surfactant	Control infants	p-value
1 and 2	7	17	<0.01
3 and 4	4	3	NS
Total	11	20	<0.01

NS = not significant

Intraventricular haemorrhage is often a complication of RDS, and it would seem that the milder forms were prevented by the surfactant treatment, whereas the more severe forms were seen equally often among the treated and the control infants (Table 19.1).

Natural surfactant of bovine origin, used in our study, in the first report on successful surfactant supplementation[27], and in a recently published study on the baboon[28], has demonstrated its efficacy. Human surfactant, another natural product, is also clearly effective[29]. Thus the soundness of the principle of supplementing a pulmonary surfactant that is inadequate has now been given strong support. Most likely it will become possible to use a synthetic surfactant that completely mimics the surface properties of the natural product.

It can be concluded that the principle of surfactant supplementation prior to the first breath is feasible, and probably the best way to prevent RDS when the infant is born prematurely. However, the opportunity for such early treatment will often be lost. It remains to be seen what the price would be if the treatment were delayed until the first symptoms of RDS had developed, and also if infants born at a later gestational age would benefit.

Acknowledgement

This work was supported by Medical Research Council of Canada Grant MT-4497.

References

1. Avery, M. E. and Mead, J. (1959). Surface properties in relation to atelectasis and hyaline membrane disease. *Am. J. Dis. Child.,* **97**, 517–23
2. Clements, J. A., Hustead, R. F., Johnson, P. P. and Gribetz, I. (1961). Pulmonary surface tension and alveolar stability. *J. Appl. Physiol.,* **16**, 444–50
3. Clements, J. A. (1962). Surface phenomena in relation to pulmonary function. *Physiologist,* **5**, 11–28
4. Clements, J. A. (1962). Surface tension in the lungs. *Sci. Am.,* **207**, 121–30
5. Watkins, J. C. (1968). The surface properties of pure phospholipids in relation to those of lung extracts. *Biochim. Biophys. Acta,* **152**, 293–305
6. Fujiwara, T., Adams, F. H. and Scudder, A. (1964). Fetal lamb amniotic fluid: Relationship of lipid composition to surface tension. *J. Pediatr.,* **65**, 824–30
7. Robillard, E., Alarie, Y., Dagenais-Perusse, P., Baril, E. and Guilbeault, A. (1964). Microaerosol administration of synthetic β-ɤ-dipalmitoyl-L-α-lecithin in the respiratory distress syndrome: a preliminary report. *Can. Med. Assoc. J.,* **90**, 55–7
8. Chu, J., Clements, J. A., Cotton, E. K., Klaus, M. H., Sweet, A. Y. and Tooley, W. H. (1967). Neonatal pulmonary ischemia. I. Clinical and physiological studies. *Pediatrics,* **40**, 709–66
9. Normand, I. C. S., Olver, R. E., Reynolds, E. O. R., Strang, L. B. and Welch, K. (1971). Permeability of lung capillaries and alveoli to non-electrolytes in the fetal lamb. *J. Physiol.,* **219**, 303–30
10. Tierney, D. F. and Johnson, R. P. (1965). Altered surface tension of lung extracts and lung mechanics. *J. Appl. Physiol.,* **20**, 1253–60
11. Enhörning, G. (1964). The surface tension of amniotic fluid. *Am. J. Obstet. Gynecol.,* **88**, 519–23

12. Enhörning, G. and Kirschbaum, T. H. (1964). Surface tension of the respiratory tract fluid in fetal guinea pigs. *Am. J. Obstet. Gynecol.,* **90**, 537-45
13. Enhörning, G. and Adams, F. H. (1965). Surface properties of fetal lamb tracheal fluid. *Am. J. Obstet. Gynecol.,* **92**, 563-72
14. Enhörning, G. (1977). Pulsating bubble technique for evaluating pulmonary surfactant. *J. Appl. Physiol.,* **43**, 198-203
15. Enhörning, G. and Robertson, B. (1972). Lung expansion in the premature rabbit fetus after tracheal deposition of surfactant. *Pediatrics,* **50**, 58-66
16. Enhörning, G., Grossman, G. and Robertson, B. (1973). Tracheal deposition of surfactant before the first breath. *Am. Rev. Respir. Dis.,* **107**, 921-27
17. Enhörning, G. (1977). Photography of peripheral pulmonary airway expansion as affected by surfactant. *J. Appl. Physiol.,* **42**, 976-79
18. Wallin, A., Burgoyne, R. and Enhörning, G. (1977). Oxygen consumption of the newborn rabbit treated with pulmonary surfactant. *Biol. Neonate,* **31**, 245-51
19. Enhörning, G., Robertson, B., Milne, E. and Wagner, R. (1975). Radiological evaluation of the premature rabbit neonate after pharyngeal deposition of surfactant. *Am. J. Obstet. Gynecol.,* **121**, 475-80
20. Jobe, A., Ikegami, M., Glatz, T., Yoshida, Y., Diakomanolis, E. and Padbury, J. (1981). Duration and characteristics of treatment of premature lambs with natural surfactant. *J. Clin. Invest.,* **67**, 370-75
21. Nilsson, R., Grossman, G. and Robertson, B. (1980). Pathogenesis of neonatal lung lesions induced by artificial ventilation: evidence against the role of barotrauma. *Respiration,* **40**, 218-25
22. Ikegami, M., Hesterberg, T., Nozaki, M. and Adams, F. H. (1977). Restoration of lung pressure-volume characteristics with surfactant: Comparison of nebulization versus instillation and natural versus synthetic surfactant. *Pediatr. Res.,* **11**, 178-82
23. Metcalfe, I. L., Enhörning, G. and Possmayer, F. (1980). Pulmonary surfactant-associated proteins: their role in the expression of surface activity. *J. Appl. Physiol.,* **49**, 34-41
24. Metcalfe, I. L., Pototschnik, R., Burgoyne, R. and Enhörning, G. (1982). Lung expansion and survival in rabbit neonates treated with surfactant extract. *J. Appl. Physiol.,* **53**, 838-43
25. Enhörning, G., Shennan, A., Possmayer, F., Dunn, M., Chen, C. P. and Milligan, J. (1985). Prevention of neonatal respiratory distress syndrome by tracheal instillation of surfactant: A randomized clinical trial. *Paediatrics,* **76**, 145-53
26. Liggins, G. C. and Howie, R. N. (1972). A controlled trial of antepartum glucocorticoid treatment for prevention of the respiratory distress syndrome in premature infants. *Pediatrics,* **50**, 515-25
27. Fujiwara, T., Maeta, H., Chida, S., Morita, T., Watabe, Y. and Abe, T. (1980). Artificial surfactant therapy in hyaline-membrane disease. *Lancet,* **1**, 55-9
28. Vidyasagar, D., Maeta, H., Raju, T. N. K., John, E., Bhat, R., Go, M., Dahiya, U., Roberson, Y., Yamin, A., Narula, A. and Evans, M. (1985). Bovine surfactant (surfactant TA) therapy in immature baboons with hyaline membrane disease. *Paediatrics,* **75**, 1132-42
29. Hallman, M., Merritt, T. A., Jarvenpaa, A.-L., Boynton, B., Mannino, F., Gluck, L., Moore, T. and Edwards, D. (1985). Exogenous human surfactant for treatment of severe respiratory distress syndrome: A randomized prospective clinical trial. *J. Pediatr.,* **106**, 963-9

Discussion

Dr B. Smith	I would be less sanguine than you about the rather unfortunate sex distribution in your study. I think all of us who are planning trials should probably think about stratifying for sex.
Dr L. B. Strang	How many patients did you consider for treatment but not actually have an opportunity to treat for some reason?
Dr G. Enhörning	I can't give you the exact figures but it was around double the number actually treated.
Smith	To return to the question of reporting complicated data in this kind of trial, one of my questions, which probably relates to both these chapters, is that many of these data use non-parametric scoring systems, yet in both cases I saw non-paramatic data reported with standard error bars which made me wonder if your statisticians had really thought about the issue of continuous versus discontinuous variables.
Enhörning	I put in the standard error bars before the statisticians educated me, and I don't think you saw any standard error bars in the latter part of our second trial.
Dr C. J. Morley	We did use non-parametric statistics and perhaps we shouldn't have shown the results with t tests: but we did it both ways and the significance of the differences was never lost with non-parametric statistics.

20
Mechanical Ventilation: The Role Of High-Frequency Ventilation

A. C. BRYAN

INTRODUCTION

Mechanical ventilation of the lung has two functions: to produce cyclic volume exchange and to increase the mean lung volume. The volume exchange is primarily to eliminate CO_2 by manipulating tidal volume and frequency. This function is a mechanical substitute for respiratory muscles which can't or won't perform their accustomed task. The second function, increasing mean lung volume, is an attempt to open up closed or flooded units to decrease shunt. To accomplish this the strategy is much less clear-cut. It can be achieved by altering peak pressure and rate as in the first function, but it can also be achieved by increasing end-expiratory pressure or reversing the I:E ratio. Here the ventilator is being used as a mechanical strut. One of the real problems with mechanical ventilators is that these two functions can become inextricably tangled so that the optimum setting for O_2 exchange may not be the optimum setting for CO_2. The unique advantage of high-frequency ventilation is that it separates these two functions; the 'high frequency' uses novel fluid dynamic principles to eliminate CO_2 without cyclic volume exchange while oxygenation is controlled by continuous positive pressure.

This review will be confined to experience with high-frequency oscillatory ventilation.

CO2 EXCHANGE

It is now well accepted that excellent gas exchange can be achieved during high-frequency ventilation (HFV) using tidal volumes less than the volume of the dead space. Because this apparently defies the well-established laws of pulmonary ventilation, the fluid dynamics of HFV have been extensively studied. Gas transport appears to be the result of a variety of mechanisms the relative importance of each being unknown:

1. Bulk convection – even with a small tidal volume there will be direct alveolar ventilation of short path length units.
2. Pendelluft – at high frequency, distribution becomes highly dependent on time constant inequalities. Asynchronous motion of the lung (the Disco lung) has been observed, and this must stir the gas around[1].
3. Asymmetric velocity profiles – the inspiratory velocity profile is more skewed than the expiratory profile, particularly at bifurcations[2]. It has been suggested that because of this asymmetry, even with a symmetrical oscillation, there will be a net forward flow[3].
4. Taylor dispersion – when radial diffusion is superimposed on axial convection the effective dispersion of gases can be substantially increased[4].
5. Molecular diffusion – as in normal ventilation, this probably still dominates the flux in the terminal airways.

There have been a number of attempts to define an 'optimum' frequency/tidal volume combination, for gas exchange. This doesn't exist. Rather CO_2 elimination appears to be a function of $VT^x f$ with x being[5] of the order of 2 and, not surprisingly, differing between species[6]. Because of the more powerful effect of tidal volume, we operate at a fixed frequency and control $PaCO_2$ by manipulating the tidal volume. This allows one to develop a valuable visual clue about the adequacy of chest wall motion; if frequency is altered this clue is lost. It should be stressed that $PaCO_2$ is very easy to control, the usual problem being an overshoot into hypocarbia. If the $PaCO_2$ starts to rise it is usually some minor obstruction in the circuit, the endotracheal tube or the airway. The only conditions where CO_2 is difficult to control are diseases involving the airway. Although there is no optimum frequency for gas exchange, there may be one for barotrauma (see below).

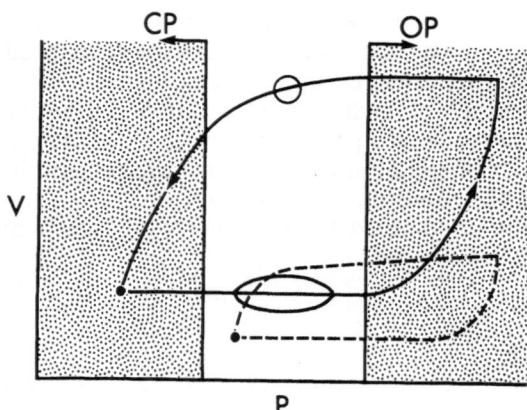

Figure 20.1 Schematic pressure–volume curve of surfactant deficient lung (solid line) bounded by zones of opening and closing pressure. Dotted line from a lung with hyaline membranes showing loss of hysteresis and rise in both opening and closing pressure

OXYGEN EXCHANGE

Because it is possible to 'shake' CO_2 out of the lung, it is sometimes naively assumed that O_2 can be shaken in. This is true of the normal or near-normal lung, but it is not true for acute diffuse hypoxic lung disease characterized by extensive atelectasis or flooding. In these cases the whole strategy must be directed to the recruitment of lung volume, and this strategy is illustrated in Fig. 20.1. If the mean airway pressure (MAP) is increased along the inflation limb of the P–V curve, there will be no volume recruitment until opening pressure is reached, and this pressure is often quite high. A better approach is a modest increase in MAP, followed by a sustained inflation (SI) for about 10 s (as the P–V curve has a third dimension: time) and then return along the deflation limb of the P–V curve to the original MAP[7]. This often results in a dramatic increase in lung volume and PaO_2. Whether or not this improvement will be maintained depends on whether the MAP is above or below closing pressure. If the improvement is not maintained we increase MAP and SI again, and repeat this process until the improvement is maintained. This strategy works very well in early RDS, i.e. when the infant has had little or no preceding mechanical ventilation. In late RDS, when there is extensive hyaline membrane formation, the P–V curve has lost much of its hysteresis and SI produces little volume gain and hence only a small increment of $P aO_2$. Further, as closing pressure has increased, it is difficult to maintain even this modest gain. In practice the SI strategy is not much use in late RDS. This is not to say that HFV is useless in late RDS; it is particularly useful if there is difficulty in controlling $P aCO_2$ or there are air leaks, but it is a passive waiting game.

Thus HFV is really CPAP with a novel way of getting rid of CO_2, and is akin to the approach of Pesenti et al.[8] who use apnoeic oxygenation with CO_2 removal through an extracorporeal membrane lung.

BAROTRAUMA

Application of large phasic pressures to an immature lung with a non-uniform distribution of compliance must lead to local overdistention, and it is overdistention which leads to air leaks[9]. According to Macklin[10], the highest stress is at the alveolar base where it is tethered to a blood vessel, and the commonest site is in alveoli juxtaposed to areas of atelectasis, as would be predicted from the theory of alveolar interdependence[11]. As the large phasic pressure swings which produce bulk flow are not present with HFV, air leaks may be less common. They will still occur because the continuous distending pressure can also cause alveolar rupture.

Of greater importance is the role of ventilator pattern in the genesis of hyaline membranes. It is now well established that there is epithelial damage to a surfactant deficient lung within minutes of starting conventional ventilation[12]. Further, it has been shown[13] that the damage did not occur in a lung ventilated with liquid. It was argued that an air–liquid interface was formed in terminal airways. Pressure applied to these interfaces caused overdistention of the terminal airways and disruption of the epithelium. The normally tight epithelial junctions are opened and there is a protein leak into the lung[14]. This protein, and the shed epithelial debris, form the hyaline membranes. It now appears that the lesion may be more complicated than this. In the hyaline membranes there are a striking number of granulocytes. If an animal is depleted of granulocytes, rendered surfactant-deficient and then ventilated, there are few, if any, hyaline membranes. Thus granulocytes appear to play a major role in the genesis of the injury by releasing toxic products: oxygen free radicals, proteases and arachidonic acid products. The central role of the neutrophil in the genesis of the lung injury is important in the development of bronchopulmonary dysplasia (BPD). It has been shown that there is a sustained high level of both neutrophils and neutrophil-derived elastase in the tracheal lavage fluid in infants with BPD compared to both RDS and control babies[15]. These levels are significantly elevated by the third day of life, and that means that whether or not the infant develops BPD depends on what happens to the infant in the first 72 hours of life.

The argument for HFV is that by avoiding large phasic pressure swings barotrauma might be reduced, but the evidence to support this is still somewhat inconclusive. In adult rabbits rendered surfactant-deficient, by lung lavage, HFV was dramatically successful in almost totally preventing hyaline membrane formation that was invariably present after conventional ventilation[16]. However, in premature lambs there was a similar degree of epithelial necrosis and hyaline membrane formation on both forms of ventilation[17]. The lavage model leaves the lung architecture and the type II cell intact, with the possibility of repletion of the surface film. In contrast the premature lamb has a primary surfactant defect.

An optimum frequency may exist for the reduction of barotrauma. To deliver a given volume to the alveoli, the minimum pressure excursion will occur at the resonant frequency. In the normal infant resonance[18] is between 3 and 7 Hz, but in the infant with RDS the resonant frequency[19] is in excess of 40 Hz. Thus there are compelling theoretical reasons for operating at much higher frequencies than are being used currently.

CONTROL OF BREATHING

High-frequency ventilation leads to apnoea at normocarbia, both in animals and in humans. This apnoea is not simply that breathing has become unnecessary; it is a reflex inhibition of breathing. One pathway is vagal: fibres from slowly adapting receptors entrain to the high-frequency rate[20] and rapidly adapting receptors increase the firing rate[21]. In most dogs made apnoeic by HFV, breathing is resumed after vagotomy[22]. The fact that some dogs did not resume breathing suggests a secondary inhibitory pathway. Vibration of the chest wall is known to inhibit breathing through the muscle spindles, so it is possible that this also occurs with HFV. Certainly curarization, which blocks muscle spindle activity (as well as many other things), restarts respiration as measured from the phrenic neurogram[23]. In trained dogs, HFV produces prolonged apnoea or near apnoea in the quiet awake or quiet asleep states, but breathing is present during phasic rapid eye movement (REM) sleep[24].

Infants on HFV behave very much like trained dogs. In the immediate post-natal period, when behavioural state is indeterminate, they are apnoeic most of the time with occasional bursts of irregular breathing occurring in REM sleep. As they get older their predominant behavioural state is REM, and breathing is more continuous, interrupted by periods of apnoea. Continuous breathing for prolonged periods is a cause for concern as it indicates some additional respiratory drive. This may be due to a rising $PaCO_2$ or the presence of a pneumothorax.

References

1. Lehr, J., Barkyoumb, J. and Drazen, J. (1981). Gas transport during high frequency ventilation. *Fed. Proc.*, **40**, 384
2. Schroter, R. C. and Sudlow, M. F. (1969). Flow patterns in models of human bronchial airways. *Respir. Physiol.*, **7**, 341–55
3. Hazelton, F. R. and Scherer, P. W. (1980). Bronchial bifurcations and respiratory mass transport. *Science*, **208**, 69–71
4. Fredberg, J. J. (1980). Augmented diffusion in airways can support pulmonary gas exchange. *J. Appl. Physiol.*, **49**, 232–8
5. Chang, H. K. (1984). Mechanisms of gas transport during ventilation by high frequency oscillation. *J. Appl. Physiol.*, **56**, 553–63
6. Watson, J. W. and Jackson, A. C. (1985). Frequency dependence of CO_2 elimination and respiratory resistance in monkeys. *J. Appl. Physiol.*, **58**, 653–7
7. Kolton, M., Cattran, C. B., Kent, G., Volgyesi, G., Froese, A. B. and Bryan, A. C. (1982). Oxygenation during high frequency ventilation compared to conventional mechanical ventilation in two models of lung injury. *Anesth. Analg.*, **61**, 323–32
8. Pesenti, A., Kolobow, T., Buckhold, D. K., Pierce, J. E., Huang, H. and Chen, V. (1982). Prevention of hyaline membrane disease in premature lambs by apneic oxygenation and extracorporeal carbon dioxide removal. *Intensive Care Med.*, **8**, 11–7
9. Caldwell, E. J., Powell, R. D. and Mullooly, J. P. (1970). Intersitial emphysema: a study of physiologic factors involved in experimental induction of the lesion. *Am. Rev. Respir. Dis.*, **102**, 516–25
10. Macklin, C. C. (1938). The site of air leakage from lung alveoli into the interstitial tissue during overinflation in the cat. *Verk Anat.*, **85**, 78–82
11. Takishima, T., Mead, J. and Leith, D. (1970). Stress distribution in lungs: a model of pulmonary elasticity. *J. Appl. Physiol.*, **28**, 596–608
12. Stahlman, M., Lequire, V. S., Young, W. C., Merrill, R. E., Birmingham, R. T., Payne, G. A. and Gray, J. (1964). Pathophysiology of respiratory distress in the newborn. *Am. J. Dis. Child.*, **108**, 375–93
13. Schwieler, G. and Robertson, B. (1976). Liquid ventilation in immature newborn rabbits. *Biol. Neonate.*, **29**, 343–53
14. Jobe, A., Ikegami, M., Jacobs, H., Jones, S. and Conway, D. (1983). Permeability of premature lamb lungs to protein and the effects of surfactant on that permeability. *J. Appl. Physiol.*, **55**, 169–76
15. Merritt, A. T., Cochrane, C. G., Holcomb, K., Bohl, B., Hallman, M., Strayer, D., Edwards, D. E. and Gluck, L. (1983). Elastase and alpha-proteinase inhibitor activity in tracheal aspirates during respiratory distress syndrome. *J. Clin. Invest.*, **72**, 656–66
16. Hamilton, P. P., Onayemi, A., Smyth, J. A., Gillan, J. E., Cutz, E., Froese, A. B. and Bryan, A. C. (1983). Comparison of conventional and high frequency ventilation: oxygenation and lung pathology. *J. Appl. Physiol.*, **55**, 131–8

17. Solimano, A., Bryan, A.C., Jobe, A., Ikegami, M. and Jacobs, H. (1986). Effects of high frequency and conventional ventilation on premature lamb lung. *J. Appl. Physiol.,* **59,** 1571-7

18. Wohl, M. E., Stigol, L. C. and Mead, J. (1969). Resistance of the total respiratory system in healthy infants and infants with bronchiolitis. *Pediatrics,* **43,** 495-509

19. Dorkin, H. L., Stark, A. E., Warthammer, J. W., Strieder, D. J., Fredberg, J. J. and Frantz, I. (1983). Respiratory system impedance from 4 to 40 Hz in paralyzed intubated infants with respiratory disease. *J. Clin. Invest.,* **72,** 903-10

20. Man, G. C. W., Man, S. D. P. and Kappagoda, C. T. (1983). Effects of high frequency oscillatory ventilation on vagal and phrenic nerve activity. *J. Appl. Physiol.,* **54,** 502-7

21. Wozniak, J. A., Davenport, P. W. and Koch, P. C. (1983). The response of pulmonary afferents to high frequency oscillation. *Fed. Proc.,* **43,** 106

22. Thompson, W. K., Marchak, B. E., Bryan, A. C. and Froese, A. B. (1981). Vagotomy reverses apnea induced by high frequency oscillatory ventilation. *J. Appl. Physiol.,* **51,** 1484-7

23. England, S. J., Onayemi, A. and Bryan, A. C. (1984). Neuromusclar blockade enhances phrenic nerve activity during high frequency ventilation. *J. Appl. Physiol.,* **56,** 31-4

24. England, S. J., Sullivan, C., Bowes, G., Onayemi, A. and Bryan, A. C. (1985). State related incidence of spontaneous breathing during high frequency ventilation. *Respir. Physiol.,* **60,** 357-64

Discussion

Dr B. T. Smith	Is there a physiological way of determining the best mean airway pressure?
Dr. A. C. Bryan	We are now in a position to measure repeated compliances by the method described by Mortola in Chapter 9. This should provide a guide to the best pressure.
Dr J. P. Mortola	From your data, as well as Dr Robertson's in Chapter 17, I get the impression that the comparison between high-frequency ventilation and standard ventilation is a little unfair. As you said at the beginning, the main trick is to keep the mean lung volume extremely elevated. You just don't give time for the lung to deflate. If that is so, what is the difference between high-frequency ventilation and standard ventilation with an extremely high end-expiratory pressure (PEEP)? Why not use standard ventilation with very high PEEP and avoid the danger of the high pressures which accompany high frequency ventilation.
Bryan	The problem is CO_2 elimination, because if you work at a high PEEP you need a very high peak pressure to get enough volume exchange to get the CO_2 out. There are other ways around this problem, such as Reynolds' (1971) technique[1] which allows very little time for expiration and so doesn't give the lung time to deflate.
Dr E. A. Egan	When you run these high volumes and mean airway pressures, do you get a significant afterload on the right ventricle?
Bryan	This happens only if the lung opens up and then I would be dropping the mean airway pressure. We've never had problems with the cardiovascular system.
Prof L. B. Strang	Many years ago Cournand et al [2] showed that positive pressure ventilation in an adult animal with a closed chest produced a fall in cardiac output due to reduced diastolic filling. Have you any idea what happens to cardiac output with your type of high-frequency ventilation?
Bryan	Both in the normal dog and in the dog with pulmonary oedema there is no difference in cardiac output between oscillation and mechanical ventilation at the same mean airway pressure.
Dr D. V. Walters	Would Dr Clements speculate on what might be the 'alveolar' surface tension during these long periods of ventilation when the lung is not volume cycled?
Clements	Exactly 27 mN/m! I assume there would be at least a small amount of surface-active material in those lungs, and that at a given time it would find its way into the interface. There it would reach its equilibrium surface tension rather than the value it would have as a compressed film.
Dr C. L. Gaultier	Can you comment on the fact that high-frequency ventilation can sometimes induce apnoea?
Bryan	The apnoea is not just passive. It is not that you stop breathing because you don't need it, but rather an active inhibitory response mediated partly through the vagus. Animals, if oscillated to cause apnoea, mostly start breathing again when the vagi are cut. However, not all animals start breathing after vagotomy. There may be another inhibitory pathway, which could be vibration of intercostal muscle spindles, because if we paralyse the animal being oscillated with pancuronium, he starts producing rhythmic phrenic nerve activity. Besides, in REM sleep when the

293

	Herring–Breuer reflex is extinguished and the intercostal muscle spindles are out of action, the animal continues to breathe even during oscillation
Mortola	What do you think of the attempts by Dr A. Zidulka[3] to produce high-frequency ventilation by oscillating the chest wall with a jacket on the outside of the chest?
Bryan	The problem is how to achieve a mean airway pressure of 15–18 cmH$_2$O without intubation. Theoretically it could be done with a negative pressure device, but it would require a neck seal capable of sustaining large negative pressures which might pose an insuperable problem.
Dr W. Seeger	Have you tried to apply high-frequency ventilation alone or in combination with surfactant replacement in the late phase of hyaline membrane disease?
Bryan	I have a feeling it probably wouldn't work. Surfactant replacement in the late stage of the disease is not going to be very effective, and could not dissolve the hyaline membranes. Oscillation may lessen lung damage but it's not going to have a dramatic effect except early in the course of the disease.
Dr Senterre	It appears from the presentations we have heard that the prophylactic use of surfactant and high-frequency ventilation are both beneficial. As a practising neonatologist I would like to know if we can be given more information about the oscillator and about surfactants coming on the market.
Egan	As Dr Enhorning's assistant, I would like to answer the part of the question relating to surfactant. Ross Laboratories is investigating a surfactant both in Europe and in the United States in a clinical trial. It is also being compared, I understand, to the surfactant extracts that Dr. Enhorning and I have used experimentally. Extensive clinical trials still have to be done, at least in the United States, before any of these products will be considered for marketing.
Dr M. Hallman	It should be possible to get enough natural human surfactant from the amniotic fluid of normal, term elective Caesarean sections to treat all cases of severe RDS. This is the basis of ongoing trials in Helsinki and San Diego, where there have been more than 120 patients involved in a trial.
Strang	If I might make a final comment relating to the treatment of newborn babies with respiratory disorders, we would all agree that treatment has to start very soon after birth. This just adds a voice to the others which tell us that the separation of treatment units and places of delivery should be eliminated whenever possible. These matters are not usually decided by scientists or paediatricians but by politicans and administrators, and we need to draw their attention to the importance of these requirements.

References

1. Reynolds, E. O. R. (1971). Effects of alterations in mechanical ventilator settings on pulmonary gas exchange in hyaline membrane disease. *Arch. Dis. Child.*, **46**, 152–9
2. Cournand, A., Motley, H. L., Werko, L. and Richards, D. W. (1948). Physiological studies on the effects of intermittent positive pressure breathing on cardiac output in man. *Am. J. Physiol.*, **152**, 162–74
3. Zidulka, A. (1983). Ventilation by high-frequency chest wall compression in dogs with normal lungs. *Am. Rev. Resp. Dis.*, **127**, 709–13

Index